MASSAGE

a career at your fingertips

THIRD EDITION

The Complete Guide To Becoming A Bodywork Professional

MARTIN ASHLEY

ENTERPRISE PUBLISHING

Copyright © 1999 by Martin Ashley

Published by Enterprise Publishing
P.O. Box 179 / 208 Nichols St.
Carmel, NY 10512
(914) 228-0312

courtesy of Bancroft School of Massage Therapy, Worcester, MA
All other illustrations by Lorrie Klosterman
Cover design by Adventure House, New York, NY
Typesetting by PDS Associates, Allenhurst, NJ

Library of Congress Catalog Card No. 98-96462

Publisher's Cataloging-in-Publication Data

Ashley, Martin
   Massage: a career at your fingertips : Martin Ashley. — 3rd ed.
   p. cm.
   Includes index.
   ISBN 0-9644662-6-0

   1. Massage—Vocational guidance. 2. Massage—Practice.   I. Title.

RA780.5.A75 1999   615.8'22'023

10 9 8 7 6 5 4 3 2 1

Printed and bound in the United States of America

Contents

I: An Overview of the Profession
& What It Takes to Succeed in It

II: Career Options, Strategies and Tactics

III: Sex, Gender and Touch

IV: Business, Practical and Legal Information
for the Practitioner

Acknowledgements

First, my gratitude goes to my wife, Deborah Fay, for her invaluable suggestions, additions, editorial advice, and design assistance, in both the Second Edition and this Third Edition. The ideas to include Chapters 11 and 19 were hers, and she has provided many textual and aesthetic improvements. I want to thank Doug Brodeff, who originally gave me the idea to write this book. I also extend my gratitude to Pete Whitridge, who took the time to read the original manuscript and give me many helpful criticisms and suggestions. Thanks also to Kathleen Batko for proofreading the text.

In addition, the following massage and bodywork practitioners all contributed to the writing of this book by allowing me to interview them, or by furnishing useful information about reference material. Thank you all.

Paul D. Arneson
Lauren S. Bain
Ann W. Bertland
Wes Boyce
Gordon E. Bradford
Alberto Breccia
Iris Brown
William T. Bunting
Sharon Callahan
Robert Calvert
Norman Cohen
Karen E. Craig
Paul Davenport
Jo Anne Davies
Patrick Dempsey
Doug Deyers
Bob Fasic
Adeha Feustel
Andre Fountain
A. Ann Gill
J. Joy Gottus
Roy Gottus
Ruth R. Haefer
Susanne Setuh Hesse
Pamela Hodgson
Stuart Holland
Sita Hood
Shirley Hooker
Jeff Hopkins
Jeffrey Kates
Deborah A. Kimmet
Bob King

Apara Kohls
Shivam Kohls
Scott Lamp
Mae Leone
Glenn Lloyd
Jerrine F. Manders
Danila Mansfield
Charles Mardel
Maureen A. Miller
Artie Mosgofian
Ginann Olmstead
Grieg A. Osmundson
David Palmer
Cindy Patterson
Laura Perna
Anna Pekar
Chad Porter
Cate I. Rainey
Deeta Rasmussen
Kay E. Richey
Dennis Simpson
Timothy Starbright
Christiana Stefanoff
Bruce Stephens
Kathy Tanny
Debbie Thomas
John "Shane" Watson
Dana S. Whitfield
Sherri Williamson
Carl S. Yamasaki
Etelka M. Zsiros

Introduction
Who This Book Is Written For

When I was embarking on a massage career, there was no source to turn to for information about the field, educational programs, and equipment. That was 1982, and a lot has happened since then.

My idea in creating this book was to provide you with everything you need to know to consider, plan and execute a career in massage or bodywork. This book will not only help you decide whether to get into the field, but will guide you to the best massage or bodywork school for you, and help you make the choices that bring you a rewarding career. No other source contains the information you can find in this volume.

For the novice:

For someone contemplating a massage or bodywork career, this is truly one-stop-shopping for all the essential information you will need. First, you will find an overview of the field and what a career in the field will be like. Next, you will be guided through choosing the specializations you may want to practice, finding a job or acquiring a clientele, and opening an office. Business skills, book-keeping, record-keeping, massage laws nationwide, how to file income taxes, how to receive insurance reimbursement, and even saving for retirement are all covered. Finally, there is a reference section that includes hundreds of equipment manufacturers and distributors, 62 forms of bodywork, and 572 massage schools arranged in a state-by-state format.

For the massage student:

If you are already enrolled in a massage school, this book will expand on your school's courses in business, law, ethics and marketing, or it may be your school's textbook for the Business and Professionalism course.

The practical information about career strategies, bodywork modalities, marketing your services, opening a massage office, billing insurance companies, legal issues, taxes, professional associations, and professional politics, as well as sample forms, will be useful to you for years to come.

For the practitioner:

If you are already a trained and practicing massage therapist or bodyworker, you will still find much of value in this book to help you expand your practice and be more successful. The sections on marketing and taxes may give you much useful information, and Chapter 20 can get you started billing your services to insurance companies. You may also be interested in bodywork training programs, schools teaching different modalities, and requirements for practice in states you might move to.

You may also want to have this book in your library for the time when an aspiring massage therapist asks you how to get started in the field. It could save you a lot of time!

Browse the table of contents and see if you aren't interested in learning more. And whether or not you choose to enter the field, enjoy...

Introduction to the Third Edition

The First Edition of this book was published in 1992. At that time, massage was a rapidly growing field, but it was still widely regarded as being on the fringe of society, and not a part of the mainstream.

The Second Edition, published three years later, documented incredible growth in the field. The number of massage schools in the country increased from 190 in the First Edition to 316 in the Second Edition, an increase of 66%.

Three years later still, as we enter 1999, the growth in the massage field has not only continued, it has accelerated. There are now 572 massage schools, plus branch locations. This is an 81% increase in the last three years, and a 300% increase since 1992!

For the first time, one can get a college degree in massage. Seven massage schools now offer Associate, Bachelor or Master's degrees. (See page 219.)

The growth in massage schools reflects the acceptance of massage as part of our modern society. Newspaper and broadcast stories about the benefits of massage appear regularly, and Life Magazine's cover story in August, 1997 was about the health benefits of massage. 14% of Americans had a massage during the past 12 months.

Scientific studies at the Touch Research Institute and other institutes have dramatically increased the scientific documentation of massage's health benefits. In one study, massage given to premature infants shortened their average hospital stay by six days, resulting in a savings of $3,000 in hospital costs per infant. (See Chapter 19.)

Twenty-seven states and the District of Columbia now regulate the practice of massage, and others have legislative activity in the works (see Chapter 17). The increased regulation of the profession makes physician referral and insurance reimbursement more common.

Over 31,000 massage therapists have taken and passed the National Certification Exam, and the combined membership in the major professional associations is well over 70,000.

This field has been growing briskly for several decades, and the growth shows no sign of slowing. Most Americans have yet to experience their first professional massage. If you are considering a career in the field, it's a great time to be getting into it. The profession is still evolving, and if you join the field, its future will be in your hands.

This book is dedicated in loving memory of my father
Sam Ashley

I

An Overview
of the Profession
&
What It Takes
to Succeed in It

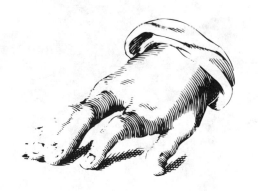

1 Is a Career in Massage for You?

Massage can be a delightful career. Your clients regard you as the person who gives them relaxation, helps relieve their pain, and assists then in improving their health. You have freedom to set your own schedule, and can earn a good living with a clear conscience.

Massage can also be a frustrating career. You have great skills and desire to help, but clients are not calling, bills are piling up, and a client has asked you for sex at the end of a massage. You may wonder whether the whole thing is worth the effort.

If you are considering pursuing a career in massage or bodywork, it is worth your while to spend a little time now examining what lies ahead and whether it is what you want. You will find information throughout this book that will help you get a fuller picture of what it is like to be a massage professional. However, certain pros and cons should be set out at the start.

First item: Money.

Many people are lured to the idea of a massage career by some simple arithmetic. The local massage therapist is charging $55 per hour. Eight hours a day times $55 per hour comes to $440 per day, or $2,200 per week. Eureka! How can I get into this!?

It is true that there are *a few* massage therapists whose economic picture is like the one in the last paragraph, but they are the exception and not the rule. The vast majority of massage professionals have a very different story to tell. And it has been my experience that those who enter the field *for the purpose* of making a lot of money are not happy in the field. They either do not succeed in massage, or are unhappy in their careers even though they earn large amounts of money.

The people in the field who are financially successful *and happy* are those who got into the field out of a sincere desire to help other people, who have good skills and who have the determination necessary to achieve success.

Second item: Drive and motivation.

What massage has in common with other professions — such as law, medicine and accounting — is that the professional has to attract a following, a clientele, in order to earn a living.

True, there are limited circumstances in which you can work for an hourly wage or on commission, but these situations are usually regarded as "entry-level" positions, or situations in which you can gain experience before you are truly established in the field. Jobs where some person or institution brings you a clientele are seldom well-paid jobs; your employer might take up to 70% of the amount paid for your services.

Therefore, to succeed in the long run, you will need to establish yourself as an independent professional with a substantial client base. Every client is an individual who could choose any massage practitioner, but chooses you because of what you have to offer. To be worth choosing and to be well-known and respected take time, dedication, and organization. Know before you begin that this is the path you are choosing for the long run when you choose a career as a massage therapist.

Third item: Commitment.

From reading just this far, you are getting the idea that massage is not a field you just drift into and easily start making money. You can get started more easily if you have substantial experience in a related hands-on therapy field, or a solid reputation in your community. Otherwise, you can expect that during your first couple of years after massage school you will have a limited income from massage, and will be spending a fair amount of time promoting yourself in an attempt to become established.

Therefore, make a commitment to your massage career. If you approach the field in a mature way, it will be a rewarding choice for you. However, if you approach it with a half-hearted commitment, you will likely flit from place to place without staying long enough to reap the reward of the seeds you sow.

Making a commitment to your career means making some commitment to a place. That is not to say you must settle down in the first place you practice massage, but ultimately you should make a pledge to yourself to spend at least three years in a location as a massage therapist. If you don't take that step, you don't do justice to your chances to have a successful career in the field.

Still interested?

If none of this scares you off, you probably have a good chance of making it as a massage therapist. Other chapters will provide you with strategies and techniques that will enable you to minimize your frustration and maximize your success as a professional. If you are making the decision to undertake a career as a massage professional, may I extend a warm welcome to you, and a wish that you enjoy all the ups and downs and in-betweens that await you...

2 The Massage and Bodywork Field
Its Time Has Come

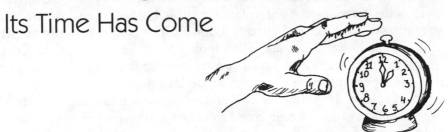

Massage is an ancient art that has been having a renaissance during the last 50 years in the United States. Many types of massage have been developed, and many types of closely and not-so-closely related therapies have evolved in recent times. In an attempt to clarify this sometimes confusing picture, I offer the following discussion of massage and definitions of various terms.

What is massage, anyway?

In one sense, the term "massage" deserves to be many words, because one word cannot be stretched enough to include the various therapeutic techniques practiced by people who call themselves massage therapists. Consider these categories:

- **Wellness massage,** for preventative general health;

- **Sports massage,** for training, preparation and recovery from exertion during sporting events;

- **Relaxation massage,** to remove the results of stresses of daily life;

- **Pain relief,** to relieve muscle soreness, minor injury pain, headaches, or the like;

- **Transformational or psychotherapeutic massage,** to explore emotional or psychological issues or to produce shifts in consciousness;

- **Medical massage,** as an adjunct to medical treatment for illness;

- **Rehabilitative massage,** for recovery after physical injury such as broken bones;

- **Chiropractic adjunct,** to enhance the effectiveness of chiropractic adjustments;

- **Pampering (or beautification) massage,** to provide a sensuous, pleasurable indulgence or as an adjunct to beauty services.

"Bodywork" and massage

Confusing the matter still further, many people also include "bodywork" in the term massage. Such hands-on therapies as shiatsu, Trager, Rolfing, polarity, and at least 60 other forms of bodywork now available are sometimes referred to under the umbrella term "massage," especially in the Western United States.

In order to make the information in this book easier to organize and use, I have drawn a distinction between "traditional" massage, and other newly-formed kinds of hands-on therapies. With apologies to those who prefer a definition of "massage" that includes a broad spectrum of bodywork styles, I have settled on the other, perhaps more conservative, definition.

In this book, the term "massage" is used to mean traditional "Swedish" massage, or systems very much like it. Swedish massage is characterized by the five strokes effleurage, petrissage, friction, vibration and tapotement. Other systems that work with the body are called "bodywork." The following definitions are offered for clarification.

Definitions

Please note: There are no "official" or widely accepted definitions of the terms "massage" and "bodywork." These definitions are offered to clarify the meanings of these terms as used in this book.

Massage. The application of touch by one person to another, using manual techniques of rubbing, stroking, kneading or compression (effleurage, petrissage, vibration, friction or tapotement), when done to produce relaxation, pain relief, injury rehabilitation, athletic preparedness or recovery, health improvement, increased awareness, or pleasure.

Bodywork. The application of touch by one person to another, to produce relaxation, pain relief, injury rehabilitation, health improvement, increased awareness, neuromuscular re-education, or pleasure, using any techniques other than those used in massage (see definition of massage, above). Bodywork does not include chiropractic, osteopathy, or any other system which has an organized licensing structure and grants the title "doctor" to its practitioners. (See the Bodywork Organizations and Trainings Directory starting on page 193.)

Massage Practitioner. Any person who publicly offers massage in return for money.

Massage Therapist. A massage practitioner who has received training in the theory and practice of massage, and is competent to use massage as a means of promoting pain relief, injury rehabilitation or health improvement.

Bodyworker. Any person who publicly offers bodywork in return for money.

The following definitions clarify the meaning of several words used in the above definitions:

"Compression" does not include static pressure applied to one spot (as in shiatsu and trigger point therapy), but does include pressure that increases and decreases or moves along the body, such as tapotement and friction.

"Health improvement" includes mental, psychological, emotional and spiritual health, as well as the health of the body's immune system, or any other system of the body.

"Pleasure" means the enjoyment of the sensations in the body, but does not include sexual arousal or stimulation of sexual organs.

Recent growth of massage — factors involved

In 1960, the average American had one of two associations for the word "massage." It was thought of either as a prelude to sex or a health club rub-down, heavy on the "karate chops." These images still remain for many people, especially older people whose experience of massage has been one or the other of these types. However, the last 40 years have seen tremendous growth of legitimate, therapeutic and scientific massage. Today, massage is considered a conventional treatment for stress reduction, pain relief, treatment of medical conditions and emotional and physical well-being.

Several societal trends have facilitated the rediscovery of the ancient art of massage. The hippie movement in the 60's, and related consciousness-raising activities, opened doors for massage as a tool for self-exploration and personal transformation.

The explosion in fitness activities during the 70's and 80's brought acceptance for massage as both a wellness modality and a sports training aid. This acceptance of massage by the general public has allowed the development of chair massage, (also called on-site or seated massage). Chair massage has gone into the workplace, the shopping mall, storefronts, airports, street fairs, health fairs, and many more locations. It has been a major factor in making the general public aware of the benefits of massage, and making it more available to a mass market.

As a result of all this growth, massage schools have proliferated (one person described it as an "algae bloom"), the membership of massage organizations has skyrocketed, and in short order massage is changing from a service for the wealthy to a service accessible to the general public.

The change is happening at a different pace in different places. In some parts of the West coast, massage has been popular for so long that there exists a surplus of massage therapists. In contrast, many remote or rural locations still have very little activity in the massage field. However, in most of North America, large numbers of people are just now learning the benefits of massage, and most areas are seeing a steady, even dramatic rise in the popularity and availability of massage.

What does the future hold?

People have been doing massage for many thousands of years. Massage was something people were doing before surgery was ever performed or medicine was prescribed, before science was even conceived, before almost any other human activity you can name. It has lasted these thousands of years because it is good. Much like gold has been the investment of choice throughout much of history because of its inherent value, massage is a part of human culture that has stood the test of time because it has real value for people.

Because massage is a service with inherent value for people, it does not need to have a market created for it in order to be in demand. Instead, massage is naturally in demand as soon as people release the artificial barriers they have against using massage services.

People's barriers to massage

These barriers are (1) anxiety about nudity and about one's own body, (2) fear of making contact with another person or oneself, (3) a belief that spending money on oneself is indulgent or wasteful, and (4) fear of the unknown.

These are significant barriers, but they are the sort of things people tend to outgrow. The more sophisticated our society becomes, the more irrelevant these barriers will seem to the general population. The general societal and scientific acceptance of massage will help these barriers continue to come down in the years to come.

Another issue is affordability. The 1980's saw an increase in income for many, and facilitated the growth of massage in part by creating a larger group of people who could afford it. Price is a factor for many people. The economy will play a role in how widely massage is accepted, and the profession can aid the growth of massage by not pricing itself out of reach of most people.

Finally, the payment for massage services by insurance companies, if widely available, would open a whole new market for massage services. A large number of potential massage clients will receive massage only if it is covered by their medical insurance policy. Currently, insurance reimbursement plays a minor role in the overall picture of massage therapy, but that factor might be poised to increase sharply. Whether that will change in the near future is one of the topics touched on in the next chapter.

3 Current Professional and Political Issues

This is a very lively time in the life of the massage and bodywork profession. If you liken the massage field in the U.S. to a growing person, it is currently a late adolescent or young adult.

The 1960's saw the birth (or re-birth) of massage as a sophisticated profession worthy of widespread acceptance in society. The 70's, 80's, 90's were a time of phenomenal growth, and a time when the profession as a whole went in many different directions looking for a sense of identity, or for its personality. Massage expanded into many different contexts, and related forms of bodywork grew up by the dozens.

Now, at the end of the century, the profession has some sophistication, some muscle, and a lot of energy. State regulation of massage exists in over half the states, and in many towns, cities, and counties. The National Certification Exam has been in existence for some years now, and many states have adopted it as their written licensing exam, facilitating therapists moving from state to state.

Mainstream America has realized that massage is not sex, and that it is a scientifically-proven health modality. Related forms of bodywork have evolved and blossomed into a rich tapestry of touch therapies that present almost unlimited choices for the practitioner and for consumers. The profession has really taken its place on the American scene. It has reached a level of maturity from which it can spread more completely into the fabric of modern life.

The purpose of this chapter is to set out the main political and professional issues currently confronting the industry. Understanding this information may not be essential to your career as a massage or bodywork practitioner, but you might find it helpful to have a broad understanding of the political issues in your chosen field. Some of this information may help you decide which school or schools to attend, and which association or associations to join. Participating in the political process in your chosen profession may also help you avoid unpleasant surprises in the future.

What is at Stake in Political Issues?

The following scenarios are drawn from real-life experiences. Most massage practitioners will not experience the problems indicated by these examples, but some will. These scenarios are meant to alert you to a few of the real-life situations that create some of the motivation for governmental regulation of massage and bodywork:

- You have a successful private massage practice. One day, your mail carrier delivers a certified letter from the State Board of Physical Therapy, ordering you to cease and desist practicing massage unless you can prove that you have a license to practice physical therapy or chiropractic.

- You want to move to a new state, but on investigation, you learn that your educational training is considered inadequate under that state's licensing law, and you must attend school at a massage school in that state from start to finish, and then take that state's licensing exam.

- You are working with a car-crash victim who could benefit from massage therapy. She asks you "are your services covered by my medical insurance?"

- You are attempting to establish a referral relationship with a physician and when you say you do "medical massage" she says she has never heard of that and asks what credential you have that allows you to practice.

This chapter will give you an overview of the current political situation and some of the conflicting views that are being advanced, and will suggest some directions for progress in the future.

Governmental Regulation of Massage

Massage is the newest member of the group of regulated professions. Dentists, doctors, psychologists, nurses, lawyers, physical therapists, and chiropractors, among many others, have all gone through the process of establishing procedures to regulate who can and can't practice the profession. That regulation process has begun in the massage and bodywork field, but is far from over.

At present, 27 states and the District of Columbia have laws regulating massage. The requirements differ from state to state. Texas, for example, requires 300 hours of educational training. Most states require 500 hours. Ohio requires 600, New York 605 (increasing to 1,000 on 1/1/00), New Mexico 650, New Hampshire 750 and Nebraska 1000. Some of these states have licensing, two have certification and two have registration. Some use the National Certification Exam as their written test, others do not.

The 23 states without regulatory laws require *zero* hours, and do not restrict the practice of massage. Although some municipalities and counties in those states regulate massage, most practitioners in those 23 states do not have to answer to anyone.

Why regulate the practice of massage and bodywork?

Why not just let people do what they want, and let the free marketplace take care of who succeeds and who fails? Many in the profession believe that's the best approach and for that reason oppose governmental regulation of massage in those states where it has not yet been enacted.

Proponents of governmental regulation put forth several arguments in favor of governmental regulation of massage:

First, the public deserves protection.

When a state agency regulates the practice of massage, they maintain a hearings board or grievance board to consider complaints by members of the public about how they were treated by a practitioner. In this way, the profession gives the public a quick and easy remedy against a practitioner who is incompetent or unethical. This inspires trust and confidence on the part of the public and enhances the respect of the entire profession.

If there is no agency regulating massage in a state, it is much harder for an injured party to get satisfaction from the practitioner who injured her. The only remedy available is to hire a lawyer and pursue a lawsuit, which is usually a very lengthy, traumatic and expensive undertaking.

Second, state licensing protects the massage profession from other professions that claim *they* are the only ones with the right to do massage. Physical therapists in Maryland made a concerted effort to restrict the practice of all massage therapists in that state. They instituted legal proceedings against massage therapists, charging them with practicing physical therapy without a license. Similar challenges have taken place in Oregon and the District of Columbia. State regulation of massage prevents this kind of headache — the state, by regulating the field, ensures the right of massage practitioners to practice.

Third, governmental regulation of massage helps in getting rid of those who offer sexual gratification as part of a massage. Where massage is regulated by the government, there is a quick and easy process for suspending the license or registration of one who is unethical. However, where massage is not governmentally regulated, the only remedy against unethical practitioners is the criminal justice system, which is notoriously slow and inefficient. Therefore, in areas where massage is not regulated by the government, it is much harder to stop those who offer sexual massage.

Finally, some believe that state regulation of massage encourages mainstream society and the medical profession to take massage practitioners seriously. The desire for acceptance as a mainstream health care provider has been an undercurrent in the licensing and certification debate for a number of years.

Why Some Oppose Attempts to Create State Regulation

Some people are against governmental regulation on principle — they are suspicious of government and don't want any outside authority taking control over their lives.

Others oppose regulation because the situation in the practice in their location does not need improvement. Perhaps the profession is well-established, unlicensed practitioners are able to receive insurance reimbursement, and there is no lack of respect and acceptance for massage and massage practitioners. Governmental regulation adds expense, burdens and restrictions. If there is no problem to be solved by regulation, then regulation is unnecessary.

During the last two years, I have subscribed to an internet discussion group for massage and bodywork practitioners. Governmental regulation of massage has been the most frequently debated topic on the list, and has evoked some of the most strenuous debate. The majority of those expressing an opinion favor not regulating massage. They don't want the red tape, the governmental control, and the "big brother" factor of having someone looking over their shoulder.

Another area of controversy in the debate, however, concerns not whether licensing is a good idea in principle, but *the way* in which the attempts to enact licensing laws are sometimes made.

Specifically, some groups within the massage profession keep legislative proposals secret, propose legislation without consulting the majority of practitioners in the state where the law would be in force, and propose legislation that favors the members of the group sponsoring the legislation, as opposed to considering the interests of all practitioners in the state.

Many groups are interested in the outcome of legislative efforts. However, two national professional organizations have some of the strongest interests concerning these issues. These organizations, the AMTA and the ABMP, sometimes have different ideas about how the licensing process should proceed. From published articles and magazine editorials about licensing issues, the following seems true of the current situation regarding attempts to create governmental regulation for massage:

The AMTA (American Massage Therapy Association) initiates attempts to create new state licensing, but does not necessarily advocate licensure for every state.

The ABMP (Associated Bodywork and Massage Professionals) is not against licensing, nor is it against the AMTA, but it opposes unilateral attempts to impose massage licensing without input from the majority of practitioners who will be affected by the law.

Currently, the ABMP is maintaining a network to alert practitioners about attempts to enact laws regulating massage. The ABMP's goal is to be included in the process of formulating the law, so the law will be responsive to all groups within the profession. In some states, AMTA representatives have invited the members of other groups to join in a coalition to formulate legislative proposals acceptable to all.

One additional note is that some state laws require practitioners to get their massage education at a school accredited by COMTA, which is an arm of AMTA (see page 131)(West Virginia formerly required attendance at a COMTA school, but that provision was removed by the legislature). Creation of laws with this requirement has been one of the sources of discord between competing groups in the industry. In addition, there is a potential legal argument that it is improper for a state government to officially favor the accrediting agency of one professional association over another.

Licensing, Certification and Registration

These terms can be confusing. They do not mean the same thing. In order to properly understand the political issues in the massage and bodywork field, you should understand the differences between these three terms. Once you read the following, their meanings will come clear to you.

First, ask yourself this question: Are you concerned with what a government is doing or what a private group is doing?

Governments can create any of the three kinds of regulations mentioned — licensing, certification or regulation.

When a government requires a *license* to practice massage, then practicing without a license is a criminal act. The license law sets out the requirements for obtaining a license and establishes a procedure by which qualified individuals can apply for a license.

When a government *certifies* practitioners, that is usually a voluntary procedure that carries some benefit. For example, in Maine, certified practitioners may use the title "Massage Therapist" and non-certified practitioners may not. In Delaware, certified practitioners are exempt from the "Adult Entertainment Law" but non-certified practitioners fall under its authority.

When a government *registers* practitioners, they generally do not restrict the practice, but keep track of practitioners by requiring them to submit certain information to the government. (However, Texas requires registration as a mandatory condition to practice massage, so registration operates much the same as a license in that state.)

Private groups can give *certification*. They cannot give a license or registration. Private groups that give certification are giving an individual their official approval, or are certifying that the person has completed specified requirements for certification, such as a training program.

While certification of a private group is never a legal requirement to practice massage, some forms of bodywork are protected by trade-name or service-mark protection. As to those forms of bodywork, permission from the owner of the name is required to use that name in connection with your work.

Now that you know this much, I have to tell you that the National Certification Exam complicates the picture by being a little bit "certification" and a little bit "license."

The National Certification Exam (NCE) is a standardized written test that is created by a private group (not by a government). However, it has been adopted as the *written exam* by governments in most of the states that regulate massage. (See page 131.)

These states have other requirements, such as educational requirements, licensing fees, and sometimes character references. However, in these states the government has chosen to adopt the National Certification Exam as the written exam for state regulation of massage.

Those states that require the National Certification Exam as their written test do not require individuals to comply with other aspects of National Certification, such as continuing education. Once an individual passes the test and obtains a state license, the individual's subsequent activities regarding National Certification are not of interest to state licensing authorities.

Therefore, the National Certification Exam is kind of a hybrid — part private certification, part governmentally-required exam. A brief history of the creation of this exam is the subject of the next section.

A Brief History of the National Certification Exam

During the late 1980's, the AMTA announced its plan to create a voluntary, nationwide certification exam for massage. It was initially to be an AMTA project, and was to be a Swedish massage certification exam. Although the exam was to be voluntary, many therapists became concerned that it would nonetheless become a practical requirement, since the goal of the exam is to standardize the qualifications of professional massage therapists.

Some non-AMTA massage therapists became resentful that a standard was being created without their input, which could damage their ability to earn a living. Some were angered that this action was being taken without consultation with any industry leaders outside the AMTA.

In the wake of this initial controversy, some organized attempts at reconciliation took place, without much success. As time went on, AMTA decided to make the certification project separate from the AMTA. When it was launched as an independent organization, the certification project was funded by a loan from the AMTA, and seven of the nine members of the steering committee were AMTA members. These connections to the AMTA caused some non-AMTA members to believe that the project was still an arm of the AMTA.

After the exam had been created, the steering committee was dissolved and replaced by the National Certification Board, which now administers the test. The National Certification Board is incorporated as a separate entity in the state of Virginia, and Board members are elected by mail ballot from all nationally certified practitioners.

The National Certification Exam certifies basic competence in massage, and does not test for competence in any specific area of practice, such as sports massage, medical massage, shiatsu or the like. There is no practical portion of the test, i.e., no test of manual skills is involved.

The exam is on a continuous basis at locations with interactive computer terminals. It was first administered in June 1992. As of January 1995, over 14,000 practitioners had taken and passed the exam, and as of 1998 there were over 31,000 NCE certified massage therapists.

To be eligible for the exam, a practitioner must have completed 500 hours of education in massage or bodywork. Professional experience can substitute for a portion of the educational requirement. The exam covers anatomy and physiology, clinical pathology, massage assessment and technique, business practices and ethics. Continuing education is required to maintain certified status, but not to maintain state licensure in states that use the test as their written exam. (For further information about the NCE, you can contact National Certification Board for Therapeutic Massage and Bodywork at (703) 610-9015 or on the Internet at www.ncbtmb.com.)

Suggestions for the future

It seems that individuals and organizations that are concerned about licensing will continue to work out their process state by state. I would like to offer a slightly broader perspective that could be a goal for the industry to aim toward. That is the idea of *specialized credentials* for massage therapists and bodyworkers.

The idea of a basic, or entry-level credential for massage and bodywork has received a lot of attention. State licensing and the National Certification Exam both aim to assure basic professional competence and to confer professional status to the practitioner.

In the years to come, additional states may adopt the National Certification Exam, and other states may create licensing that uses a different written exam, or no written exam. The "average" number of hours required for massage licensing is approximately 500, although that number appears to be trending upwards.

500 hours of training is enough to provide entry-level competency in massage. However, it is probably not enough to provide training both as a massage practitioner and also as a specialist in a particular branch of massage. The next issue for the profession to address is the creation of unified *specialty* certifications. Medical massage seems to be an ideal candidate for such a unified specialty certification.

Forms of bodywork that are protected by trade-name or service-mark protection perform this function by requiring that certain standards are met before an individual is allowed to use the name, such as "Rolfer" or "Trager Practitioner."

Providing a specialty certification for massage specializations will let the public know who is properly trained, and will give mainstream society some way to judge the qualifications of a practitioner who claims to be an expert in a particular field. If there were a unified medical massage credential, it would be much easier to convince physicians, hospitals and insurance carriers to use massage as a healing modality for medical patients.

The great challenge, as with national certification, is to foster dialogue among all the practitioners and educators so that a unified credential is created that appropriately represents the specialty. With this in mind, I note that the Bodywork Directory on pages 193–216 lists the massage schools throughout the nation that teach each form of bodywork and massage specialization. Anyone wishing to create a specialty certification for a kind of bodywork has a ready-made list of institutions that would be likely to take part in such an effort.

Massage in the United States has come a very long way in the last few decades. The profession has stepped into a mainstream role in American life. You, as a practitioner, will have the power to help shape the future evolution of the profession's role in society. Unless you participate in the process, you will give others the voice to speak for your future on these important career issues.

II

Career Options,
Strategies
and Tactics

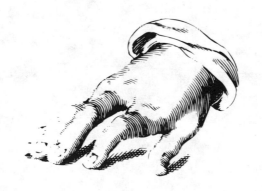

4 Your Career in Massage or Bodywork
Let's Get Organized

A surprising fact is that most massage school graduates never create a massage practice that supports them financially. They either never make an organized effort to practice massage professionally, or they give it a try but abandon their efforts before they achieve a successful practice.

The purposes of the chapters in this section are:

1. To help you gain clarity about what it is you want from your professional life in massage or bodywork.

2. To help you make a sensible plan for achieving your goals.

3. To help you follow through on that plan with a minimum of wasted effort and a maximum of success.

Common misconceptions

Many would-be massage therapists have certain wrong assumptions about the paths their careers will take. One very common expectation about a massage career goes like this:

> I will attend massage school, where I will learn everything I need to know to be a successful massage therapist. When I finish school, I will set up a practice. Clients will come to me and I will be busy and happy.

Several misconceptions are evident in this scenario. First, massage school will not teach you everything you need to know, either about giving a good massage or about operating in the business world. In fact, you should look at your first 1,000 professional massages as completion of your education as a massage therapist. Your skill level and confidence level will grow for years to come.

Second, you probably will not be in a position to set up a practice right out of school. Unless you have a very good reputation in the community, it will take time and effort to build your reputation sufficiently to establish a clientele.

Third, clients will not come to you just because you make yourself available. If you get yourself an office and say "Here I am, world!" the world will respond with a deafening silence. In order to be a busy massage therapist or bodyworker, you will need to take organized, affirmative steps to let people know you are there and make them want to take advantage of your services.

Finally, being busy and being happy are not necessarily the same thing. You want to attract those clients that most suit you. Even when you do not have enough work, there are still clients out there whom you do not want to have. Your clients will be a significant part of your life when your practice is going, so take the time to attract a clientele you will enjoy serving.

Typical career paths

In imagining what your career will be like, and taking logical steps to reach your goals, it will help you to have the benefit of the experiences of those who have walked the path before you. Numerous interviews with successful massage therapists and bodyworkers have disclosed many common elements in their career paths.

Below are capsule versions of the careers of some actual massage therapists and bodyworkers. Some are more successful than others. All are earning their sole livelihood at massage or bodywork.

"A" started his career in massage when he had a wife and a baby and was very poor. His wife was very supportive. During the early years, he did very little else to earn money, except some painting work for Christmas money. He chose this approach so that he would be fully immersed in the profession and would be forced to overcome any obstacles. It took two years to achieve a steady client load. After four years, he was so busy he was turning away clients, and now travels with world-class athletes to international sporting events.

"B" went to massage school, then went traveling in Asia for 15 months. On his return to California, he found he was seriously depressed. After three months of depression, he pulled himself out of it and began working at a health spa and promoting himself locally, working out of his home and doing house calls. Newspaper coverage of him and his Asian trip helped his practice grow, and within eight months, he was doing upwards of 20 massages per week. His business is growing, yet he plans to spend only one or two more years in the area before moving on to some other location.

"C" had a marketing background, and when she graduated from massage school, used newspaper ads, coupons and flyers to gather a practice quickly. She worked out of her home in San Diego, and had 10 to 15 clients per week within a month of starting her marketing program. After two years, she got out of massage completely, finding she was "fed up" with dealing with men who were asking her for sexual favors. She currently works as a receptionist in a wholistic health center.

"D" opened a store-front massage office in Chicago right out of massage school. She did a great deal of personal promotion in the neighborhood. Almost all of her clients in the early days were men, many of whom presented her with requests for sex. Her husband supported her financially for the first few years, and despite aggressive promotion, it took about three years for her practice to reach a profitable level, especially in light of the very high rent she had to pay for a corner store-front business location. After four years in practice, she is seeing 20 to 30 clients per week.

"E" did massage for about five years as a hobby, accepting donations, before ever attending massage school. He has been out of massage school eight years, and does 6 to 15 massages per week. The slow growth of his practice and his current pace of activity are exactly to his liking.

"F" spent quite a few years not succeeding in the massage field. He worked as a physical therapy assistant for three years, and also tried to establish a massage practice in a hair salon. Then he "took some time off" from the profession. He returned to the profession and became involved in his state massage associations. He became active in the AMTA and went into practice with a prominent sports massage teacher and practitioner. His massage practice reached full capacity within three months of starting in this office, and he has since taken on a significant leadership role in the AMTA.

"G" had 10 years experience as a swimming trainer and worked as a case manager in a chiropractor's office while she attended massage school. She did some massage in the chiropractor's office for a few months after graduation. A cardiologist who had heard of her invited her to rent an office in his tasteful, downtown practice building at a very reasonable rent. She accepted, and once there, she was able to work on some very influential community members who spread the word about her skills. Within three months of moving to the cardiologist's office, she had a thriving practice.

"H" started out in the field as a new mother, and very poor. She was always moving from one home to another in search of cheaper rent. Her main priority was to be very good at her work, and it took her several years to begin to earn a living at massage. She has now been in practice 10 years, specializes in pregnancy massage, and works at a birthing center. She sees 15 to 20 clients per week, most of whom are regulars. She would welcome having more clients.

"I" made a point of having non-massage work that supported her when she began her massage career. She was concerned that if she were financially needy, clients would sense that neediness and be put off. Instead, having her financial needs met, she could approach her clients with warmth and openness. Within one and a half years, she was seeing 20 clients per week, and only then did she quit her other job. She has kept her practice at that level ever since.

"J" did house cleaning at the beginning of her massage career to meet expenses. The first year brought only enough massage income to pay expenses such as office rent and supplies. After fifteen months, she was earning enough from massage to stop doing cleaning work. After 18 months, her client load was 10 to 15 per week.

"K" was a public school teacher. She started gathering a practice during after-school hours, and as the practice grew, she switched to substitute teaching, and eventually was able to let go of substitute teaching, and be a full-time massage therapist. The entire process took four years, which was longer than she thought it would take. She currently sees 15 to 20 clients per week.

"L" has a practice as a polarity therapist, which she took six years to build. For the first year, she kept her job as a university teacher, and saw one to three clients per week to decide if she wanted to pursue polarity more seriously. For the next three years, she held a consulting job two days per week, and built her polarity practice up to about six clients per week. She currently sees 12 to 15 polarity clients per week, teaches four yoga classes per week, and markets her own yoga instructional tapes.

"M" opened a practice in the town she grew up in immediately after finishing massage school. During the next two and a half years, she worked in at least six different locations in and around the area, gaining experience and slowly gaining a client base. She then opened an office in a charming, wealthy seaside resort town a few miles away. She coordinated this new office with a direct mail promotion and a public speaking engagement. Within weeks of moving, her practice doubled, and within two months she was seeing 30 or more clients per week.

"N" worked for four years as a physical therapy assistant and sports therapist before going to massage school. She has been supporting herself with massage work during the first year after massage school, doing house calls and working in a chiropractor's office doing massage for $14 per hour. Her goal is to be a physical therapist.

"O" worked full-time for AT&T, and practiced massage in her off-hours, doing house calls in an affluent community. After about one and a half years, she left her job and went into massage full-time. She went to work in a hotel health spa to supplement her practice, and has a busy practice.

"P" went to massage school after several years in practice as a lawyer. After graduating from massage school, he took a job teaching law, and did one to three massages per week on the side. He did this for three years, and then set out to establish a massage practice in a new location where he knew very few people. It took two years for the practice to produce enough income to meet his living expenses. He used some of his spare time to work on a book about the massage profession. After three and a half years of practice, he is seeing between 12 and 20 clients per week.

Elements these career paths have in common

The experiences summarized above display several elements that are repeated in more than one story. Consider the following:

- Those who had substantial experience in a hands-on field before going to massage school became established massage therapists much more quickly than those who had no such experience.

- For those without such prior experience, the average time needed to establish an income-producing practice varied quite a bit, but two years was about average. Some made it in a year, some took three or four years. Those taking longer than four years probably were not making an organized attempt to become established.

- Advertising was useful in building a practice quickly, but also tended to draw sexually-oriented clients.

- It appears to take longer for most men to become established massage therapists than it does for women.

Main causes of career failures

The two main ways in which would-be massage therapists sabotage their careers are moving too often, and being reluctant to promote themselves.

As you can understand from reading the career capsules above, success as a massage therapist comes only after a period of building a reputation in the community. The two essential elements in this process are (1) doing things to become known and (2) giving the process some time.

Recent massage school graduates are often very unsettled. Perhaps you are "in transition," having moved away from home to attend massage school, and not knowing where you want to settle to start a new life. Perhaps you are living in your home town, and you are apprehensive about becoming established, for fear that if you acquire a successful practice, you will never leave your home town and see the world. Perhaps you do not have confidence in your ability to give a professional massage.

If you are in such a situation, or in a similar situation that makes you unsure or reluctant about becoming established, you have at least three logical approaches you can take:

1. **The side-step.** Do some other kind of work to earn a living, and do massage on the side. This will give you the opportunity to see if you really enjoy massage work, and will give your skills a chance to slowly improve. It also will give you time to become better known in the community. If and when you decide to move to full-time massage work, you will have a stronger local reputation.

2. **The trial balloon.** Take any job you can get doing massage, such as working in a health club, resort, spa or chiropractor's office. These jobs will give you substantial experience doing massage, will give your skills a chance to grow, and may yield some contacts that can lead to a different job opportunity. While the pay usually will not be high, you retain the opportunity to leave town without sacrificing any time and energy spent in reputation-building.

3. **The leap of faith.** Act as if you have decided to stay in town for awhile. Commit yourself to staying for two or three years and take some steps to build a clientele.

If you don't know where you'd rather live, and you can't figure your life out, there is a good chance that three years from now you will either be right where you are now, or will move to a new place and still not be sure what you want to do. If you decide to take a stand wherever you are now, you may find that any major issues in your life are just as easy to wrangle with while you build a massage career as they would if you moved somewhere else or did something different.

The golden keys to career success

Having discussed what holds some people back from succeeding in the field, what is it that generates success for those who succeed? There are four keys to success in this field, and all four are indispensable. Imagine them like the four legs of a table. If any of the legs is short or missing, the table is not of much use.

The four golden keys to success in this field are:

Location   Personality   Skills   Desire

Location. You might be the greatest massage therapist on earth, but if you are in a town filled with people who cannot afford your services, or who have overwhelming resistance to trying massage, you will not do well.

Location refers also to the part of town your office is in. Neighborhoods have characters, as do streets, as do individual buildings. The character of the surroundings seeps into people's attitudes about you and your office.

Personality. Your clients are not simply coming to you for a physical treatment. They are coming to you for your presence as well as your skills. They may come in for work on the body, but it is the whole person who decides whether to come back for another massage.

Not only should your clients feel completely comfortable in your presence, they should look forward to coming to see you as a chance to be with you for an hour. Successful massage therapists develop personal, often warm relationships with their clients.

Skills. You need to have the ability to do a good treatment. The client must feel better leaving than coming in. The client must also feel there is some good reason for choosing your therapy over the competition.

In short, whatever type of massage or bodywork you practice, you need to know what you are doing and do it well. This can mean not just education, but experience. Your skills as a massage therapist will improve throughout the first few years of your massage career.

Desire. Consider whether you whole-heartedly want to succeed in your practice. If not, what is it that is holding you back? Your deepest and most honest desires deserve expression. If you honestly want to be a professional massage therapist, you will focus your efforts efficiently and effectively.

Do your best to look inside and discover what you really want from your massage career. If you have reluctance to really put yourself in the public eye and build a clientele, ask yourself why, or talk it over with a trusted friend. Understanding yourself is a valuable asset in making choices that will bring you a career you can really enjoy.

How do you rate yourself on the Four Golden Keys?

Re-read the four golden keys to success. This is the most important information in this book. If you embark on a massage career with a significant weakness in any of these four areas, you should understand that you need to work on this area in order to become successful. Before you put yourself through any needless hardship, consider very carefully your assessment of yourself and your career.

Make a commitment to strengthen your weaknesses

If any of these four keys is missing or deficient in your assessment of yourself, make a commitment to yourself that you will work on this area. Here are some suggestions for how to improve.

Location. Do some research about the town, neighborhood and building you are planing to be in. Find out about the residents' income and standard of living. Find out how well the massage therapists in that area are doing.

Generally speaking, it is more difficult to be the only massage therapist in town, because that indicates there is no established massage clientele in that area. On the other hand, if you are the first and only practitioner in an area, you will have a secure professional foundation once you do become established.

Imagine the best neighborhood, street and block for your massage office. What other businesses arc on the street? What is the look of the neighborhood? Imagine yourself as a client coming to this office. Is it difficult to get to? Is it on the way to other places you may want to go? As you come onto the block and into the building, what thoughts do you have? How do you feel?

Coming to your office is what every client will do at the start of your sessions. Evaluate the experience of coming to your office, and make sure you choose a location that makes coming to see you a pleasant and comfortable experience.

Personality. If you have an abrasive personality, make a commitment to yourself to soften it. If you are shy, make a commitment to yourself to be a little more outgoing so you can put your clients at ease.

You yourself enjoy being around people who are caring, accepting, warm and easy-going. These traits are important for the massage therapist. If you are too talkative, judgmental, sarcastic, crude or angry, these traits will tend to discourage your clientele and make it difficult for you to become established.

Of course, you cannot become someone you are not. However, you can choose to suppress the aspects of your character that would interfere with your career. Remember that the tongue often acts as a sword, so when in doubt, say less rather than more.

Skills. Understand that your skills will continue to grow for years to come. Take continuing education workshops, and professional trainings. Get massage often, not only to feel good but to learn from the skill of others. Continue to grow psychologically as well, as growth and maturity will lend their own added value to your manual skills.

Look for opportunities that match your skill level, and understand that your fees will rise with your skills and reputation.

Desire. Take steps that are consonant with your true desires for success — don't reach for the stars if you heart is not in it. You may not be ready for success today. If you are not ready, don't struggle — do something else for awhile and do massage on the side. When you have the desire that fosters organization and commitment, it will be much easier for you to get started in this profession. Be honest with yourself about what you want.

Weaknesses can be worked into strengths if you have the commitment to do so. These are the keys to success in your career. Use them well.

5 Career Options in Massage

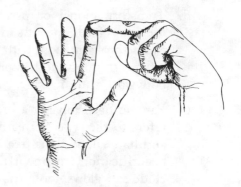

This chapter's purpose is to expose you to the broad range of options for the kinds of massage work you can do, the types of clients you can work with, opportunities for self-employment, and what you can expect in various employment situations.

Kinds of massage, types of clients

The six categories described below pretty much cover the field of massage at the present moment. Each of these types of massage attracts its own type of client, and requires its own set of skills on the part of the practitioner. You might practice several of these types of massage, but in most cases you will not practice more than one or two types in any one location.

1. Relaxation/stress reduction. The most common kind of massage, relaxation or stress reduction massage includes the types of treatments common in resorts, spas, private offices and clients' homes. This category would also include wellness massage, or preventative health massage.

2. Sports massage. This rapidly growing field encompasses athletic training massage, and massage designed to help an athlete prepare for competition and recover from competing.

3. Medical massage. Working by prescription, or in a hospital, or in a physical therapist's office, the medical massage therapist works with pathologies, pain or recovery from injury. Medical massage can also be adapted to a non-medical clientele, and practiced in a home or office setting.

4. Chiropractic adjunct. Working in chiropractors' offices is becoming more and more common, especially on the West coast. Some practitioners operate relatively independently from the chiropractor, with a cross-referral agreement. Others work by prescription of the chiropractor, working on specific parts of the body that the chiropractor designates.

5. Transformational or psychotherapeutic massage. Some massage therapists focus on shifts in awareness and psychological insight that can be brought about with massage. These therapists often work by referral from psychotherapists. They often combine another form of bodywork with massage.

6. Pampering. Probably a branch of relaxation massage, pampering refers to the type of treatment that might be found in some spas and hair salons. This treatment is usually thought of as more of a beautification treatment than a health treatment, and might include salt glows, loofa rubs, and light Swedish massage.

7. Chair massage. Massage or shiatsu done with clothing on, client seated, in any location. This can be done as an introduction to massage for clients who may not come in for an office massage, or can be a continuing form of stress-reduction therapy when done on a regular basis, as in the office setting.

Settings for the practice of massage

The following are locations where massage is currently practiced. Some of these locations are traditional locations for massage, and the arrangements establishments make with massage therapists are fairly uniform. Others are not so well established, and the arrangements may vary from place to place.

In general, the more the owner of the location provides in terms of linens, booking service and client base, the less she or he will expect to pay the massage therapist. If the location has a built-in clientele, such as a resort, the owner will usually take at least half of the fee, and sometimes quite a bit more than half.

At the other end of the spectrum, if the massage therapist brings additional business to the location, or adds a sense of uniqueness to what the location has to offer, the owner may make a very favorable deal with the massage therapist, on occasion even allowing the therapist to retain 100% of the fee.

Health clubs. Home of the "rub down" in the old days, health clubs are increasingly being staffed by well-trained massage therapists, who may practice relaxation massage or sports massage.

Some clubs will hire a therapist for an hourly wage, usually between $6 and $10 per hour. Some give an hourly wage plus a small percentage of the price of the massage, and some offer the therapist anywhere from 45% to 100% of the price of the massage.

Generally, clubs where the massage therapist has to cultivate the clientele will offer the therapist a larger percentage of the proceeds. Clubs where massage is an established part of the routine, especially where there are two or more treatment rooms, will usually pay less to the therapist, since they are supplying the clients.

Common disadvantages of health clubs are relatively low pay, noisy environments, and clients who may not have a sophisticated understanding of the value of massage.

A major advantage of health clubs, especially for newly trained massage therapists, is the chance to get lots of experience in a short period of time. If your health club will allow you to bring outside clients in, it can also serve as an office location for you while you develop a private practice, and this can be a substantial advantage.

Spas and resorts. Many of the same comments that apply to health clubs apply to spas and resort facilities. The pay tends to be low. A sampling of pay at some resorts disclosed the following: A four-star resort hotel in Washington State pays massage therapists $5.15 per hour plus 30% of the fee paid by clients; a Hilton hotel in New Jersey has a beautifully equipped spa, and pays its massage therapists 45% of the price paid by clients; a South Carolina resort pays $22 per massage (clients pay $90). A Texas therapist reports that resort hotels in his area pay therapists between 50% and 70% of the fee charged to clients; a spa in Texas pays $15.00 per hour.

The therapist in a spa or resort usually does not need to supply anything. The massage room will be equipped, and the spa or resort will do the bookings. The clients are supplied for you, but since they are vacationers, they seldom will become repeat clients for you in your local practice. They will be repeat clients only if they come back to the spa or resort again.

Spas usually have clean, comfortable and quiet massage rooms, and the clients are there for vacation or healthful relaxation, so their mood is usually conducive to enjoying a pleasant massage experience. Tips are usually good, and the costlier the resort, the better the tips are likely to be.

Hair salons. There are no reliable generalizations to make about the practice of massage in hair salons. Sometimes the service offered is a pampering-style light Swedish massage, and sometimes it is expert massage therapy.

Some salon owners expect a large percentage of the proceeds or a fixed monthly rental from the massage therapist, and some offer more reasonable arrangements to the therapist. It may depend in part on whether the salon owner sees the massage therapist as bringing new business or prestige to the salon, or simply relying on the salon's established clientele.

The salon owner will often offer a "day of beauty" or "day spa" experience which includes a massage, usually a half-hour full-body massage. The price of the package will be discounted, and the salon owner will usually expect the massage therapist to offer her services at a discount for the day of beauty clients.

Common disadvantages of practicing in hair salons are noise, noxious odors, and an approach to massage as a "pampering" or beautification service. Advantages include a strong clientele for referrals (in an appropriate salon) and an atmosphere in which massage stands out as a unique service.

Cruise ships. The big advantage of working on a cruise ship is the excitement and exploration available to one traveling the seas of the world. However, for someone principally interested in developing a massage career, it is usually not a viable choice. Working conditions are usually cramped, an eleven-hour workday is not uncommon, and pay is usually low. A sampling of cruise ship wages in

1996 found these typical pay scales: (a) $200 per month plus 15% of the gross; (b) $20 per day plus 10% of the gross; (c) 10% of the gross, increasing to 30% if the gross is over $1,600 per week.

Room and board are paid, so a cruise ship therapist will take home most of the amounts listed above, but compared to what one would make for a comparable amount of work on dry land, the pay is small.

Hiring is usually done through a separate company, or through a franchise (such as Steiner TransOcean, 1007 North America Way, 4th floor, Miami, FL 33132). In order to be hired for cruise ship work, it is necessary to be in direct contact with the franchise company that does the hiring for a ship or a fleet of ships. Once you are known to those who do the hiring, it may be easy for you to find work on a ship, as schedules are often changing, and companies are often looking for experienced massage therapists to fill in on relatively short notice.

Chair massage or on-site massage. Chair massage, also called on-site or seated massage, has grown rapidly into a substantial part of the massage industry. On October 17, 1989, the Wall Street Journal ran a front-page story about on-site massage, and its growth has accelerated ever since. On August 15, 1990, the Associated Press carried a photograph of an on-site massage session being given to a customer waiting in line at the new McDonald's in Moscow. Since then, the locations for practicing chair massage have become practically unlimited.

When practiced in the workplace, the practitioner usually offers a ten to fifteen minute session to employees. Sometimes the company hires the practitioner and provides the service as a fringe benefit, and sometimes the employees pay individually for their massages. Other locations for chair massage that are gaining in popularity are shopping centers, airports, fitness fairs, craft shows, and store-fronts (such as The Great American Backrub).

The type of treatment done is often a shiatsu-like treatment, done in a specially designed chair that supports the client's chest and face, exposing the back and shoulders.

There are two ways to approach on-site — as a practitioner, or as an entrepreneur. As with other forms of massage practice, the hardest part of the job is acquiring a clientele. In this case, that means convincing a corporate executive that your services would be beneficial to his or her workers, or arranging some other setting for a practice.

Once you have a contract to perform services in a workplace or other location, you can perform them yourself, or hire others to do so. If you establish a large number of clients, you can keep yourself and others busy, often making a percentage profit on the work done by those you hire.

Chiropractic offices. Especially in California, business relationships between chiropractors and massage therapists have become quite common. Chiropractors typically employ massage therapists to work in the chiropractor's office. The chiropractor most often prescribes massage for his or her patients, handles the insurance billing procedure, and pays the therapist either a commission or an hourly wage.

Some chiropractors pay the therapist 50% of the amount charged for massage. Some pay 50% but require the massage therapist to pay a monthly rental out of the therapist's 50%. Those who employ therapists at an hourly rate often pay in the neighborhood of $15 to $20 per hour.

Chiropractors have traditionally had great reluctance about prescribing massage for their patients. Some clients enjoy massage much more than chiropractic, or believe they benefit more from massage, and choose to stop going to the chiropractor and go to the massage therapist instead.

Chiropractors combat this by having the massage therapist in their office, and prescribing massage so that insurance reimbursement will cover the cost. The client sees massage as a no-cost added benefit of chiropractic care, and therefore has an added incentive to keep coming to the chiropractor.

The chiropractor not only gains a unique service to offer, but makes a large profit, since chiropractors can bill massage services to insurance companies at far more than they pay the massage therapist (often $80 per hour or more). The massage therapist, usually a recent massage school graduate, has a way to make a living wage and to gain a great deal of professional experience quickly.

The massage/chiropractic relationship varies greatly from state to state. In some states, like California, New York and Virginia, no restrictions exist on practice relationships massage therapists and chiropractors may enter into. In other states, some barriers do exist. Maryland and New Jersey chiropractors have all received a letter from their state boards advising them that only chiropractors can perform massage services in a chiropractic office, disrupting established relationships between chiropractors and massage therapists.

Hospitals.   Hospital-based massage is experiencing a long-overdue phase of growth. Massage programs based in hospitals have existed for about twenty years, but until recently they were few in number. One writer estimated in 1993 that 50 U.S. hospitals had one or more massage therapists working in some capacity with patients (*Massage* Magazine, March/April 1993). Three years later, in 1996, the newsletter of the Hospital-Based Massage Network estimated there were 100 to 150 hospitals using massage. That number has been swiftly rising since then. As we enter the new century, the field of hospital-based massage is expanding very rapidly, with many hospitals no longer resisting massage, and instead seeking out massage therapists who can start various kinds of hospital-based massage programs.

Several different kinds of hospital-based massage programs exist. Some involve working only on staff members, giving chair massage for stress reduction. Some involve working on the general public, usually in a wellness center, in association with the hospital. Some involve working on hospital patients by physician referral as a part of the hospital's health care team. These are sometimes paid positions, sometimes volunteer. The paid positions may be employee positions or independent contractor positions. The departments most likely to employ massage therapists are pre-surgery and post-surgery, obstetrics & gynecology, ante-partum and post-partum, neonatal intensive care, oncology, physical therapy, occupational therapy, orthopedics, cardio-pulmonary, rehabilitation, out-patient pain management, speech therapy, HIV/AIDS, and fitness or wellness centers.

The acceptance of massage in hospitals is usually the result of a good working relationship between doctors or administrators at the hospital and educators or practitioners in the massage community. The exchange of information and ideas in personal and professional relationships brings about the possibility of establishing a hospital-based massage program.

Those who wish to work in hospital settings or who want additional information about this area of practice can contact:

> Hospital-Based Massage Network
> 5 Old Town Square, Suite 205
> Fort Collins, CO 80524
> (970) 407-9232; www.HBMN.com

The Network produces a quarterly publication (sample issue $6.00). The following individuals may be hired as consultants on creating or joining a hospital-based massage program, and other consultants are available by referral from The Hospital-Based Massage Network:

> Xerlan Geiser, 9433 E. 51st, Suite H, Tulsa
> OK 74145; (918) 622-6644

> Karen Gibson, P.O. Box 1617, Glenwood Springs
> CO 81602; (970) 945-3060

> Jeanne M. Wagner, 2142 N. 51st St., Milwaukee
> WI 53208; (414) 789-8189

The following schools offer training or externships in hospital-based massage (Addresses and phone numbers can be found in the State-by-State directory): Blue Cliff School, Kenner, LA; Brenneke School, Seattle, WA; Desert Institute, Tucson, AZ; East-West College, Portland, OR; Oregon School of Massage, Portland, OR; Stillpoint Center, Hatfield, MA.

House Calls. If you talk to massage therapists about house calls, you will find that most therapists either love them or hate them. The majority seem to hate them. I personally love them.

All of the massage therapists I have talked to who hate house calls charge only a few dollars more than they charge for studio massage. Those who love house calls generally charge 40% to 50% more for a house call than for a studio massage.

Clients expect house calls to cost more. If your price is $50 for a studio massage, consider charging $75 for a house call. Another method of pricing is to start with your basic fee for massage; add $5 for carrying and setting up your table, and add 50 cents per mile for your commuting fee.

House calls have several advantages. First, there is no office rental to pay. Second, the higher fee includes compensation for your time in driving to and from the client's home. It's nice to be paid for driving time, especially if your body is feeling the effects of a busy massage schedule. Third, the client usually finds it easier to fit a house call into their schedule, and may have an easier time relaxing at home than she or he would in an unfamiliar environment. Finally, you get to visit lots of people's homes, many of which are quite interesting.

Certain disadvantages exist as well. First, you have little control over the environment. You can turn off the phone ringer, but the kids might cry, the dog might bark, the room might be cramped and it might be too hot or too cold.

Second, people dawdle more at home than they would if they came to your office. They will take a phone call, or someone will come to the door, or they will be late getting home. It is not uncommon for a one-hour massage to extend to an hour and twenty minutes. Add commuting time, and you might spend well over two hours doing a one-hour massage.

Third, carrying the massage table in and out of the car, in and out of the house, and up and down stairs can be tiring. It helps tremendously to purchase a carrying case with side handle and shoulder strap.

The real beauty of house calls comes when you can establish yourself in a community, so that you have enough business to go from one house call to another, thereby reducing your commuting time. Another advantageous situation is the couple, each of whom wants a massage. Some therapists do house calls exclusively, and when they become established can make a very good living.

Suggestion: Keep your oil bottle in a zip-lock plastic bag when traveling to avoid messy leaks and spills.

Office in your home. Home massage office practice has major advantages and major disadvantages. The advantages are fairly obvious — no commute and complete control over your massage environment. One disadvantage is the increased vulnerability of your home because of contact with the public. Another is that some zoning boards prohibit massage as a home occupation, fearing either that you will conduct a prostitution service in your home or that your business traffic will disturb the neighborhood.

A practitioner operating in a home office must have all the permits and licenses that would be necessary for any massage office. However, some communities will not issue a permit for a home massage practice, even though they would issue a permit to a dentist or psychotherapist in the same location.

In communities that refuse to permit massage practices in the home, some practitioners simply keep a low profile and hope they do not get caught violating the law. It is a shame that professionals are required to do this, but it results from local government officials who believe that massage equals prostitution. Consider organizing the home practitioner massage therapists in your town and trying to work through the governmental process to get the zoning restrictions changed. If you choose this option, consult your professional association for guidance and support.

Another potential obstacle to a home office is liability insurance, also called "slip and fall" insurance. Most homeowners' policies will not cover a home business. It may be possible to purchase a rider for your home business at a small additional cost, or you may have to purchase business liability insurance. See Chapter 16 for more information.

The challenge in a home office is to create a professional massage environment. This means no dogs barking, no music or television sounds wafting into the room. It also means keeping your massage environment separate from your living environment, and if possible, having a separate entrance so that clients do not have to walk through your living space to get to the massage room. If there is no separate entrance, the massage room should be the first or second room one comes to on entering the house.

If you are going to base your business in your home office, treat it as professionally as you would any other office space. Charge the going rate, have a separate phone line, and create the ideal massage room. Your efforts to create a professional atmosphere are just as important in a home office as in any other office you practice in.

Group Practice. Joining in practice with other massage therapists or other health practitioners can be a great way to share expenses, generate cross-referrals, and create a sense of community in which each member draws support from belonging to the group.

The disadvantage that is most often reported by members of group practices is that everyone shares the responsibility for making decisions that affect the group, so there is a need for regularly scheduled meetings in which everyone must participate. This can be time-consuming, and can take lots of energy, especially when it comes in the middle of a busy week.

Some group practices hire a receptionist, and others use the group members to answer the phone on a rotating basis. A receptionist is a substantial expense that has to be split among the practice members, so sharing phone duties substantially lowers the overhead. However, if the practice is well-established, having a receptionist can be a luxury for the practitioners who would rather not deal with telephones and scheduling. The presence of a receptionist also designates the office off as a successful and professional operation.

Entrepreneur with associates. Similar to a group practice, several massage therapists or other kinds of therapists practice in a single location. Instead of being a group venture, however, it is the business venture of one or two who lease or own the establishment. The other practitioners either rent space or pay a percentage of the fees they charge. Payment of rent is much more common than fee-splitting.

The entrepreneur can often arrange things so that the rents paid by the other therapists cover the entire expense of the building, giving the entrepreneur a rent-free office. Generally, the entrepreneur is someone with a strong reputation in the community and good business skills.

Individual massage office. In an individual office, you have complete control over your environment and your schedule. You also have complete responsibility for getting done everything that needs to be done, including paying the rent and all other expenses. You have the most freedom and the most responsibility; the most potential for debt and the most potential for large income.

Legal relationships

Any two people who have a business relationship also have a legal relationship. These relationships can apply to people in all of the categories discussed above.

Sole proprietor. When you are the only one in charge of your business, you are the sole proprietor. In the eyes of the law, you and the business are one. Business income and personal income are pooled together for income tax purposes. Most bodyworkers operate as sole proprietors.

If you work in another person's office, you will need to understand whether you are working as an employee or as an independent contractor.

Independent contractor/employee. This refers to the two different legal relationships you can have when you make an agreement to work in another person or organization's location.

The main difference to you lies in how your income taxes are handled. If you are an *employee,* your employer is responsible for paying social security tax on your earnings, and must withhold money from your pay for this purpose.

However, if you are an *independent contractor,* you are responsible for paying your own contribution to the social security system, called a self-employment tax, and nothing is withheld from your pay. This can make a significant difference to you and to the person who may have to pay social security tax on your wages.

Another difference between employees and independent contractors relates to insurance. The person you are working for will normally have business insurance that covers employees but *not* independent contractors. For this reason, some massage employers will hire only employees, so that they will be covered under the business insurance policy.

The key fact that distinguishes between your status as an independent contractor or employee is who has *control* over the way in which you perform your services. If you are in charge of setting your hours and your fees, and choosing the specifics of the treatments you give, then you are an independent contractor. If the person or organization you work for controls your hours, your prices, and your therapeutic services, then you are an employee. If this is the only company you work for, or if you do not use your own equipment or supplies, or if massage is the main business of your employer, you are more likely to be considered an employee.

If your situation has elements of both, then you have to examine it to see whether it more closely fits the description of an independent contractor or an employee. If you are really an employee but your employer treats you as an independent contractor, the IRS can charge substantial penalties *to your employer* for failing to withhold the appropriate social security tax.

6 Career Strategies

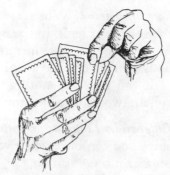

The purpose of this chapter is to help you acquire a "big picture" of your possibilities for a massage career. This chapter will examine the ways you can organize your career, from the investigation phase through the building of a practice.

The following four steps form a framework for your massage career:

1. Investigate the field — explore the field to see if you are interested in pursuing a career.

2. Go to massage school — make a choice based on geography, educational standards, or specialization.

3. Choose one of four approaches for professional growth: permanent part-time, cautious exploration, planned transition or total immersion.

4. Create a business plan and follow it through.

1. Investigate the field

This book contains some of the flavor of a career in massage, but your own experience is the most reliable guide you can consult. Use the resources and ideas you pick up from this book to find people who can complete your picture of the field. Get a professional massage. Talk to professionals about their careers. Listen to what people say about massage.

Imagine yourself in the profession. Can you? Is it easy, enjoyable and exciting, or awkward and unnatural? Ask yourself why you want to go into the field. Are your motives based in service and a desire to connect with other people, or are you thinking more about what you can get from the profession?

This is the time to be as honest with yourself as you can. Choosing massage as a career can be very rewarding for the person who wants to grow and serve. It can be frustrating for the person who does not have the determination to make a commitment and follow it through.

2. Going to massage school

Some massage schools offer evening programs so that you can go to school without changing your life. Others require full-time attendance.

If you are unsure about pursuing massage as a career, you might consider taking some adult education massage classes, or classes for the general public offered by a massage school in your area. This can be an excellent way to "get your feet wet" without risking your whole lifestyle. It may also have the advantage of making the rest of your professional education tax-deductible. (See Chapter 18).

Your choice of a massage school will set the tone for your career. The items to look at in selecting a school are:

A) Consider the licensing requirements of the states you are interested in living in.
If your chosen state has a licensing requirement, you will probably find it easiest to attend a massage school in that state. The school will be aware of the licensing requirement in its home state, and will tailor its curriculum to those requirements.

If you go to an out-of-state school, be sure their training is acceptable to the authorities in your state. The specific requirements for licensing in each state are unique. Even states with the same number of required hours of education may require study of different subjects.

B) Give yourself a strong educational foundation to support your career in the years ahead.
You might choose a 100-hour massage program, learn all you need to establish a career, and enjoy tremendous success in the field for years to come.

You might choose a 100-hour massage program, and on graduating find out that the state or locality you want to practice in has adopted a 500-hour educational requirement.

This is an unsettled time in the massage profession, and no one can tell you what the future will bring. The trend seems to be for the profession to settle on 500 hours as a "normal" amount of professional training, although that number may be trending upwards. All things being equal, it would be prudent to obtain at least 500 hours.

Of course, all things are not equal, and more training costs more time and money. You will have to gather all the information you can, and use your own judgment and intuition to make the best choice for yourself.

C) Choose a school that offers the approach to massage and the specializations that most interest you.
The State-by-State directory contains enough information to understand the emphasis, or general orientation of all the massage schools described. Almost all schools will send a brochure or catalogue upon request, which will give a more complete picture. You may find it useful to compare several schools' catalogues before making your decision.

Some schools require a personal interview, and even for those that do not, it is a good idea to visit the school before making a commitment to attend. Get the feeling of the place. See if you would expect to fit in comfortably with the students currently there, and with the overall atmosphere. Get the details of the financial arrangements, including the school's refund policy for those who leave early.

Massage school is very often a "different" sort of school than the ones you are used to. Since students practice on each other, a large part of your curriculum will consist of giving and receiving practice massages. Receiving massage can bring about emotional awarenesses and unexpected changes. Receiving massage several times a week during your massage school program can accelerate the process of change.

Many massage schools recognize this and integrate this aspect of learning into the program. In fact, many schools consider a student's personal growth an essential component of the curriculum. These schools will recognize the psychologically transforming effect massage can have for clients.

Other schools emphasize "medical massage" or the "medical model." Schools with this emphasis present Swedish massage with an emphasis on medical massage. These schools tend to minimize the focus on consciousness and personal growth.

Still other schools present a focused approach to career growth, emphasizing a strong work ethic. These schools will place a greater value on building technical skills, business skills and practical experience. Their programs will be more directed toward the goal of achieving professional competence and career placement in the most efficient way.

Think about these issues, but also let your intuition guide you to the best school for your needs. Going to massage school can be a very special and life-changing experience. Choose with your mind and your heart, and have a great time.

3. Choose your approach:
permanent part-time, cautious exploration, planned transition or total immersion

Your massage career will take some time to grow. Your skills as a therapist will mature for years after you finish massage school. Your reputation in the community will likewise take time to build. It is best to have a plan that will allow you to integrate that period of career growth into the context of your life.

Plan A: Permanent Part-Time

Massage is a career that lends itself well to part-time practice, and a great many massage therapists choose to keep their career permanently part-time.

A 1994 AMTA member survey found that the average massage therapist gave 6-10 massages per week. A 1996 practitioner survey by the National Certification Board for Therapeutic Massage and Bodywork had a similar finding, with 51.4 percent of respondents giving 10 or fewer massages per week.

Full-time massage work can be physically demanding. Repetitive strain injuries can be a problem, and giving out your energy all day can be depleting. While some practitioners can give six or seven massages per day with no ill effects, others know that they must stop after three or four massages per day in order to stay healthy.

If you can acquire either a house-call practice or an office practice with low overhead costs, a part-time massage practice can support you, and can give you the freedom to pursue your other interests as well. For parents of small children, those with other part-time jobs, aspiring writers, dancers and actors, and people in a variety of other work situations, a part-time massage career can make a lot of sense.

Plan B: Cautious Exploration

This is a low-risk alternative. The idea is to make no significant changes in your current lifestyle, but integrate massage education and exploration of massage practice into your life.

You can do this by going to a massage school that has evening or weekend classes, and using your after-hours time to experiment with doing massage professionally. You can charge for your services or not, as you see fit. (In states that require a license, you can charge only after licensure.) The idea is to gain experience, and to learn whether massage is a field you want to put some real energy into.

After exploring the field in this way, you will be in a position to know whether it is something you enjoy and can commit to pursuing for a living. At this point, you can move to Plan A, Plan C or Plan D.

Plan C: Planned Transition

This is for those who are committed to pursuing a career in massage, yet want to do it in a way that creates a minimum of disruption in their lives. It is a plan that is particularly well suited to teachers, part-time and flex-time workers, and others with substantial free time to pursue a massage career.

A teacher might build her massage practice after working hours. When it reaches a good level, she can switch to substitute teaching. When the practice will support her fully, she can quit teaching and rely fully on massage. Similarly, a waiter or waitress can cut back on hours as the massage practice grows, eventually giving up waiting tables completely.

In order to make this option work, you will need to be committed. Making a living at your "day job" can take a lot out of you, yet you need to have the energy and drive to become established in your new field during your after-hours time. In the next chapter, you will read about the many marketing techniques available to you. Make sure you will have the energy to keep your current job and also apply yourself to building a massage practice. The transition may take several years, so be sure you are prepared.

Plan D: Total Immersion

This is a sink-or-swim approach in which you quit your job, rely on whatever financial support you have, and focus 100 percent on establishing yourself as a professional massage therapist. This option requires some means of financial independence — either a bankroll, a generous spouse or benefactor, or a talent at living without much money.

Most marketing techniques require you to have an office setting for the practice of massage. To pursue Total Immersion, you should have an office. This will of course add a significant expense for which you must be prepared. Give some thought to the economics of the situation, and decide whether you could essentially go without any income for a year. There is a good chance that your first year will be a very lean one, and that your second may not be a great deal better.

Some prefer this approach because it forces the person to do everything possible to make a success of their massage career. To pursue this option requires a clear sense of commitment, and also an understanding of the balance between self-promotion and patience. You should also be prepared for some long, lonely days.

This option will be easier for the individual who has lots of contacts and a strong local reputation. Such a person will have the best chance of establishing a practice relatively quickly. It is not advisable for someone who is new in the community.

4. Create a Business Plan and Follow it Through

A business plan is like a blueprint. You can build without one, but having one is likely to make your task easier and your result better.

The specifics for creating a business plan, and a form you can use to create your own, are provided in the next chapter.

7 Marketing Yourself as a Massage Therapist

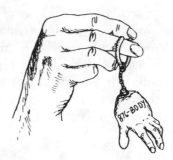

This topic mystifies more massage therapists and bodyworkers than any other. Books, marketing kits, seminars, instructional videos, and other items are on the market to teach you how to acquire a following in your chosen profession.

This guide will give you the benefit of my experiences, as well as those of many other therapists I have interviewed, as to principles and techniques you can use to market your professional services. Before examining the specific techniques you can use, however, there are a few questions you should ask yourself.

Preliminary questions

Are You Ready?

Do you feel your massage is worth $55 per hour (or whatever is the going rate in your area)?

How would you feel about having a strong clientele in the town you are now living in? Are you prepared to call this place home?

Imagine introducing yourself to a variety of people in your town. You tell them you are a massage therapist. How does that feel to you?

The above questions touch on the chief reasons that massage practitioners, even after they have gone to massage school, are reluctant to make a commitment to building a massage practice. If you are not ready to present yourself to the public as a professional deserving their time and money, take the time to grow before making a sincere effort at professional marketing.

That growth may mean gaining new professional skills. It may mean confronting issues of self-image or self-esteem. It may mean learning to be comfortable relating to a broad variety of people. Your growth on all these levels will continue for a long time, well into your professional career. You do not need to be perfect to succeed as a massage therapist — just ready.

How Long Do You Expect This To Take?

How much of a hurry are you in? Are you expecting to throw yourself into a marketing campaign for six months and then have a thriving practice? Are you willing to spend two years or longer creating a practice for yourself? If you are looking for the six-month version, you will probably be disappointed in the results. These things take time.

Consider advertising, for example. One study has shown that the average consumer will notice your ad only one out of three times you run it, and that the same consumer has to *see* your ad nine times before she is ready to purchase the advertised goods or services. Therefore, you may need to run an ad 27 times to have your client actually come in for a massage.

Word of mouth can be similarly time-consuming. A new client told me that his friend had been urging him to try my massage for two years. Two years is an exceptionally long delay in accepting a referral, but I include this example to give you the idea that some aspects of marketing simply cannot be rushed. Successful marketing involves a blend of *commitment* and *patience*.

What's your plan?

Make a plan for your career — what your practice will be like in six months, one year, two years, three years, five years. Use the form on page 45 or create your own planning form.

All sources of professional business guidance will tell you, as a business person, that a business plan is an essential part of your growth process. Advantages of a business plan are:

- It helps you know where you want your career to go;
- It helps you keep track of your progress toward your goals;
- It helps you organize your efforts toward meeting your goals;
- It gives you the clarity to express your goals to others so that they will help you find opportunities.

At the same time, it is important to stay flexible and be quite willing to depart from the plan. In fact, every few months or so, you may want to completely re-write your plan to reflect what you have learned or how your goals have changed.

For example, let's say you make a business plan that emphasizes house calls in an affluent suburb. It includes working at a health spa in that area part-time and using advertising in a community newspaper to try to break into the house call market. Midway through this project, you meet a cardiologist who offers you an office in his group practice. This is a terrific opportunity that you had not even realized was possible.

Do you pass up the cardiologist because you are in the middle of a different plan? Of course not. You change your business plan. At the same time, it was important to have the business plan even though you changed it; you might never have met the cardiologist.

When you make your plans for six months, one year, two years, three years and five years from now, be as detailed and specific as you can. Include your best predictions about all of the following:

- Location for doing massage
- Target clients
- Type of work you want to be doing
- How clients will learn about you
- Number of clients you want or expect to have
- Workshops, professional trainings and meetings to attend
- Advertising and other promotional plans
- Expenses you are likely to incur

Mark on the top of each plan the date you write it, and the target date for the goals you create. Take your plans out every few months and see how things are going. Revise your plan at least once a year.

Sample Business Plan

On page 44 is a sample business plan for Mary Jones. Mary has been out of massage school one year, and is seeing 8 to 12 clients per week. Some of these are house calls, and some are in a resort 15 miles from her home. She has a part-time job doing cleaning work to supplement her income.

Create Your Business Plan

Use the form on page 45 as a sample to create your business plan. If you feel the form does not suit your particular needs, by all means modify it to take into account the planning you need to do.

You will be creating more business plans as time goes by, so you may want to create a form that suits you and make a few copies of it. Keep your business plans in a folder and keep the folder with your other business materials, such as business receipts, client records, and professional books.

Nuts and Bolts of Marketing for Massage and Bodywork

You have examined your readiness for success, your expectations about your career path, and your plans for making your goals take shape. You now have an understanding of the larger picture that your marketing efforts will fit into.

Before discussing the specific marketing techniques you might use, there is one broad principle to consider:

Person-to-person contact is the most effective.

Because massage is a personal service, and because it is relatively expensive, people want to have a good idea that they are going to like both the person and the person's treatment before they come in for a massage. It is much harder to convey this level of confidence with impersonal contact, such as advertising, than it is with person-to-person contact.

To overcome people's natural shyness and resistance to the idea of nudity and being touched, you need to let people know enough about you to trust you, and enough about your work to have confidence in it.

Keeping this in mind, consider the following techniques you can use to promote your professional services.

A. Person-to-Person Marketing Techniques

All professions depend chiefly on referrals, or word-of-mouth, and massage is no exception. A certain amount of word-of-mouth marketing happens naturally. If you give one client a great massage, she naturally wants to tell her friends, and some of them may be curious enough to try you out sooner or later.

MARY JONES' BUSINESS PLAN   MAY 7, 2001

Goals:

To increase clientele to 25 per week at $50 per session
To keep commuting distances to a minimum
To emphasize sports massage in my practice

Target clientele:

Amateur and professional athletes
Local residents
Professionals and their spouses

Possible new locations to work in:

Hospital wellness center
Sports injury clinic
Country club

Means of reaching new clients:

Ads or feature story in country club newsletter
Person-to-person contact with physicians and attorneys in the area
Contacts with personal fitness trainers and athletic trainers in the area
Ads or feature story in local circulation newspaper

Six month goals:

Acquire a local office at a low cost where I can see clients; meet at least four personal fitness trainers or athletic trainers and give them complimentary demonstration massages; meet at least four doctors or lawyers in the area and introduce them to myself and my work.

One year goals:

Take advanced trainings in neuromuscular therapy and sports massage techniques; expand contacts with personal fitness trainers and athletic trainers; expand athletic clientele to at least 12 per week; obtain a quality office environment where I can create the ideal setting for sports and rehabilitative massage as well as doing relaxation massage.

Two year goals:

Have firmly established sports/rehabilitative massage office, seeing 20 clients per week. Supplement practice with occasional house calls for professional clientele. Work with world-class athletes in preparation for competitive events.

Three year goals:

Travel with athletes to sporting events, hire other sports massage therapists to work in my clinic when I am away.

Five year goals:

Offer sports massage trainings; employ at least one full-time massage therapist in my clinic; work exclusively with competitive athletes.

SAMPLE BUSINESS PLAN   date _____

Items to consider:
     Location for doing massage
     Target clients
     Type of work I want to be doing
     How clients will learn about me
     Number of clients I will have
     Current fee structure
     Workshops, professional trainings and meetings
     Advertising and other promotional plans
     Expenses I am likely to incur

Goals:

Target clientele:

Possible locations to work in:

Means of reaching target clientele:

Six month goals:

One year goals:

Two year goals:

Three year goals:

Five year goals:

The art of marketing yourself, however, lies in accelerating this process as much as possible. The main task to accomplish in that regard is to become widely known and accepted within as many groups as possible in your community.

The following are some proven methods for making people familiar with you and comfortable with you, and interested in trying your therapy:

1. Demonstration/lecture at health clubs, professional groups and social groups

These can be a very effective way to become known and accepted, and to increase your clientele. The idea is to present a short speech on the nature of massage, the benefits it can have, and what is to be expected during a session. This is followed by a brief demonstration on a volunteer.

If you are doing it in a place where a massage room is available, such as a health club, you might consider following it up with an offer to do a ten-minute foot massage or chair massage on anyone who is curious.

A presentation of this sort accomplishes many marketing goals all at once. As you establish rapport with the group, you become known, familiar and accepted. They learn the theory of massage and how it can help them, and they gain an understanding of the process and what to expect. Then, after your demonstration, they see and hear from your client how wonderful a person feels after one of your treatments.

For someone who is curious about massage but fearful about nudity or about being touched by a stranger, the lecture/demonstration is perhaps the only marketing tool that will give that person the confidence to try a massage. By creating confidence in yourself, taking the mystery out of the massage process, and giving the person a clear idea of what she has to gain by having a massage, you can effectively break down some strong barriers to using your services.

A therapist I know gave several lecture/demonstrations at her health club, a women-only club. She made such an impression that practically each time she went into the club for a workout after that, one or more members came up to her asking to schedule a massage appointment.

Other locations for this type of presentation are civic, professional and social groups. Ask your friends and clients about any groups they are members of, such as the Rotary, local women's club, yoga group, church group, exercise class, or toastmasters. These groups are often glad to have outside speakers, and the fact that one of their members recommends you will be an advantage.

Many people have a great fear of public speaking, and will feel it is impossible to do a lecture/demonstration in front of a group. If you can't, you can't. However, if you can't you are missing out on one of the most effective and successful marketing opportunities you can use. Remember that the group you speak to will be there because they are interested in you and in massage. They are on your side and they want to like you. Prepare in advance what you are going to say and do, and just be yourself.

A group that can help you overcome your fear of public speaking is Toast-masters International. They have regional meetings everywhere, usually early in the morning, and each participant gives short talks and receives constructive criticism. You can find your local groups by calling Toastmasters at (714) 858-8255 or writing to Toastmasters, P.O. Box 9052, Mission Viejo, CA 92690.

2. Free introductory massages for selected individuals

Anyone who is likely to be a source of repeated referrals should be cultivated as a contact. Such people are psychotherapists, medical doctors, chiropractors, acupuncturists, wholistic practitioners of all sorts, team coaches and sports trainers, dancing teachers, other massage therapists and bodyworkers, and people who are well-known and well-respected members of the community.

Any of these people, who are in a position of trust with their friends, neighbors, clients, and patients, will generally be listened to by those they know. Therefore, once they believe in you and your work, they can be a good source of referrals.

You may wish to seek out these people and try to introduce yourself, or you may wait until you meet someone in the natural course of events. Either way, offering a complimentary massage can be an excellent way of introducing that person to you and your work. Once they know you and have confidence in you they will be more willing to refer clients to you.

3. Discounts to clients for referrals

One therapist gives a ten-dollar discount on the next massage to any client who refers another client. She believes this fosters referrals, as it gives clients a motivation to spread the word about massage.

In a similar vein, one therapist offers a "buy two gift certificates, get your massage free" promotion. I have not tried either approach. My hunch is that clients have a natural desire to tell their friends and neighbors when they like you and your service. However, it is possible that a financial incentive would give them more of a reason to do so. Those of you who do try it, let me know your experiences.

4. Join the local Chamber of Commerce

Consider joining the Chamber of Commerce in your community. These are local business people who are getting together to share matters of common concern. You are such a person, and there is no reason you should not be involved in such a group.

The contacts you make in a group like this will be valuable for your career, in that these are people who know many members of the community. The more you become known and accepted as a "normal" business person, the less resistance people will have to the idea of coming to you for a massage.

5. Do on-site promotional massages

This means going where the people are and working either for free or for a small amount, doing brief treatments. You can rent a booth at a health fair, craft fair, workshop center or convention and offer five or ten minute massages. You can arrange in advance to set up at the end of a sporting event, or at a shopping center during busy times. The exposure you get from such activities may bring you clients immediately, and also may have a long-term benefit in getting you known in the local community.

6. Join as many organizations as you comfortably can

The goal is to meet large numbers of people and to become known. Don't join organizations just to accomplish a marketing goal. You won't have fun, and you may seem pushy. Join organizations you are interested in, but don't be shy about telling people what you do, and never get caught without your business card handy to give out to an interested person.

B. Person-To-Paper Contact

There are some people who are your potential clients, whom you cannot reach in person or through a personal recommendation. Reaching them through the printed word may be your only means of making contact.

Advertising is a quick way to reach large numbers of people. The difficult aspects of using advertising effectively are *avoiding* the people you do *not* want to find you, and making a persuasive impression on the people you do want to find you.

Advertising has the disadvantage of being impersonal contact. It will let people know who you are and where you are and perhaps what you offer. However, it will not tell them that they will like you, that they can trust you, that you have a great touch and tremendous skills, or that they will feel much better after one of your treatments.

Therefore, advertising will most effectively reach those clients who are already familiar with massage but do not currently have a massage therapist whom they go to. This is a relatively small percentage of the general population. However, it takes only one new regular client to make any advertisement worth its cost.

The biggest disadvantage of advertising is that it opens you to sexually-oriented massage clients. A great many men have had sexual experiences that were billed as "massage." In many areas of the United States today, it is easier to find sexual massage than it is to find legitimate massage. Though great progress has been made in legitimizing the profession in recent years, confusion persists.

Doing any general advertising virtually guarantees that you will be confronted by at least some men calling to find out if they can get sexual services from you. Every massage therapist I know finds this to be draining, degrading and infuriating. However, at this point in the history of massage, it is an unavoidable side-effect of using advertising as a tool to build your practice.

Suggestion: In any person-to-paper advertising you do, consider including a photo of yourself. This will do several things. First, it will help dispel any idea that you are offering sexual massage. Second, it will convey some information about you — it is the best substitute available for personal contact. Finally, it is an eye-catcher. In a print medium, a photo tends to draw attention, and it can help clients see an ad they might otherwise miss.

1. Flyers and Business cards

Flyers and business cards are best used after you have made person-to-person contact, to further explain your work or to serve as a reminder about you and your services.

Most therapists who have tried leaving flyers for the general public and posting business cards in places like health food stores and supermarkets find that the results are poor. The main people you are likely to reach by posting your business card are the other therapists who see your card when they post theirs.

One flyer that worked was the one used by Wes Boyce in southern California. That is reproduced on the following page. Wes used this flyer as part of his plan to become established quickly from the ground up. This flyer brought him 100 clients within seven months, and at that point he canceled the promotion. His promotion had raised $1,000 for Meals On Wheels.

He did not make much money directly from these massages, although some clients tipped him, and a few became paying customers. However, he was able to get a lot of practical experience in a short time, and also generated a great deal of public awareness about himself and his work.

2. Direct mail

This refers to those packets of ads and coupons we all get in the mail from time to time. Some massage therapists have used these very effectively to build their practices.

These direct mailings generally go to 10,000 homes at a time. The cost to have your ad or coupon included will usually be a few hundred dollars. This may sound like a lot of money, but consider that one weekly client will repay the entire cost of the promotion in two to three months.

Two useful approaches to direct mail are to use it when you open a new office, and to use it at holiday times to advertise gift certificates. It can also be used as a major promotion to boost an existing practice.

To get in touch with direct mail companies, look in the mailers for their phone number and address, or check the Business-to-Business Yellow Pages if there is one for your area (available from your local phone company's business office). Look in the listing for "Marketing Programs and Services."

The direct mail sales person will help you design your promotion. Most such promotions include a special offer, such as an introductory massage for new clients at a reduced price.

3. Yellow Pages

All of the massage therapists I interviewed who have yellow pages listings agreed that the listing more than paid for itself with the business it generated. However, they also agreed that the quality of calls that came from the listing was poor. A large percentage of these calls are from men seeking sex, and a significant amount of time and energy is taken in screening these calls.

Some localities have two listings in the yellow pages — one for massage, and one for massage therapists. The idea behind the distinction is to tip off the sex-

Treat Yourself!...
Treat the Senior Adults of North County

Receive a **FREE One-Hour MASSAGE** if you donate a minimum of $10.00 to the Senior Adult Services - North Coast - Meals On Wheels program.

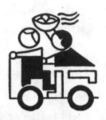

 WES BOYCE, M.S., Ms.T., is an experienced, state certified Massage Technician licensed in the City of Encinitas. He is offering a **FREE**, one-time, **Full-Body Massage**, normally valued at $40.00, when you support Meals On Wheels. Your $10.00 donation will feed one senior for two days — meals delivered by M-O-W volunteers.

If you are in need of ENHANCED ENERGY, BODY RELAXATION, STRESS REDUCTION or SPORTS MASSAGE, contact Wes. He'll help to relieve your stiffness, aches and pains, in the neck, back and shoulders. Treat yourself and/or a friend to this unique opportunity and experience the wonders of massage.

You'll feel better — for supporting a worthwhile cause and for giving your body the freedom from tension that it deserves.

Call Today for an appointment
(619) 436-1569

seekers that those listed as massage therapists are legitimate. Unfortunately, the sex clients either don't see the distinction, or figure that you're really offering sex massage and you put the listing under "massage therapist" to fool the police. If your listing has the word "massage" in it, you can count on sex calls.

You can help create the image you want by carefully selecting the name and information you present in the yellow pages. One practical option is to choose a business name at the beginning of the alphabet, since you will get more calls if you are listed first.

Another practical option is to choose a name like "wholistic health center" to generate a minimum of sex calls. The business name you choose for your yellow pages listing need not be the same as the one on your business cards or bank account. The people who publish the yellow pages will accept most any business name you supply.

Yellow pages ads are expensive. A basic listing with no more than name and phone number will cost around $15 per month, or $180 per year. A small block ad with some basic information can cost around $50 per month, or $600 per year. Larger ads can cost a great deal more. This will be more economical for a group practice than for an individual.

Getting into the yellow pages requires some planning in advance. In my area, the deadline for new orders is in March, and new books are distributed in July. If you are opening a new office, or changing locations, you may want to coordinate your move with the schedule of the yellow pages publisher to minimize the disruption in your practice.

4. Newspaper coverage of you and your practice

One way to become better known is to have a local newspaper reporter write an article about you, about massage, and about any particular aspect of you or your work that is unique or interesting.

Make contact with a reporter for your local newspaper, and give her or him a massage. Discuss anything about yourself or your work or training that may be of interest, and let the reporter decide what angle might serve as the basis for a story.

After the story appears in the paper, frame it and put it on your office wall. Your clients will be gently reminded that you are a special person worthy of respect.

5. Placing ads in newspapers

Many successful massage therapists have never advertised in newspapers and never will. Others have found newspaper advertising to be a way to shorten the time needed to build a practice to a self-supporting level. Others have advertised and been so frustrated by the clients who responded that they have burned out on massage as a profession. The following information about newspaper advertising should help you make the most of newspaper advertising.

Two types of newspaper ads — classifieds, display ads

Two types of massage ads are available in newspapers — display ads and business classified ads. Display ads (also called block ads) appear in the body of the paper, with the news and features articles, and therefore are seen by more readers than business classifieds. Display ads are larger and substantially more expensive than business classifieds. Display ads make sense in small-circulation newspapers, when you are trying to break into a new market. In larger newspapers, massage ads almost always run in the business classifieds.

Business classifieds

Business classifieds is a separate section of the classifieds, devoted to business services such as painting, carpentry, cleaning and hauling. While these ads are much cheaper than display ads, they cost a great deal more than a normal classified ad.

The response to advertising in the business classifieds tends to be immediate. If the response to your classified ad is going to be good, you will know within the first few days. Start with a short run for your ad, so that if the response is not good, you have the opportunity to try a different newspaper.

Generally speaking, business classified advertising is cost-effective for massage therapists. In other words, you will generally make more money as a result of placing the ad than you spend on the ad. The other question, however, is how much grief you will have to put up with in the process.

Display advertising

Display advertising is quite different from business classified advertising. Someone looking up massage in a business classified is ready for a massage — today, if possible. Someone just reading the news or features, who sees your display ad in the newspaper, was not thinking about massage until she saw your ad. She may not be ready for massage for quite a while.

In fact, it may take many exposures to your ad before this person feels you are sufficiently "familiar" to give you a try. After seeing your ad a few times, she will begin to get the idea that you are not just a passing fad, but a true fixture in the community.

The more times a person sees your ad, the more familiar and accepted your name will be to that person. After five to ten exposures to your ad, the person may be sufficiently comfortable with your print image that she would consider trying a massage. The more nervous the person is about massage, the longer it may take for her to begin to feel comfortable about you by repeatedly seeing your ad.

Therefore, display advertising is generally best used in small circulation newspapers, where you have a particular desire to break into a new market that you feel has a good potential for your practice. Choose your newspaper and plan to place your ad many times. Keep your ad the same each time you run it, so that the "familiarity" factor works best. Use a picture of yourself in the ad — this will be an eye-catcher, will help the person feel she knows you and will give more of a sense that you can be trusted.

Types of Newspapers

Many types of newspapers exist, and you can use each differently in aid of your marketing goals. The different types of newspapers are general circulation dailies, special interest newspapers (usually weekly or monthly), and local or regional papers (usually weekly).

General circulation newspapers

These are the daily newspapers read by the general population. The general circulation newspaper I advertised in is the Asbury Park Press, which serves a region within about a 25-mile radius of Asbury Park, New Jersey. Their business classified directory includes a listing for massage, and at the top of the massage listing each day is the following notice:

> ATTENTION ADVERTISERS: The only copy permitted in a massage ad is: name, address, phone number, rates & hours. The only exception is a licensed spa listing their facilities (sauna, steam room, etc.)
>
> The terminology 'Professional or Licensed' can be used if customer sends copy of certificate from a school of massage prior to ad running.
>
> Ads must be paid in advance.

This notice appeared for the first time shortly after the same newspaper ran a story about a prostitution ring that had operated through the massage classifieds. The management placed the notice at the top of the massage listing in an attempt to prevent the use of its massage ads for prostitution.

I advertised in this listing immediately before and immediately after the story about the prostitution ring operating through the massage classifieds. Despite the notice at the top of the listing, and despite the story in the same newspaper about prostitution arrests, roughly ninety percent of the calls I received from this ad were men looking for sexual massage. This percentage did not seem to change as a result of the prostitution story or as a result of putting the notice at the top of the massage listing.

Phone calls at 7:00 a.m. and 11:45 p.m. in response to my ad were not uncommon. I chose to answer my own phone, although some therapists who advertise leave the answering machine on and selectively return calls. I found that, in general, people calling at unusual times were looking for unusual massage services. My first name (Martin) indicated I was a man, and my ad apparently attracted a great many gay or bisexual callers. Calls for sexual massage dropped off dramatically after the first week.

Most of the clients looking for sex had the sense to stop trying when I explained in no uncertain terms that my massage was completely legitimate and did not include any sexual contact. A few, however, apparently regarded that as a challenge and made appointments anyway.

These men would wait until the end of their massage, or in some cases until their second or third massage, to verbally or non-verbally make their wishes known. This was quite a growth experience for me, as I had to learn how to deal with my own feelings of anger and resentment in such a situation.

My growth brought me to a point where I could comfortably take charge of the situation. I learned to discuss any suspect signs of arousal immediately, carefully watch the client's attitude about the subject, and terminate the massage immediately if the client was being inappropriate. Once I realized that I had control of the situation, my emotional response lessened dramatically.

The several regular clients I acquired through this advertising exposure are lovely people whom I appreciate very much as clients, and who never would have found me without the ad. The total expense for the ads I ran was about $250 over a period of several weeks. Despite the irritation factor, on the whole it was well worth doing.

Special interest newspapers

There may be newspapers for special interest groups in your area that can be good sources of massage clients. Such papers include:

- New age or wholistically oriented newspapers
- Religious or community-oriented newspapers
- In-house newspapers for institutions such as retirement communities and hospitals

Two such newspapers I have advertised in are written for the Jewish community.

The cost involved is usually low, and the response level probably will also be low. However, such exposure can be useful in gaining entry into a new market. In my case, my small ads in two Jewish newspapers generated enough new business to at least pay for the ads, and also served to gain some name recognition.

Local and regional newspapers

Many communities have small local papers, which are published once or twice a week. These are sometimes mailed to all households in the community at no charge. These papers often have a "business classified" section similar to the one in general circulation newspapers.

Before advertising in one of these, get the flavor of the other ads in the paper. If a massage ad would seem distinctly out of place in comparison to the other types of ads that are currently running, it may not be a good idea to place your ad in that paper.

As with special interest newspapers, the circulation of local papers will be small, as will the cost to advertise. One advantage is that you can be sure that any potential clients who see this ad will be close to you and able to conveniently come to see you.

C. Broadcast Media

Radio, broadcast television, and direct access cable television are also possibilities for massage marketing. Generally speaking, the cost of commercial advertisements on radio and television is too great for a massage practice.

Direct access cable, however, can provide opportunities for exposure. A pair of chiropractors in my area produced a multi-part feature on wholistic health modalities for showing on direct access cable. One segment was on massage, and the therapist they chose for that segment received significant exposure at no expense to her.

D. Ethereal Marketing Techniques

"There is more to the world" says Shakespeare, "than is dreamt of in your philosophy." Many successful practitioners believe there is more to making contact with another person than operating in the world of the physical senses.

These are some of the unorthodox marketing tips used by some successful massage practitioners:

- Visualize an open field, and see clients coming across that field to you.
- Meditate, tell the universe you are ready for people to come into your life.
- Imagine that you have a dial you can turn to control the flow of your practice. Turn it up to become busier, turn it down when you need freedom from your practice.

If this sounds like so much hocus-pocus to you, don't bother with it. You may find, at some point, that it has meaning for you. For example, several therapists have said that when they find themselves feeling frantic and wishing they had spare time instead of appointments, their clients often call in and cancel.

A skeptical person can always see something like this as coincidence. It is not scientific and cannot be proven. If it intrigues you, simply suspend disbelief. Allow the possibility that it is hogwash and allow the opposite possibility that it is a real phenomenon. Then stay with your experience, see how things go and form opinions later.

E. Fostering Repeat Business

The first goal of your marketing efforts is to get potential clients to try you out. The next goal is making them realize they should come back and make massage a regular part of their lives.

The two main ways you can foster repeat business are to create an understanding of the benefits of massage, and to stay in touch with your clients.

Create an understanding of the benefits of massage

After receiving a massage, the client's body will understand how healthful it is, but the person's mind may not. Many people guide themselves primarily by their mental processes, and unless these people have an understanding of the value of massage, they may not become repeat clients.

You can help them understand the process by honestly explaining how massage benefits people in general, and how they specifically could benefit from a regular program of treatment. It can be helpful to give them a brochure or other printed material setting out the health benefits of massage therapy. There is no need to be a salesman, or to be pushy. If you are honest and forthright, people will respect your professionalism and appreciate the information — they want to take care of themselves once they understand how.

Stay in touch with your clients

Some therapists call their clients a day or two after their first massage to ask how they are feeling. This is especially appropriate with clients who have come in for relief from a specific condition.

Other ways to stay in touch with clients are:

- Send birthday cards
- Photocopy an article of interest about massage and send it to all your clients with a short note
- Send holiday greeting cards at Christmas or Rosh Hashanah
- Send a flyer or post card reminding clients that you offer gift certificates at holiday time
- Send flyers or post cards advertising any special offers you are making on your services
- Send announcements to your clients when you begin working in a new location or take on an associate in your office
- If you have a seasonal clientele, send thank-you letters to your clients at the end of the season for their patronage.

If initiating contact of this type feels unnatural to you, do not bother with it. If it is a genuine expression of your interest in your clients, they will take it as such and respond positively.

For further information about marketing

A book that will expand on several of the concepts in this chapter is *Guerilla Marketing* by Jay Conrad Levinson, published by Houghton Mifflin (The sequel, *Guerilla Marketing Attack*, is not as useful). This book emphasizes the creative, low-budget techniques and principles you can use in marketing. Much of the information is inapplicable to marketing professional services such as massage, but it is worth looking through if you are seriously interested in marketing yourself. It is widely available at libraries and bookstores.

Other marketing aids tend to be expensive, and you should be cautious about using them. The best marketing devices you can obtain are education and motivation — these turn you into your own best resource. I have included reference to *Guerilla Marketing* because, as I have tried to do in this chapter, it educates you so that you can understand and use effective marketing techniques. It is more worthwhile to invest in training yourself about marketing than it is to buy the expensive videos and packets you may see advertised.

8 Opening a Massage Office

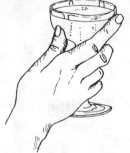

Opening an office is a big step. It is the mark of maturity of a massage career. It requires confidence in your professional skills, your business ability, and your commitment to your practice.

When the time comes in your career to open your own office, it should be a joyous venture. It will bring you the chance to make a better living and have a clear professional identity. This chapter will help you be fully prepared and ready to take this step, and will give you the basic information you will need to make the best choices in bringing your office to life.

The topics covered in this chapter are Governmental requirements, practical requirements, and business decisions. Business decisions include subjects like measuring your readiness to open an office, choosing a location, and negotiating a lease. In addition, you will find a checklist for office opening, and discussions of opening a group practice and buying an existing practice.

Governmental Requirements

You are becoming a local business owner, and as such you are taking on a new identity in the eyes of your local government. One of the main functions of local government is to regulate the operations of businesses. By the same token, one of the chief sources of revenue for local government are the license fees and taxes paid by local business owners.

So you are in a two-way relationship with your local government. On one hand, the government wants to exert its authority over you to make sure you do things to their liking. On the other hand, the government wants to see you succeed, so that you will make money and share it with the government.

Your first step is to visit your local government, whether it is a town hall, city hall, municipal complex, or village governmental center. Bring a note pad and pen. Ask for assistance about the following items:

1. Massage licensing law

Most towns and cities do not have laws regulating the practice of massage, but many do. These laws often were written more to guard against prostitution than to realistically regulate massage practice. You may find that the local law regulates

massage quite heavily. Some local laws prohibit massaging members of the opposite sex. A few towns prohibit the practice of massage completely.

If your town has a restrictive law, you will have to choose (1) meeting all of
the restrictions, (2) giving up the idea of practicing there, (3) fighting to have
the law changed, or (4) practicing there and risking being penalized for violating
the law. If you think you may choose number 4, it is probably not a good idea to
march into city hall and identify yourself as a way of getting information.

2. Practitioner license, establishment license

If the town has a licensing law, it will probably have two parts to it. One will
give the requirements for a massage practitioner license, and the other will give
the requirements for a massage establishment license.

The practitioner license applies to your right to practice massage within the
town, and the establishment license applies to the office in which you will practice massage. Each will have a separate procedure and a separate fee.

3. Zoning requirements

Almost all towns have zoning laws, which regulate the types of "uses" that may
take place in different "zones." In other words, zoning laws restrict the kinds of
businesses you can operate in different neighborhoods. Certain neighborhoods
are set aside for residences only. Others may be zoned for industrial uses, such
as factories and warehouses. Others will be for stores or professional practices.
A sample zoning map appears on the following page.

Before committing to a particular location for a massage office, you should be
sure that the location has the proper zoning for use as a massage business.

Different communities will use different zoning classifications for massage.
Some will call it a personal service. Others will call it a profession. Others will
call it a health service. Still others refer to it as "adult entertainment." What they
call it will have an effect on which zones you will be allowed to locate in.

The town clerk can direct you to the zoning map for the city. If the zoning
board can tell you exactly which category massage is considered to be for zoning
purposes, you can check the map to see which neighborhoods are open to you
for an office location. If there is doubt about which category they consider massage, you may need to go before the zoning board to get a definitive ruling before choosing your office location.

If you are opening a home office, the zoning board may require a hearing before deciding whether to allow you to operate a massage practice in your home.
They may consider factors such as the burden placed on neighborhood parking,
the percentage of space in the home devoted to your business, and whether you
will be the only one who performs massage services in your home. If you need to
appear before the zoning board, consider consulting an attorney beforehand for
advice about how to proceed.

4. Health, police and fire department inspections

Inquire of the health department, police department and fire department what
their policies are about inspecting a massage office before it opens. Ask about

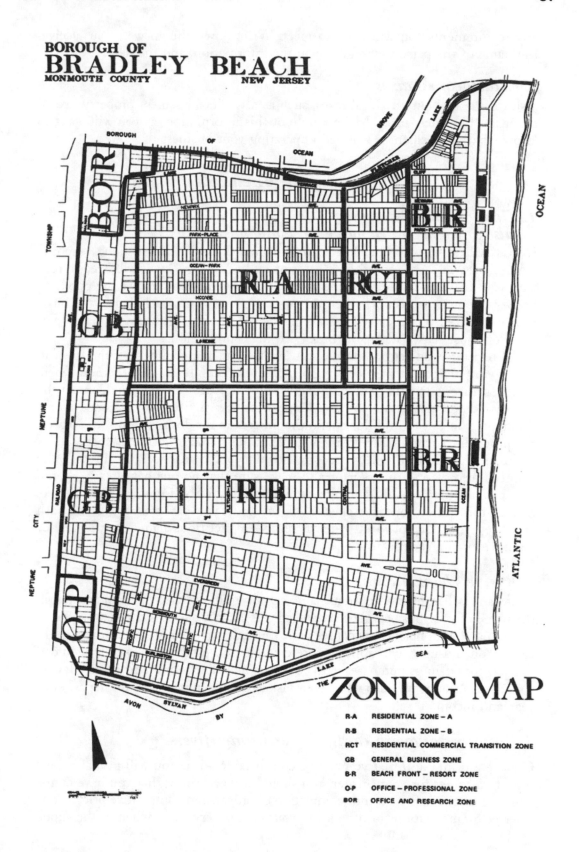

BOROUGH OF
BRADLEY BEACH
MONMOUTH COUNTY   NEW JERSEY

THE ZONING MAP

R-A	RESIDENTIAL ZONE – A
R-B	RESIDENTIAL ZONE – B
RCT	RESIDENTIAL COMMERCIAL TRANSITION ZONE
GB	GENERAL BUSINESS ZONE
B-R	BEACH FRONT – RESORT ZONE
O-P	OFFICE – PROFESSIONAL ZONE
BOR	OFFICE AND RESEARCH ZONE

any requirements you will need to meet. Write down the answers you receive, the name of the person who gives you the information, and the date.

5. Local business taxes

Ask the clerk about any local taxes, such as sewer tax, business property tax, or other local business taxes. Make a note of this information, as you will want to know what your expenses will be in operating your business.

Practical Requirements

1. Fictitious name statement (also called "assumed name" or "doing business as")

If you will give your business a name other than your own name (such as "Wholistic Massage Center" or "Beams of Light Massage") you will need to register your fictitious name with the county government. This allows the public to know who owns a business when the owner's name is not included in the business name. This certificate does not give you exclusive rights to the name. For that you must seek trade-name or service-mark protection.

To register your fictitious name, you must go to the county seat, the town in your county that houses the county government offices. If you do not know where that is, someone in your bank or city government office can tell you. Contact the county clerk, and find out the cost for registering a fictitious or assumed name, the hours you can go and do so, and the procedure for doing so. In some places, the procedure includes advertising your fictitious name in local newspapers.

In most cases, you will be required to do your own checking through the county's records of business names to make sure that no one has already chosen that business name. This can take awhile, so give yourself enough time to take care of this. After you have checked the records, you pay your fee (bring cash and keep your receipt) and you will receive a "fictitious name certificate" (or "assumed name certificate").

2. Business bank account

Your bank will require a fictitious name certificate in order to open an account in the name of your business. It is a good idea to have a business checking account, and to pay for all business expenses with your business checks (or business credit card). Your business will appear more credible and established than it would if you pay for business purchases with your personal checks or credit cards. Having a separate account will also make your task easier when it is time to prepare your year-end income taxes.

3. Business stationery, cards, gift certificates, flyers

Choose a print shop that you can be comfortable with. You will probably be a repeat customer for your printer. You should have a printer that you have confidence in, as to quality, prompt completion of orders, and competitive price. Consider recommendations of others and your own observations when in the shop.

The bare minimum you will need to open your office is business cards. Consider whether to also invest in customized gift certificates and business stationery.

Also consider: A rubber stamp with your business name and address, a rubber stamp with your bank account number to endorse the back of checks, flyers that describe you and your business, a printed coupon for purchasers of pre-paid series of massage, and promotional items to publicize your office.

Business Decisions

1. Can You Afford an Office?

Before you open a massage office, you should calculate what income you can reasonably expect, and what expenses you will have to bear. In the sections that follow, you will learn how to determine your projected income and expenses so you will know what financial resources you will need to see your new office through its initial phase.

Start-up costs

First consider that you will need some money up front in order to open an office. You will need money for office furnishings, first month's rent, security deposit, telephone and utility deposit, printing needs and advertising or other promotional costs. If you have established credit, you may be able to get a loan. Otherwise you will need to use your savings to meet these start-up costs.

As a guideline for planning purposes, the following figures probably come close to the amounts you will need to spend on start-up costs:

Massage table	$500	First month rent	$400
Desk	175	Security deposit	400
Table or shelf	80	Phone deposit	150
Hamper	35	Utility deposit	75
Phone/ans. mach.	75	Printing	100
Music system	250	Ads/promotion	300
Sheets/towels	200	Miscellaneous	100

Any of these items can be more or less than the amounts shown, depending on your particular circumstances. The start-up costs in the sample above total $2,840.

Next examine your ability to meet the continuing financial obligations of operating a professional office.

Estimated Monthly Business Income

Perhaps you work in a health club, hair salon, or doctor's office. Would most of your clients stay with the new massage therapist who replaces you or would they follow you to your office?

Take an honest look at your client list, and imagine the first month in your new office. How many clients do you expect, and what would your total income for the first month be?

Consider, also, that once you have an office of your own, it may be easier for you to create new growth. First, you will have strong motivation to do so. Second, you will have a location that is conducive to the kind of work you want to do. Third, you will have an established office that will serve as the focus of your marketing efforts — promotional ideas such as direct mail, lecture/demonstration and advertising will be more open to you than they would be if you were working in an employer's space.

Make an estimate of your first month's income. If in doubt, choose a lower figure for planning purposes. For purposes of making a sample financial projection, we will assume you can start in your new office with an income of $1,200 per month. This is your "estimated monthly business income."

Other Monthly Income

Calculate your other sources of income, apart from your business. Include any sources of income you know you can count on, such as interest, alimony, dividends, pension, or the like. Total all this income, and figure how much you receive in an average month. For purposes of this example, we will use the figure $150 per month for your "Other Monthly Income."

Total Estimated Income

Add your "estimated monthly business income" ($1,200) to your "other monthly income" ($150). In this example, the total is $1,350.

Estimated Monthly Business Expenses

Calculate the amount you must spend each month for your office rent, telephone, and yellow pages. Also include a twelfth of your annual business expenses, such as advertising, oils and linens, business taxes, professional association dues, accountant fees, insurance costs, and the like.

The total of your monthly business expenses is likely to be between $300 and $1,200. This is the amount you need each month to support your business. We will use the figure of $600 per month as an example of "estimated monthly business expenses."

Estimated Monthly Personal Expenses

This is the amount you need to live on each month, for such essentials as home rental, food, automobile, health insurance and taxes. One way to calculate this is to look through your checkbook for last year. Add up all the money you spent on personal expenses, plus your best guess for how much cash you spent, and divide by 12. Another way is to add up your fixed expenses and then add an estimate for your spending money.

Let's say you come up with a total of $1,000 per month for your "estimated monthly personal expenses."

Estimated Total Monthly Expenses

Add the "estimated monthly business expenses" of $600 per month to "estimated monthly personal expenses" of $1,000 per month to find your "estimated total monthly expenses." This is the amount you will need to earn each month in order to support your new office and your current lifestyle. In our example, this is $1,600.

These estimated figures are summarized in the chart below.

New Office Financial Projections

INCOME

Estimated monthly business income	$1,200
Other monthly income	150
Total estimated income	1,350

EXPENSES

Estimated monthly business expenses in new office location	600
Estimated monthly personal expenses	1,000
Estimated total monthly expenses	1,600

NET DEFICIT $250   per month

This projection shows expenses will be higher than income. Subtracting income ($1,350) from expenses ($1,600) shows an estimated deficit of $250 per month for this person's overall lifestyle after opening the new massage office.

If your financial planning estimate shows a net deficit per month, you should plan to have a reserve of at least one year's worth of deficits before you decide to open your office. It may take a year for you to see any significant increase in your business, so plan to start with the ability to sustain your practice at its current level for at least a year.

In this example, that would mean you should have a capital reserve of $3,000 (12 months × $250/month) to supplement your income for the first year.

Consider choosing a larger figure for your capital reserve, since it is possible your second year may also produce a net deficit.

Additional Reserves For Business and Personal Expenses

In addition to the predictable expenses, you should ideally be prepared for the unforeseen ones as well. For example, your car's transmission falls out. You need $600 to fix it. You decide it would help business to do a direct mail promotion. You need $400 for the cost of the mailing.

This kind of expense can come up without warning, so you should plan on at least another $1,000 to draw on for such emergencies.

Calculate Your Financial Readiness

Add your Start-up Costs ($2,840), your first year's Net Deficit ($3,000), and Additional Reserves ($1,000). This is what you need in the first year to open your office and supplement your income. In this example, the total is $6,840.

If your skills, personality and location are good, and you approach your marketing with commitment and organization, you should find that after the first year you begin to see some increase in your practice. You may still have a net deficit each month in the second year. If you proceed with organization and commitment, you should have a net profit after the second year, and have a net operating profit for the rest of your massage career.

2. Location

There is an old joke in the real estate business:

Question: What are the three most important factors in the value
                of real estate?

Answer: Location, location and location

This expresses a basic truth about the business world. Location counts for a great deal in business. Choose a location that is central, easy to get to, enjoyable to go to, and that conveys a positive image for your practice.

WIZARD OF ID

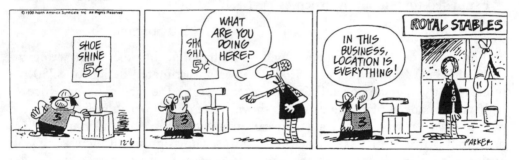

Take your time finding a location. Consider a broad range of questions.

Consider the town:

- Is the town one that can support a massage therapist?

- Are any massage therapists currently earning a living in this town?

- Will I be in direct competition with them or will we draw on different client bases?

- Is there another town in the area that would afford a better image or a more receptive client population?

Consider the neighborhood and building:

- What is the ideal location within my town for my particular practice?

- Will this location be one my clients are comfortable coming to? One they will look forward to coming to?

- Is the building attractive and well-maintained?

- Is the building visible to large numbers of people on a daily basis?

- Are the other offices in the building ones whose images fit comfortably with the image I want for my practice?

- Is the neighborhood safe and pleasant?

- Is parking convenient?

- What other businesses are nearby?

- Will this location support my plans for future growth?

- Do I feel comfortable thinking of this as "my" office?

Your choice of an office location can make your whole professional life easier or more difficult. Do yourself a favor, and make the selection of an office your highest priority. Investigate, think, feel and take some time with this decision. Your efforts will pay great dividends for years to come.

3. Negotiating a Lease

Look for items in a lease which give you flexibility and control and avoid items which give power to the landlord and obligate you excessively.

For example, your lease should include a statement that the office provided will be suitable for use as a professional massage office — as to noise level, temperature control and good repair of all fixtures. This gives you a legal right to complain if the landlord fails to provide you with a quiet and warm massage environment.

If you have any doubts about the zoning for the location, put in the lease that it becomes void if the city refuses to approve zoning for a massage business at that location. Otherwise, you could be stuck with a lease on an office in which you cannot open your business. Also consider making the lease conditional upon being granted a local massage practitioner license and a massage establishment license.

You also may want to negotiate for a lease that is renewable at your option. After all, you do not know for sure that you will succeed in your business, or that you will like the location. Give yourself the option to leave after a year. At the same time, give yourself the option to renew for a second and third year at the same rental (or a small increase) so that you know you will be able to enjoy the reward for your efforts if your practice is very successful.

Spell out in the lease any other items that you consider of special importance to you, and make sure you understand all of the provisions of the lease you sign. As a precaution, it is good practice to show the lease to a lawyer or experienced business person to get an informed opinion before signing.

One further thing to keep in mind is that, while your lease gives you legal rights, these may not amount to anything in practical terms if you wind up having a conflict with your landlord. If you need to hire a lawyer and file a lawsuit,

LEASE CONTRACT

This contract is entered into this 15th day of January, 1988, between Martin Ashley (Martin) and Anthony Marzarella, doing business as Anthony Louis (Anthony). The parties agree as follows:

1. Anthony will furnish a massage room in Le Club salon on Route 88, Brick, New Jersey. He will also furnish a receptionist to take appointments for massage and to collect clients' payments for massage. The receptionist selected shall be a courteous individual who presents a positive image of massage and of the massage therapists employed to work at Le Club.

2. Martin will pay a monthly rental to Anthony of $400.00 per month, payable on the 1st day of each month. Martin will also pay Anthony 17% of the cost of advertising which advertises massage at Le Club.

3. This contract shall be for a period of three months, and shall be renewable at Martin's option for additional periods of three months, up to a total of one year. In addition, after the first year, the contract shall be renewable for an additional year at a monthly rent not to exceed $500 per month.

4. Anthony shall obtain a Brick massage establishment license, and Martin shall obtain a Brick massage practitioner license. All massage therapists employed by Martin at Le Club shall have Brick massage practitioner licenses. Martin shall have the right to transfer or sell his rights under this contract to any other individual who has a Brick massage practitioner license.

5. Permanent improvements to the premises made by Anthony shall be the property of Anthony, and furnishings placed in the massage room by Martin shall remain the property of Martin.

6. Collection of the amount due to be paid for massage shall be the responsibility of Anthony. The receptionist shall collect payment from massage clients.

7. Liability to clients and customers for any accidents or injuries shall be Martin's if the accident or injury occurs within the massage room, and Anthony's if the accident or injury occurs elsewhere on Le Club premises.

_____	_____
date	Anthony Marzarella
_____	_____
date	Martin Ashley

your expenses in suing will almost certainly be more than you would recover even if you win. You can sue in small claims court if you meet the local requirements. However, even that takes preparation, time, energy and expense. While your lease should afford you legal protection, steering free of conflict is worth much more than having right on your side.

The lease on page 66 is the one I signed when I moved into a massage office in a beauty salon. It's not perfect, and the rent was too high, but it will serve as an example of the kinds of items you might want to include in a business lease.

4. Taking Credit Cards

Consider taking Visa and MasterCard in payment for your services. The disadvantage is the cost — there are setup costs, either purchase or rental, and transaction costs for each charge. If you process a small amount of business on credit cards, the setup fees will make it too costly for you. But if you process a large amount of charges on credit cards, these costs are spread out over many transactions and will not be that much of a problem.

In order to take credit cards, you first need to establish a "merchant account", and you next need either software or hardware that will allow you to process credit transactions. Hardware (the "swiper" and printer) can be purchased or leased, but these items are relatively costly. There may also be a monthly minimum processing fee from your service provider. There may also be a per-transaction fee, as well as a percentage of each sale taken as a processing fee. Shop around, as prices vary considerably from company to company.

A suggestion is to find a company that will let you use the old-fashioned imprinters that move back and forth over the credit slip. These are much cheaper than the electronic ones, and may make it feasible for a small practice to take credit cards.

Practically all clients find it convenient to write a check or pay cash, but you may find that there is some business you would not do without taking credit cards. Credit cards make it very easy for clients to buy gift certificates — they can order them much as they do flowers from a florist. An office that takes credit cards also presents a very established and professional image. This can be an asset to a massage office, which is susceptible to being thought of as outside the mainstream of the business world.

To investigate taking credit cards in your business, go to the bank where you have your business checking account, and ask for assistance. You can also do some comparison shopping — call other local banks and ask them about their arrangements for credit cards. AT&T has begun offering low-cost merchant accounts to AT&T customers (call the Rand Company at 1-888-217-3757) and Costco offers low-cost merchant accounts to executive members (1-888-474-0500). Also, check the Yellow Pages and the Business-to-Business Yellow Pages under "Credit Card Equipment and Supplies" for other companies that issue merchant numbers and credit card equipment.

5. Furnishing Your Office

The furnishings you choose for your office will reflect your personality and your preferences for a setting in which to practice your particular type of work. You might choose pastels and crystals if you lean toward the ethereal, and whites and stainless steel if you lean toward the clinical. Only you know the atmosphere you want for yourself and your clients.

- In general, you should keep your office spacious and un-cluttered, as this generally promotes a more comfortable and relaxed feeling.

- Arrange for lighting that is not harsh. Avoid ceiling lights, as these will be too bright for clients when face up. Dimming switches are inexpensive and easily available. One type installs in the wall switch and another screws directly into the bulb socket. Also consider stained glass lamps designed to hold low-watt bulbs and night lights that plug into wall sockets.

- Your diplomas will add an air of professionalism to the walls. Consider also some artwork to create an appropriate atmosphere.

- Keep a desk in your office. The desk is the place for your telephone and answering machine, phone books, schedule book, client files, and business card collection.

- Linens can be kept on a shelf, in a cabinet, or under the massage table. Choose your linens after you decide on a color scheme for the office, or use white linens, which can go with any office colors.

- Have a mirror available to your clients.

- Give your clients ample hooks for their clothing. Create a private space for dressing and undressing or leave the room while clients are dressing and undressing. Have a table or counter where clients can put their jewelry and personal belongings.

- Have a computer, word processor or typewriter in the office so you can do paperwork between appointments if necessary.

- Have your business cards out in a spot where clients will see them and can take one.

- Consider having bottled water available for you and your clients in your office.

Checklist for office furnishings

massage table	mirror
linens	desk
hamper	table or counter space for client's use
oil	telephone and answering machine
chair	
clothing hooks for clients	typewriter
business card holder	lighting system
bottled water cooler or other dispenser	artwork, diplomas or other decorations for walls

6. Telephone Reception

One advantage of a group practice is that the group can pool resources to either hire a receptionist or rotate duties on phone reception. This assures that callers will reach a person who can answer their questions about massage and schedule an appointment.

If you are practicing alone, it is much more difficult to answer your own phone. Hopefully, you will be too busy doing massage to be serving as your own receptionist. The choices available to you are hiring an answering service or using an answering machine.

Practically all therapists, faced with this choice, choose an answering machine over an answering service. The service may seem to have the advantage of presenting the caller with a live human to talk to, but the person who works for the answering service is not likely to be familiar with massage. Therefore, she or he cannot answer the potential client's questions about your services. The answering service can take messages for you, but that is about all.

Answering machines have one major drawback — a great many people simply hang up when an answering machine answers a call. A person who has a strong desire to reach you will leave a message. However, someone who has been given your card, or who has seen an ad, may not go to the trouble to leave a message. For this reason, having a live human being answer the telephone is a significant advantage.

Caller I.D.

This feature that lets you know the phone number, and sometimes the name, of the person calling you. The service costs a few dollars per month, and requires a separate caller ID device costing around $60. Some phones and answering machines now have caller ID capabilities built in.

After two rings, the caller ID device displays the phone number of the person who is calling you. The machine also stores the numbers of the last twenty or so people who have called your number. When making an appointment for some-one for the first time, you can say to the person "Can I call you at 555-3456 to confirm?" The fact that you know their phone number will be a strong deterrent for any sex clients who may be calling you.

Checklist for office opening

The items in this checklist are arranged in chronological order — in other words, do number one first, number two second, etc. Begin this process three to six months before your target date for opening your new office.

Three to six months before opening:

1. Contact local government for information about zoning, and any regulations of health, fire and police departments

2. Contact direct mail company to learn the date of their next mail-ing; contact phone company to learn deadline for next yellow pages listing

3. Consider possible locations and look at offices for rent

4. Negotiate a lease for your office location, select starting date with enough lead time to make all preparations

5. Obtain all necessary governmental approvals, licenses and permits

Two to four weeks before opening:

6. Register fictitious name with county

7. Establish business checking account

8. Contact telephone company to connect new service

9. Order stationery, business cards and any promotional items you plan to use to publicize your office's opening

10. If appropriate, plan an advertising push when you open to create an increased clientele for your new venture

11. Shop for office furnishings

12. Notify all your clients of your new office opening and any intro-ductory promotions you may be having

13. Get to know the neighbors in your new location and use any opportunities to gain clientele through your neighbors

Opening a group practice

Group practice refers to several massage therapists or related professionals sharing a suite of offices. Group practices have some significant advantages over individual practices, as well as some disadvantages.

The two main advantages of group practices are shared expenses and cross-referrals. The main disadvantage is the group decision process.

Renting an office suite and sharing the cost usually results in a lower price to each member than she would have to pay for a similar office space rented individually.

A group practice has the potential to become well-known as a center, thereby attracting a larger clientele through the reputation of the group practice. Once such a reputation is established for a group practice, it will generate a significant walk-in trade, and all the group members will benefit by having additional clients.

The disadvantage of a group practice is that decisions must be made by the group as a whole. This usually means devoting one evening per week to the process of group decision-making. After a busy week of massage, an evening of group process can seem like a burden. However, if you choose carefully which other practitioners you associate with, these group meetings can be an opportunity for learning, socializing, and professional support.

Buying an Existing Massage Practice

Occasionally, practitioners sell their practice. You may have an opportunity to purchase an existing practice. This may seem like an appealing way to have a ready-made practice. However, buying an existing practice is very risky, and you should be extremely careful if you choose to do so.

Ask yourself several questions:

1. Why is this person selling her practice? She may not be giving you the real reason. Ask to see her appointment book, and take a minute to look at it. See how busy the office really is.

2. Will she take any of her clients with her? This can be a problem if the selling therapist plans to stay in massage and to stay in the area. You may find you have paid for a practice that evaporates as soon as you arrive.

3. Will her clients like you? It was the selling therapist's style of massage and personality that attracted her current clientele. If your massage and your personality are different from hers, her clients may be dissatisfied with you and may leave to try other therapists.

If I were buying an existing practice, I would want to first become an associate, and work in the office on a part-time basis. By so doing, I would get the feel of the clientele, and know whether they would accept me, and whether I would feel comfortable working with them. I would also have the opportunity to see first-hand how busy the practice is.

Ask the seller if such an arrangement is possible.

You could try it for a couple of months, at which time you would decide whether to buy the practice for a pre-set amount of money.

The real value of an established practice is the client base, the group of people who are in the habit of coming to this practice for massage on a regular basis. The client base can be a valuable asset if you are new to a community and want to become established quickly. I suggest you base a selling price on the number of clients you believe will stay with you after you take the practice over. You will need to make your best estimate of this.

If the client base will give you only enough income to meet the office rent, it is not worth much to you. On the other hand, if you will be able to step in and immediately earn enough to meet expenses and take home an income of $500 per week, that is worth a great deal.

Figuring the value of an existing practice is tricky, but consider this formula. Project the income you expect to earn immediately after taking over the office. To do this, you must have some basis for knowing how many clients will stay with you after the selling therapist leaves.

Assume your projected income for the first month is $1,300. Next, total the expenses you will have for rent, phone, yellow pages, insurance, taxes and supplies. Assume this is $750 per month. Subtract the expenses from your expected income. You can project your estimated profit to be $550 for the first month.

Offer the seller three to five times the amount you expect to take home as profit for the first month. If your assessment is correct, you will be able to recover your investment within a year or so, and you will then have a successful practice with a minimum of marketing effort on your part.

The figure you offer will probably be less than the seller was hoping for. The seller may hope for a figure that represents a year's profit. If the business is very attractive and you can afford it, you may want to agree to such a price. However, you should only offer what the business will be worth *to you*. If you were buying a store that sold brand-name goods, the established trade would be reliable. In your case, the value of this business depends very much on how much it will change after you take it over.

III

Sex, Gender
and Touch

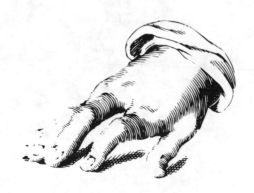

9 Sex and Massage

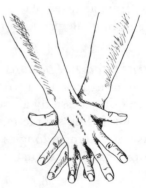

About halfway through my massage school course, I began to wonder when we would have the class about sexuality and massage, to help us understand and deal with sexual feelings that may arise for the client or the therapist during a session. I kept waiting for such a class, but it never arrived.

When I set up a practice in the "real world," I encountered sexual issues that deserved to be discussed in schools. While some schools now include a discussion of sexuality and massage in their programs, it is still relatively rare for a school to give its students any meaningful preparation for what they can expect in the "real world."

Differences in approach

The approach I suggest for a professional massage therapist or bodyworker is to set up clear boundaries for the therapeutic session. Any sexual intention by the client or the therapist is outside those boundaries. A client who presents sexual intentions should be confronted, and if the client acknowledges sexual intentions, the treatment should be ended.

Some authors and some educators differ with that approach, and regard a client's sexual desires not so much as a problem, but as an opportunity to foster the client's growth by exploring the psychological issues he has concerning sexuality. Be aware that if you choose such an approach, you are crossing the line between massage and counseling. If you have psychological training and the therapeutic skills needed to work in that way, there is nothing wrong with doing so. I don't, and most massage therapists don't. Therefore, my advice is to simply terminate a massage when a client presents the wish for sexual gratification.

Clients who want sexual massage

Occasionally, a woman massage client attempts to initiate sexual contact, either with a male or female massage therapist, during a massage session. Instances in which men attempt to initiate sexual contact, either with a male or female massage therapist are, unfortunately, much more common.

Since you should expect to deal with clients who attempt to initiate sexual contact, the following are offered as guidelines for what to expect and how to deal with what takes place. Since the great majority of sexually oriented clients are men, the male pronoun is used throughout this chapter.

Arousal need not be considered a problem

A few men experience a partial erection at some point during a massage. These men are not necessarily after sex, and may actually be somewhat embarrassed by their arousal. The simple fact of a male client having an erection should not be seen as a problem, as long as the man's attitude is appropriate and he presents no verbal or nonverbal sexual expressions.

Arousal plus inappropriate action is a problem

Signs to watch for if a male client has an erection are: touching the genitals; grinding the hips into the massage table; moving the hips in any way; using muscular contraction to flex the penis.

These activities should alert you that this client will probably present a request for sex. You should confront him immediately about his arousal. Unless he can explain his actions to your satisfaction, terminate the massage immediately.

Other, subtler signs to look for are very shallow breathing or sighs of appreciation or pleasure. If you have some experience with clients who want sex, you will learn to "feel" that desire coming from them. It may be a subtle change in the mood in the room, or a change in *your* breathing or thinking that you cannot explain.

If in doubt, confront

If a client has an erection and you perceive signs that lead you to believe this client wants sex, ask your client questions to find out if you are right. Mention that he seems to be aroused and ask his feeling about that.

If the client's response tells you his attitude about the arousal is one of enjoyment, terminate the massage immediately. If the client continues to make any voluntary movements of a sexual nature, such as grinding the hips or touching the genitals, terminate the massage.

Your massage room is your environment, and you are in control of what does and does not happen there. Do not allow a client to threaten that control. Do not be afraid of losing business — any client who is sexually oriented is a client you want very much to lose anyway.

If you are alone in your office, you may want to have a phone number handy for someone you know you can reach in an emergency. I have never heard of a massage client actually becoming aggressive, but it may help you to feel more at ease to know someone is available to help you just in case.

Understanding the big picture

Sex and massage have undoubtedly been linked for thousands of years. One explanation for the persistent connection between the two has been offered by

David Lauterstein, co-director of the Lauterstein-Conway School of Massage in Austin, Texas:

> ... we rather awkwardly encounter the one good reason massage and prostitution were ever associated. Both address people's need for love. However, prostitutes simply don't deliver — selling sex as love is robbery. That's a good reason why it's illegal. Massage therapy recognizes that underneath each person's tension, stress, even illness and injury, is an unmet need for energetic nourishment, i.e., love.

Unfortunately, many men are not aware of the distinction Mr. Lauterstein refers to. They *think* that what they need to be happy is sex, and there are plenty of "practitioners" who are willing to indulge them in their illusion.

In some parts of the world, a manually-stimulated orgasm is the normal and accepted conclusion of a professional massage. In many parts of the United States, a sexual massage is more common and easier to find than a legitimate massage. In some areas (San Diego, for example) the sexual massage ads in the yellow pages completely overwhelm the few listings for massage therapists.

In recent years, newspapers have carried stories of "acupressure" parlors fronting for prostitution in Los Angeles County, California, and massage parlors fronting for prostitution in the Oyster Bay area of Long Island, New York. The New York parlors were closed only after a march by licensed massage therapists, who announced plans to hold a press conference in front of their local senator's office unless action was taken.

Millions of men have had sexual massage experiences, and continue to have them today. As such, it is understandable that they would have some confusion about what it is you do. That is why you should be (1) non-judgmental and (2) completely clear in your communications before beginning a massage.

Screening new clients

It is a good practice to ask anyone who calls you how they heard about you. First, you want to be able to thank clients for referrals, and keep track of how successful your various promotional activities have been. Second, if the person does not come as a referral from a trusted client, you want to be able to make sure the person does not have the wrong idea.

Most sex clients will find you either through the yellow pages or through a newspaper ad. With male callers who have located me through advertising, I make a point of stating at the beginning that my massage is strictly non-sexual. I may use terms like "legitimate" or "therapeutic" to reinforce the message. I then ask them if this is the type of massage they are looking for, and pause to give them an opportunity to answer.

Massage clients understand the need for such an explanation, and are not put off. Most of the sex callers will hang up at that point, but some persist. During the conversation that follows, I have learned to watch my breathing. If my own breathing becomes shallow, and my heart starts beating fast, I have learned that this means my unconscious is getting the message that there is something dishonest about the caller.

Clients looking for sexual massage will try to find out what they can get without saying anything incriminating. Typical questions the sex caller may ask, in an attempt to find out if he can get a sexual massage, are these:

Is this a nude massage?

Is this a "complete"?

What will you be wearing during the massage?

Is tipping allowed?

Are there extras?

Can I get a release?

What else is included?

Does a girl give the massage?

If you hear any of these questions, politely tell him he has the wrong office, and hang up.

To minimize sex clients, get a first *and last* name for any first-time clients, and a phone number you can call to confirm the appointment. Try to avoid same-day appointments with first-time clients, and phone to confirm the appointment the day it is to take place. If any difficulty or confusion results from your attempt to confirm the appointment, be prepared for a no-show or a client who may be using a wrong name.

One Massage Therapist's Story

The following essay is one of four essays in a work called Massage Portraits, originally published in 1984 in CoEvolution Quarterly/Whole Earth Review, issue No. 43. It is written by Anneke Campbell and is reprinted with her permission. I include it here because it captures well many of the aspects of dealing with a client seeking sex.

CHIP

It was nine in the evening when the phone rang, and a male voice asked if he could come for a massage. "How did you find out about me?" I asked, always cautious. "Connie usually works on me when I'm in town, but she's out for the evening."

I knew Connie did good work, so I relaxed. "My old football injury is acting up," the man continued, "Could you see me tonight?" "Well…" I didn't much feel like it, but my rent was due at the end of the week. "Alright then." "I sure do appreciate it."

The fellow who walked in my door was a massive six-foot-four, dark-haired, jowly. I was going to have to work for my money. Chip had played football at college in the sixties, and nearly gone pro. Partly due to his back problem, he had opted for business, and was doing quite well, if he did say so himself. He also told me he was divorced. He took off all his clothes with bravura, as if to let me know he had no hang-ups about his body, not him.

His back was a sheet of lumpy, tight muscle. I stood close to the massage table and leaned all my weight into my hands. I began by pushing on the bunched-up erector spinae, and to my surprise, they softened up right away. Chip was responsive. I concentrated with my fingers on the vertebrae, which were buried in fibroid connective tissue. While I worked, Chip told me about the injury which had left him with some weakness in the sacral area. He had experienced both numbness and aching in his legs for years.

"There's nothing I can do about nerve impairment, if that's what the problem is," I explained, "but your entire back is a mess, probably due to compensating for the injury. And I can do something about all these tense, bunched-up muscles." I used long, firm strokes down the erector spinae and up the latissimus dorsi. I kneaded the well-padded abdominal obliques and trapezius. I worked so hard that the muscles in my own arms started aching, and drops of sweat ticked at the small of my back.

After about forty minutes, he began to moan. I was feeling pleased with the results of my work; his back was definitely less rigid than when I started. "Doesn't it feel better?" I asked. "It does, oh yes, but you're not getting to where most of the pain is." "Which is?" "Lower down."

I chased an uncomfortable thought from my mind, and moved my hands down to his sacrum and pelvic brim. I focused on the tiny muscles that lie over the sacrum; they were mushy in texture, a mushiness I associate with damage, and I could see that these could well be the source of his "weakness." Underneath, my fingers discovered some cyst-like formations. Here I worked carefully, but thoroughly. "Lower," he said.

I ignored the request. Chip's heavy body seemed suddenly disgusting to me. "Massage my thighs, that's where the problem is, on the inside of my thighs." "I've only a few minutes left." "How about another hour?" "I don't work two hours in a row," I lied.

I did some long, firm strokes down the length of his legs, trying to ignore the slight grinding of his pelvis into the massage table. I moved up, and took his bullish neck into my hands. Muscle like rock. He needed another hour, that was clear, but he wasn't going to get it from me.

"My masseuse in Florida, she does a full-body massage." I felt a sudden stab of hatred for the masseuse in Florida. "Yep, but she's a strong lady," Chip continued, "bigger than you are. You're just a little thing, aren't you. Well, what this lady does, it doesn't take much strength really."

I remained silent, kneading away at his sterno-cleido-mastoids. "She massages me down there, you know…" "I don't do that kind of massage." "I'll give you fifty dollars." "Thank you, but no," I say, clear I would never do such a thing. "One hundred dollars then." "I don't do that kind of massage," I repeated, thinking, good Lord, one hundred dollars for a hand-job, he must be filthy rich.

"Please," he said, "One hundred and twenty?" Half a month's rent, I thought. Is it really that different, rubbing his penis or rubbing his trapezius? What's a little come on my hands? And what difference would it make to anyone but me?

"No," I said, and left the room. As I washed my hands, I noticed they were shaking. I felt a little sick to my stomach, and worried about being alone in the house with this huge man. I sat down in an easy chair in the living room. After a while, Chip appeared, fully dressed. He handed me a twenty-dollar bill. "Thanks," he said, "my back feels a hell of a lot better."

For the first time in that hour, I looked him fully in the eye. The cringing I saw there took away my fear. He was obviously embarrassed, but more to the point, terribly lonely. I knew what he needed was not sex, but warmth, contact, friendship. I nearly wished I could help him, but I had no desire to be his friend. "I'm glad your back feels better." I said, getting up. I opened the door, and extended my hand. Chip held it between his for a moment. "Good hands," he said.

Therapists who have sexual feelings toward clients

Very likely, at some point in your career, you will feel sexually attracted to a client on your table. It is your responsibility to your client and to your practice to work with your own feelings and control your thoughts and actions.

Your touch transmits your thoughts

Your touch communicates an unbelievable amount of information to the person you are touching. If you are viewing them with sexual intention, they will feel that in your touch. They may not be consciously aware of what they are feeling, but the communication will take place nonetheless.

If you have ever had the experience of receiving a massage from someone who had sex on their mind, you know what I mean. You can feel it in their touch. It is a totally different experience than being treated by a therapist.

Transmitting sexual feelings in your massage can sabotage your practice. The client whom you approach sexually will feel uncomfortable, and is not likely to become a repeat client. He or she is also likely to communicate to others a feeling of discomfort, uneasiness, or general dissatisfaction with your massage.

Monitor your own thoughts and feelings. If you start to slip into sexual thoughts about a client, try to determine whether these are originating with you or the client. If you find that you are responsible for originating these feelings, simply choose to stop. Remind yourself of your therapeutic intention, and focus your thoughts on your techniques and therapeutic goals for this client.

Never initiate sexual contact with a client

Occasionally, stories are reported about professionals, including massage therapists, who sexually accost their clients. This is damaging to the profession as a whole, and disastrous to the lives of the therapists involved.

It is one thing to decide to date a client, to become friends, and then to have whatever personal relationship you both decide to have. That presents no particular moral or ethical problem.

It is another thing to attempt to initiate sexual activity with a client *during* a professional massage. This is immoral, unethical, and illegal. The massage relationship involves trust on the part of the client, who becomes vulnerable to the therapist. In this sense, the relationship resembles that of a doctor and patient, or priest and penitent. The trust placed in you by your client gives you a greater responsibility to be honest and above board in your dealings.

If you feel a desire to initiate sexual activity with your clients, seek professional help. You may be able to learn something about yourself in the course of working with this desire. If you are unable to control this desire, your best course of action may be to stop practicing massage, or to limit your practice to men only or women only.

10 For Men Only

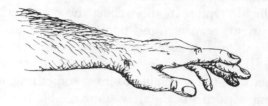

The challenge for a male massage therapist

In the massage field in general, attracting clients and becoming established is more difficult for a man than for a woman. This is not true in certain specialties, like sports massage, on-site massage, Rolfing, Trager, polarity, and other forms of bodywork that do not involve nudity and stroking. It is also not true in some other countries, such as Germany, where men tend to be accepted as massage therapists more easily than women.

However, in the field of Swedish massage in the United States, experience shows that most clients prefer having a woman give them a massage. Most women are shy about becoming undressed and being touched by a man they are not intimate with. Many also have self-image issues and are embarrassed to have a man see their bodies. Many men feel uncomfortable being touched by another man, and prefer the nurturance they receive from a woman's touch.

Some groups of clients that prefer male therapists

Some men prefer a male therapist because they want to avoid any possibility of arousal. Such groups include Catholic priests, orthodox Jewish men, and men with strong moral principles.

Many gay men prefer a male therapist, apparently because they are more comfortable in the company of men.

Many athletes and very muscular men prefer a male therapist, having the belief that most women lack the strength to give them a satisfyingly deep massage.

Some clients are gender-neutral

A certain number of clients do not care whether their massage therapist is male or female, but choose a therapist on personality and skill level. Such clients are a minority. Generally speaking, such clients are probably more common in cosmopolitan areas and in the Western United States.

The task for a male massage therapist

Because the available client pool for men is smaller, men have to try harder, be better, and have more patience than women when establishing a massage practice.

Men can and do succeed in the field, and some men become tremendously successful. Do not allow the challenge to discourage you. Knowing the situation in advance will allow you to better plan your career and focus on target groups which are likely to produce clients for you.

The male as pursuer

Societal conditioning, and perhaps instinctual patterns, result in men generally pursuing women sexually and initiating sexual contact in relationships. As a result, men tend to be in the habit of seeking sexual encounters.

One very successful male therapist told me that he considers it a great advantage to him that he is married. His desire to couple is focused on his wife, and he feels much more relaxed than he otherwise would about working with his women clients.

If this issue is a problem for you, there is no magic solution. Simply be honest with yourself, and exercise your will and creativity to avoid confronting your clients with sexual energy that will create problems in your professional life.

11 Working with Survivors of Childhood Sexual or Physical Abuse

Recent years have seen a dramatic increase in society's awareness of childhood abuse as a prevalent social problem. Those who have been abused as children may or may not remember being abused, may have been abused sexually or non-sexually, and may or may not have begun the journey of healing the effects of that abuse.

As a massage practitioner, chances are you will come in contact with a number of clients who experienced childhood abuse. Some of these clients will have normal reactions to massage — they will appreciate your services, and will pose no difficulty to work with. Others may have extreme reactions that include terror, convulsions and withdrawal. It is these other clients, who may have dramatic reactions, that are the subject of the cautionary advice in this chapter.

Because your touch may reactivate childhood trauma, there are certain fundamental things you should understand in order to work with these clients without doing additional harm to them. This chapter seeks to give you the basics you need to know to avoid doing harm and to serve these clients to the best of your ability.

Most massage clients are women, so the female pronoun is used throughout this chapter. Be aware, however, that many men have also experienced childhood abuse, both sexual and nonsexual.

I wish to thank Mary Ann DiRoberts, who provided substantial assistance in the preparation of this chapter, and also Diana Lonsdale and Anya Seerveld, both of whom provided information for use in this chapter.

Childhood abuse and the damage that results

Children have natural mechanisms to deal with stress, but extremely strong experiences can overwhelm these mechanisms. Sexual or physical abuse is too much for the child to deal with, and it can prevent the normal integration of the psyche as the child matures.

One aspect of this process is numbness, or dissociation. Minor dissociation is a natural part of life for most people, taking the form of spacing out, daydreaming, or similar behaviors. However, more significant dissociation can result in a state in which the person is not aware of the physical sensations of the body, or is not consciously present in the experience of the body. In extreme cases, multiple personalities are created and the person lives a life as different personalities who may not even know each other.

Psychologically, childhood abuse destroys the child's sense of safety and trust, and drastically violates the child's boundaries. The child may grow into an adult who has difficulty trusting and is confused about boundaries. One who experienced childhood sexual abuse may have guilt about the sensations she had during the abuse, feel shame or responsibility for the abuse, and have terror buried in her body from these childhood experiences. As an adult, she may feel like "damaged goods" and may believe that sex is all she is good for, or that she is not even good for that.

While you should not attempt to diagnose someone psychologically, certain traits can clue you in that childhood abuse *may* be an issue in someone's life. Signs to look for include depression, lack of emotion, extreme changes in emotion, feelings of being different or defective, dysfunctional relationships, irresponsible sexuality, anorexia, bulimia, obesity, childishness or excessive vulnerability, inability to take care of one's self, workaholism, alcoholism, compulsive rituals or other compulsive behaviors, and anxiety attacks.

It is important to remember that unless you are trained as a mental health professional, you should not attempt to be a psychotherapist for a person who experienced childhood abuse. In fact, unless you have specialized training in practicing massage with abuse survivors, you should consider declining to practice massage with such a client. Without the understanding and skills necessary to work with such clients, you may do more harm than good by giving a massage.

The intake interview

When initially interviewing a client, do *not* directly ask if she experienced childhood abuse. Asking this question violates the client's boundary; it requires her to either lie or disclose something she may not wish to share with a person she does not yet trust.

It is better to ask generally whether bodywork brings up feelings for her. You may tell her orally or in your printed information that you invite her to let you know if she is in psychotherapy. However, avoid probing too deeply, as this violates a client's boundary. It is better to carefully listen and watch for signs that may alert you to a history of abuse.

During the massage

The abused child has been dis-empowered, has had trust violated, and has not had boundaries honored. When massaging this adult client, be careful to empower her and to operate with clear boundaries. Be scrupulous about giving control of the session to the client. Be clear about your permission to touch in specific places or in specific ways. Check in often with your client to be sure she is comfortable with the session and is present in her body.

Even a client who is not an abuse survivor will appreciate being empowered, respected, and given control. Since you likely will not know that a particular client is a survivor, consider these guidelines with all clients.

It is especially important to check in often during the massage with a client who has a history of abuse. When your touch triggers an emotional response or a memory of abuse, this client may be unable to tell you what is happening. The abusive experience often includes training in "not telling," and when a memory of that experience is triggered, the training to be silent may prevent the client from letting you know what is happening.

If a client recalls a portion of the abusive treatment during a massage session, it can be extremely upsetting for the client and a difficult situation for the massage therapist. A "flashback" can feel to the client like a flood of terrifying feelings. She may dissociate from current time and reality and be completely immersed in an experience of the childhood events. She may shake with terror, convulse, go into tetany, curl up in a ball, or shout at the perpetrator.

If you as a therapist find yourself with a client having such an experience, remember that this person is re-experiencing a terrible event from her past. If you can, talk to her in simple language, telling her where she is and what is happening in the present moment. Suggest that she open her eyes and describe the room you are in, or make eye contact with you, or change her position to sitting or lying on her side.

If she tells you about her experience, let her know you understand what she tells you by rephrasing it in your own words. Maintain boundaries and give her control over what happens, and assure her that you will stay with her and keep her safe as long as she needs you. After the experience has passed, she may still need your support and attention. Help her make specific plans for the rest of the day, and encourage her to use whatever support is available in her life. If the client is not in psychotherapy, this would be a good time to make a referral to a qualified practitioner.

Because flashback experiences can be so very unsettling, it is advisable to assure that a client with a history of childhood abuse has a psychotherapist if she is going to work with you doing massage. Because of the likelihood that your work will bring up such an intense experience, the client should have the services of a professional who can help process such an event if it occurs. If you intend to specialize in working with clients with histories of childhood abuse, you should have additional training in this area, be in supervision, and have done your own psychotherapy.

One survivor's experiences with massage

The following is excerpted from an article that appeared in The Journal of Soft Tissue Manipulation. Written by Tess Edwards, it describes the experiences of a woman who experienced ritual satanic abuse as a child, and became a massage therapy client as an adult.

Her descriptions of various massage experiences and suggestions for therapists have great value. As you will see from reading the following, Tess is a client who dissociates during massage. Her massage therapist practices safe touch work, which requires specific training to do.

I wish to express my gratitude to Tess and to the Journal of Soft Tissue Manipulation for permission to reproduce this essay.

One trauma survivor's experience of massage
by Tess Edwards

I believe strongly in the importance of massage for survivors of child abuse. I feel very lucky that I am one of the few survivors I know who can both afford and tolerate a weekly massage.

In my search for healing, I saw an applied kinesiologist who told me that my trauma has settled mostly in the muscle and skeletal systems instead of the organs, as is more common. So for me, I believe that massage is crucial to the healing process because the toxic effect of the trauma is lodged in my muscles. Even when the toxic effect of abuse is primarily in the organs, I believe that massage is essential to the healing process — not only because safe touch is an important and unusual experience for most survivors, but also because trauma is held in the body.

Dancers talk about muscle memory — that is how they learn the intricate moves they must make on stage. We all have muscle memory. I have never been comfortable placing my arms above my head — I have never been able to paint a ceiling or hang curtains without going into a state of panic. Similarly, I usually postpone washing my hair for as long as possible. I always called myself lazy, stupid or other nasty names because I could not do these tasks. And I never understood that this had any meaning.

I now understand that many of my worst life experiences took place while my hands were tied above my head for long periods of time. I still have trouble with this. In fact, as the memories surface, difficulty with these tasks has increased. Now even in aquabics class I have tears rolling down my face when I try to do the above-the-head arm exercises. This is typical. As the memory surfaces, the symptoms intensify.

I've always thought that massage would help me, but it has been a long battle to allow myself to afford it and to learn how to tolerate it.

For three or four years, I got massage treatments about three times a year. For the most part, I don't think they helped me at all because I simply left my body during them. Touch of this type is really a re-enactment of the original abuse and in fact gives me even further to go in my healing journey. In one case, the massage I received was truly a re-enactment of the abuse and for months undermined the healing work I was doing.

One massage therapist really upset me when she was giving me her new-age philosophy about how we all choose our lives — have choice even about abuse in childhood. One of the hardest things to recover from is the guilt and shame that every survivor I've met feels about the abuse. Hearing their stories, I have noted that in most cases, the abuser blames the victim: "You're too sexy." "You make me do it." "You love it." "You know you want it."

"You're making me evil" was what my father used to say to me and he even taught one of my personalities to beg him for intercourse at an early age. So for my massage therapist to tell me that I chose either to come back in this life as a victim of child abuse, or that I as a child had some choice in the matter, pushes all my shame and guilt buttons. If I'm lucky, this makes me very angry. If I'm not, I feel despair.

My biggest difficulty with massage, although it took me a long time to realize it, was that any touch was triggering. Two years ago, a group of four survivors of sexual abuse started a self-facilitated group based on giving and receiving safe touch. In our weekly five-hour sessions, we would ask for what we wanted that night — anything from getting a back rub, to being rocked while we sang lullabies, to massaging just a hand, to building a protective igloo with pillows, to brushing hair. Any activity involving touch that the survivor could accept that evening.

During these sessions two of us began retrieving new memories of abuse while in the group. Instead of being a group for safe touch, the group became, temporarily, a group for memory retrieval. The memory work triggered by the touch was so intense for the other two members of the group that they asked us to stop. We then formed a group specifically for memory retrieval, which has been going on for over a year now and from which I have benefited enormously.

Another survivor I know began the process of retrieving memory when she began to receive massage. This is why I feel that massage is so very important and so very tricky for survivors.

Currently, I see a massage therapist once a week, and it is helping enormously. Three nights ago, I had a dream that my body turned from metal into flesh. Last Sunday in my memory retrieval group, I was able to feel and express many more of the feelings that I felt as a child than I have before.

The massage is still hard sometimes. We're still trying to develop a system so that I can ask her to stop. We haven't found a good way yet because when I need her to stop, I'm in a child part who was trained not to speak; stopping wasn't an option, no matter how desperately she wanted to. It's hard for my massage therapist to help when I go there because the signs are subtle to non-existent. This is partly because I received tons of training on how to pretend everything was alright.

I think my massage therapist is learning my body enough to notice when I hold my breath or, more often, when my flesh just feels dead or uninhabited. I don't know how she does it. She checks with me a lot, which for me is great because it can sometimes give me permission to say that I am in trouble.

I have learned to set some boundaries. We do not work on my bum. I allowed her to work on my upper legs once and got so badly triggered that I was unable to say so until a week later. During that week, I wandered around in flashbacks. My inner thighs are now off limits.

My massage therapist tells me a lot of things about my body which are very useful to me because I've spent most of my life outside of it. She is helping me to learn about my body, making it easier to reside there.

There are a number of things I feel that a massage therapist should do when working with me. I am sharing these ideas so that other massage therapists might learn about how to help someone who has been abused.

- First and foremost, I am more important than your technique. If I can't lie face down, I need you to accommodate me. Maybe massage me while I'm on my side, even if it means you can't give me what you feel is your best work. Give me what is best for me, not your best work.

  If I leave my body, you can make my circulation shoot around better, but that's it. For me, the purpose of massage is to get more into my body, not leave it more. If I'm not present, I'm not getting what I need. I need to learn to feel pleasure in my body. Pleasure is something that has never been safe for me.

- Be creative. If I can't tolerate lying down, you could have me sit on a chair with my arms on the table and do just my head and neck. If I need to keep my clothes on, figure out how you can help me with my clothes on. Encourage me to bring my teddy bear if I am terrified.

- Help me to feel safe and comfortable. I love to be rocked and so do my inner kids. I love to be warm and adore my massage therapist's heating pad and the warm blankets she covers me with.

- Find out what you need from me in order to help me. Find out my other support systems. You can't be all things for me. You're not my therapist and you're not responsible for my healing or the bad things that happened to me. If you sense that my support structure is weak, be careful if you trigger memories that you can't take me through.

- Respect me and my process. I know best about me, just as you know best about you.

- One of the skills I value the most in my massage therapist is her understanding of emotional release. It is wonderful to know that she can handle anger, grief or terror as they come up and work with them, instead of being terrified by them. She has a big bucket with a pillow on it for resting my hands on when I am on my front or hitting if I need to release some anger.

- Learn to detect the difference between re-enactment and release. Re-enactment and release can look the same but have an opposite impact on the survivor. Both re-enactment and release can cause the survivor to show physical symptoms of grief, fear or anger. However, in re-enactment, the survivor is lengthening the work she has to do. She has yet one more incident of feeling powerless and victimized to recover from. In release, she is letting go of some of the abuse and actively reclaiming her life.

Being placed in a re-enactment can help enormously if I am ready for it and I choose it. I went to my massage therapist once after a particularly nasty memory where my hands were tied. I specifically asked her if she could work on my wrists and as she did, it felt as though hundreds of wrist restraints fell off as I cried. The relief was wonderful.

- Learn about triggers: what they are, how they work and how to cope with them.

- Please refer me if you are uncomfortable working with me. Don't sabotage my courageous act of attempting to find safe touch and learning to re-inhabit my body.

To me, my healing process involves recalling my life and integrating the sensory information that I blocked or dissociated from my awareness. This includes my emotions, my spirituality and the events, sights, sounds, smells, tastes, textures that I have been unable to allow into conscious awareness. I want to experience my life as a whole.

One of the most useful parts of healing is massage. To be touched without sex, without violence, is a first for me and a great gift. To learn that it is safe to allow someone into my space is incredible. To begin to release the trauma is a relief.

IV

Business, Practical and Legal Information for the Practitioner

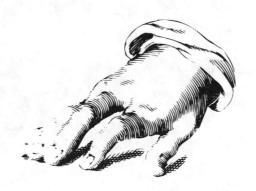

12 Business Basics and Practice Pointers

Practicing massage means operating in the business world. If you have no significant experience doing business, certain expectations of the business world may not be familiar to you. The purpose of this chapter is to give you enough information to avoid pitfalls and facilitate your success.

The subjects covered in this chapter are Steps You Can Take Toward Professionalism, What to Expect From Clients, and Pricing Your Services.

A. Steps You Can Take Toward Professionalism

1. Communicate Clearly and Keep Agreements

The business world operates by mutual agreement. In order to run smoothly, agreements must be unambiguous, and both parties must be able to rely on the other to keep the agreement.

In practice, this means you and your client should have no confusion about where or when appointments are to take place, how long they are for, how much they cost, and what sort of therapy the client is expecting you to provide. Keeping your agreement means arriving on time to all appointments with all the equipment you will need.

If an appointment is tentative, make sure both of you know when you will speak again to make it definite. If there are any questions in your mind about an agreement, speak to the client about them. The chances are that your client also has questions.

2. Present a Well-Groomed Image at Work and After Work

Most massage therapists understand the need to present a professional image at work. Your physical appearance announces who you are, and if you are proud of your work the image you present should convey that pride.

As a community member, you will see and be seen by your clients after working hours at unexpected times. Your appearance and your actions at these times will also have an effect on your clients' perceptions of you. While you need not constantly look over your shoulder, keep in mind that anything you do in public reflects on your professional character. If you have a wild side, you might want to keep it indoors.

3. Answer Your Phone in a Businesslike Manner

Even if you have separate office and home phone numbers, you should answer both your home and office phones in a polite way. You never know who is calling with what opportunity, and it is a shame to spoil an opportunity by creating a poor first impression.

4. Return phone calls promptly

Make a point of returning your phone calls as soon as you can. Keeping people waiting for a return call will train them to expect you to be hard to reach; they may think twice about calling you next time. You also run the risk that the person who is trying to reach you will find someone else to meet her needs, and you will have missed an opportunity.

5. Make Cleanliness a Priority

Massage clients are very sensitive to the issue of cleanliness. If they find you or your office unclean, they will not tell *you*, but they will tell others.

Since massage is such a personal service, clients will want to be sure the linens are fresh, the carpet is clean, and your clothing and body are clean. If in doubt, go overboard, as some clients have a very critical eye when it comes to hygiene.

6. Avoid Talking Too Much During a Massage

If your client wants to talk, let her talk. It's her massage and her hour. However, do not use the massage as a time to talk about yourself, your problems and your opinions. If your client is being quiet, then you should be quiet as well, unless your conversation concerns an issue related to the massage session.

Several of my clients have told me they left their previous massage therapist because he or she would not keep quiet during a massage. Notice that they did not tell the talkative therapist — they told their new therapist.

7. Watch the details of client comfort

Show concern for your clients' experience. Their perception of their entire experience with you is important, not just the result of your hands working their muscles.

On a physical level, make sure your clients are warm enough. Be aware of any modesty issues. Avoid getting oil in their hair, and offer to towel off excess oil. Avoid causing any pain during the massage, unless you and your client both agree that aggressively working a body part is the best thing to do.

On the level of emotions and boundary issues, make sure you honor the right of your clients to reveal or not reveal facts about themselves, to have portions of their body worked or not worked, and in general to be in charge of their session.

For example, ask permission to work the abdomen unless you know your client will not mind. You do not know much about your client — he or she may have experienced sexual or physical abuse, and your careless touch may trigger a very painful experience. Don't let your desire to give override the client's wishes about what to receive.

8. Finish on time

Clients are often on a busy schedule. You may want to do that extra five or ten minutes, but your client may feel it's more important to be on time for her next meeting. If you need to go over the agreed time, get the client's permission beforehand.

9. Get to know the other therapists in your area

Become acquainted with as many massage therapists, fitness trainers, physical therapists, bodyworkers, chiropractors, acupuncturists, psychotherapists and medical doctors as you can. The more people who know you, the more opportunity there is for them to assist you in your professional growth.

Remember that you are becoming a service professional. Allow yourself to assume membership in the community of those who are serving others' health needs. Knowing a large number of health professionals gives you a broad perspective on the field, and on the level of activity in your community. Be as involved in the total picture as you can.

10. Foster Your Own Personal and Professional Growth

As one therapist told me "There are massage therapists, and there are massage therapists, but the ones who make it are the ones who are working on themselves."

Examine what it is you offer your clients — what benefits your work gives them, and what kinds of difficulties your work helps them get through. Chances are, you are offering your clients help with the kinds of issues you also face in your life.

Acknowledge that you are also a client. Practice what you preach. Nurture your own growth through finding therapists and healers and teachers who help you grow. In the process, you will also learn new techniques that you can incorporate in your bodywork. The process of growth has no end.

B. What To Expect From Clients

1. Cancellations

Clients will cancel; plans change. It is an unavoidable fact of life. You can create a cancellation policy to protect yourself, so long as you communicate it to your clients. One fair cancellation policy is to require 24 hours advance notice, and to charge a penalty (such as $20) for canceling on shorter notice. A notice on your desk or office wall, where it can be seen by your clients, is adequate to communicate your policy, or you can mention your policy at your first session with each client.

2. Great expectations

One lesson I have learned over and over is not to place any importance on statements by clients like "I'm going to get a massage every week" or "I've got half a dozen friends who have been looking for someone like you." If I had the fee I would have charged all the people who told me they were coming in for a massage, I'd be considering retirement by now...

I'm sure they mean it when they say it, but the fact is people talk about getting massage much more than they actually follow through. Once you are an established therapist, these "great expectations" are not of great importance. However, if you are seeing four clients a week and needing the rent money, it can be harder to keep this sort of thing in perspective.

3. No-shows

Some clients make an appointment, do not cancel, and do not show up. This is about as frustrating a situation as you can get practicing massage, and there is very little you can do about it.

The great majority of no-shows are clients who have never been to see you before, and who learned about you either through the yellow pages or a newspaper ad. One way to control the problem is to require that all people making appointments give you first and last name, and a phone number where they can be reached to confirm the appointment.

If you call the number and they never heard of the person, don't be surprised if he does not show up. If you call the number, and they sound shocked that the person is getting a massage, don't be surprised if he never arrives. With experience, you will learn to evaluate the likelihood of the person showing up for the appointment based on your experience in calling to confirm.

When a first-time client fails to cancel or to show up, let that person go. This is a person you will not hear from again, and it will not do you any good to try to track him down. Put your energy into those who want and need your services.

The decision what to do when a regular client fails to cancel or to show up for an appointment is more difficult. It helps to have an announced cancellation policy, but if you do not you will need to decide whether to charge your client for the missed appointment or simply reschedule.

4. Angels

Once in a blue moon, you will get a client who takes it upon herself to be your fan club, publicity agent, networker and marketing strategist. Say a prayer of thanks.

An angel is someone who thinks so much of you and your work that she is inspired to do anything she can to help you succeed. This person will be thinking about you and talking about your work many times a day. Some are able to do more than others, but all act out of a feeling of love and caring.

My angel is one of my less affluent clients, and as a gesture of my appreciation, I have never raised his rate from the low introductory rate I was offering when he first became my client several years ago.

5. Constructive Critics

Most clients will not let you know that you caused them pain, or that they were too cold or too hot, or annoyed about something in your massage room. Although they will not tell you, such unspoken dissatisfactions cause many clients not to return for another massage.

That is why you should be grateful for the very few clients who ask you not to do a certain stroke, or complain about the temperature, or ask you to change this or that about your massage or the surroundings. In all likelihood, these clients speak for many others as well.

One such client of mine is a chef with a very acute sense of smell. One day while I was seated and working on his face and head, he asked me to please breathe to the side. Apparently, he was able to identify just what I had eaten several hours ago.

Until this time, I had not realized that I have a tendency to breathe through my mouth, and to exhale onto my clients' faces. Most clients probably did not notice any breath odor, but they probably did feel my breath on their faces. Either way, I no longer breathe on people's faces. Unless my constructive critic had spoken up, I would never have realized what I was doing.

C. Pricing Your Services

Pricing your services can be a difficult issue. This discussion is meant to give you guidance in selecting the most appropriate price for your services.

Several factors enter into a decision about pricing. The factors to consider are the "going rate" in your community, your expenses involved in providing the treatment, the price you feel comfortable charging, and the effect your price will have on your clients' ability to come to you.

1. The "going rate"

This refers to the customary charge for your kind of services in your area. The "going rate" for a one hour massage may be as low as $30 in some areas, and as high as $90 in other areas. Usually, there is a variation of $5 or $10 between the low and high ends of the "going rate." In my area, for example, the price for a one-hour massage ranges from $50 to $60.

Consider that the "going rate" is the rate charged by established professionals who have a clientele. A time-honored custom among newly-trained professionals is to slightly undercut the going rate when they are first attracting a clientele. To the cost-conscious consumer, the lower fee is an incentive to try this therapist. In addition, the lower fee is an acknowledgment that a newly-trained professional is still learning, and has not yet acquired fully mature skills.

If you choose a rate *far* below the going rate, for example $15 per hour, people will become suspicious that you are not really a trained therapist, and it may actually be harder for you to attract clients than if you charged a fee nearer the going rate.

As your skills and reputation grow, you will naturally raise your rates to a level that reflects your growth. Your clients will adjust to your new rates without much difficulty, especially since your new rates will be in line with the rates established therapists are charging. While some clients may find it hard to accept a rate increase after becoming accustomed to a lower price, most clients who know and like you will not leave you when your rates rise to the "going rate."

2. A price you are comfortable with

For you to be comfortable with the fee you charge for your services means at least two different things. It means, first, that you are comfortable asking your client to pay your fee — you believe your service is as valuable as the money you receive for it. This touches on issues of self-worth. Your fee should be one that you can ask for and receive without mixed feelings.

Second, being comfortable with your fee means that it creates an income for you that meets your needs. You should feel that it compensates you for what you have given in your therapy session, and that it provides you with the means to have the material things you need to keep your life and practice going. If you feel you are not being nourished in your professional life, you may find yourself resentful and unenthusiastic about your work.

3. Effect of pricing decisions on clients

One massage client told me "If massage costs $40, I'll come in twice a month. If it costs $55, I'll come in once in six months." I suspect this client speaks for many others.

Massage clients are generally quite cost-conscious. Many people would like to have massage on a regular basis, but feel they cannot afford it. Compared to items like a bag of groceries, a movie ticket or a tank of gasoline, massage is an expensive item to fit into a budget.

Even the wealthy are often quite cost-conscious. Many wealthy individuals either do not believe they have enough money, or resent people trying to charge them a premium because they are wealthy. They will shop for the best price, and reject a therapist who charges what they consider too high a price. This may not apply to a celebrity clientele, or the enormously wealthy, but the run-of-the-mill millionaire often watches prices very closely.

Therefore, your pricing decision may well affect the amount of business you get, the ease with which you generate new business, and the frequency of your repeat business.

4. Working on a "sliding scale"

Sometimes meeting all the goals mentioned above with one set fee is not possible. In some cases, you may need to make exceptions to your price or work on a "sliding scale." This means that you charge some clients a lower fee because that is all they can afford.

Some clients refuse to pay a reduced fee, as a matter of pride. Others may ask you directly for a reduced fee. If you are comfortable working at a reduced fee for those with a financial need, there is nothing wrong with doing so. Charge a fee they can afford and you can comfortably accept. Do not price your work so low that the client no longer places a value on it, or that you become resentful of the imbalance in the relationship.

My normal fee is $60. For clients with financial hardship, I will reduce my fee as low as $35. If I worked for less than $35 I would feel taken advantage of.

5. Discounts for series purchase

A common device therapists use is to offer a discount to clients who purchase several massages in advance. For example, if the cost of one massage is $45, a therapist may sell a series of five massages for $200 ($40 per massage).

This benefits both parties. The client saves $25, and the therapist has the use of the money in advance for any necessary expenditures. The client has the option of giving one or more of the series massages to a friend, which brings a potential new client to the office.

To offer a series, you can have a coupon printed up and sell the coupon. It may have five places to punch holes, or five numbers to cross off, or any system you prefer for keeping track of when the massages are used up. You can also create a system without coupons, by keeping track in your record book, or in a separate ledger.

6. Other discount arrangements

Create any discount arrangement that serves a business purpose. This can include discounts for those who refer new clients, or promotions in which you give a free massage to someone who buys two gift certificates, or any other such idea that makes sense to you. One discount I offer is $10 off the second massage in one week for any client.

Sometimes it is appropriate to offer a discount to a client for becoming a "regular." Take the example of Ray, one of my clients. Ray came for massage an average of once a month. Sometimes he would come more often, sometimes less often.

At the end of a massage, I asked Ray if he would come in regularly if the price were lower. He said he would, and we discussed possible agreements.

We decided that he would like to come twice a month, and could afford to do so if he paid $30 per visit instead of the $40 I was then charging. This seemed advantageous to both of us, and we agreed to adopt this plan. Ray began coming in twice a month. He enjoyed receiving more massages and I appreciated the added business and income.

I would not make this offer to most of my clients. It felt right to do so with Ray, in part because Ray did not know any of my other clients, so I knew I would not be presented with multiple requests for the same arrangement. I offer this as an example of the creative marketing you can come up with to fit a particular situation.

7. *Barter for goods or services*

Barter — exchanging your service for the product or services of another — can be a means of gaining clients who would not otherwise receive massage. It can also be a good way for you to receive valuable goods or services without a cash outlay. In addition, clients with whom you barter may refer cash clients to you.

Barter can be done on an equal basis — one hour for one hour. It can also be done on an unequal basis. For example, if you barter with your physician, you may have to give more massage time than you receive from your doctor. On the other hand, if you barter for housecleaning, you may receive more housecleaning time than you give in massage service. One starting-point for negotiations is to compare the hourly rate for your services and the services you are bartering for, and adjust your barter arrangement accordingly.

Massage therapists who use barter find they can receive some great products and services through barter. You are limited only by who you are willing to barter with. Following is a list of services and items therapists have reported bartering for:

> Accounting services, advertising banner, airline tickets, auto repair, Barbie clothes, bodywork & massage, candles, chiropractic, computer equipment, contact lenses & eye exams, decorated cake, dentistry, dinners, electrical work, facials, gluten-free bread, graphic design, hair styling/haircuts, house cleaning, landscaping, legal services, linens for the office, manicures, medical services, office shelves, office sign, opera tickets, pedicures, prayers, printing services, psychic readings, sewing, stained glass, status as official massage therapist at local fitness center, sweet corn, swing, teddy bears, trip to Cancun, voice coaching, waxing, wedding flowers & wedding cake, wristwatch.

You should be aware that the IRS treats barter as a taxable transaction. You are required to include the fair market value of the goods or services you receive as "income" when you file your year-end tax return, and pay taxes on it. It is true that the lack of a paper record of the transaction makes it difficult for the IRS to prove, but their policy is to prosecute those who do not report barter transactions when they can. In 1997, the pop artist Peter Max pled guilty to tax fraud, partly as a result of having bartered his artwork in partial payment for several homes without paying the proper taxes.

Another concern about barter is the issue of dual relationships. If you do work of a psychotherapeutic nature, barter may be an inappropriate way to interact with your clients because of boundary issues in the therapeutic relationship. Most psychotherapists will not barter for massage for this reason. However, in most cases, there is no ethical problem with barter for massage professionals.

You can barter on a private basis, where the arrangement is solely between the individuals, or you can use one of many barter exchange networks to supervise the transaction. Some resources are: International Trade Exchange (10300 SW Greenburg Rd., Suite 370, Portland OR, 97223, (503) 244-4673); Business Exchange International (333 N. Glenoaks Blvd., #400, Burbank, CA 91502, (818) 563-4966); National Association of Trade Exchanges (27801 Euclid Ave., Suite 610, Euclid, OH 44132, (216) 732-7171).

13 Staying Healthy in a Demanding Field

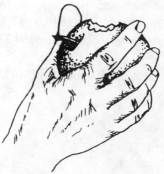

Every successful massage therapist I have spoken to has had to deal with some kind of physical or psychological problem that resulted from doing the work.

The most common physical problems are wrist injuries, back strain, neck and shoulder pain, and nodules (ganglia) in the fingers. In addition, some therapists suffer depression, some take on pain in places where their clients have it, and some "burn out" from the stresses involved in a massage practice.

There are practical ways you can avoid these problems. Successful therapists offered these tips from their experience:

Body Mechanics

Watch your body mechanics. Don't bend over when you work. Keep your spine straight and bend your knees. Let your force come from your hara, your abdominal center. Use the minimum number of muscles necessary for any particular motion. Make your body mechanics your first priority, even above the quality of work you do on your clients.

Exercise

Do yoga, tai chi, aikido, stretching, jogging, swimming, aerobics or some other exercise to improve your own bodily well-being. This helps not only to keep your body in good condition, but also to reduce the effects of stress.

Introspection

Involve yourself in psychotherapy, or meditation, and have a support group you can turn to in times of need. This will help you release your emotions, help you stay healthy, and promote your own growth.

Diet

Eat a balanced diet and drink plenty of water. You depend on your body as you would on a professional tool. You put good gasoline in your car, and keep the oil changed. Treat your body at least as well.

Attitude

Learn to let go. Life in the business world will bring you ups and downs, rewards and frustrations. Learn how to let go of the painful aspects. Letting go is not the same as denial or repressing your feelings. Accept people and situations as they are, let your emotions flow, and move on.

Receive Massage

Get massage on a regular basis. Three reasons: It promotes your overall health and well-being; you will learn techniques and awarenesses from receiving massage that will make you a better massage therapist; your credibility with your clients will be better if you "practice what you preach."

Specifics of Body Maintenance

Keep your wrists straight as much as possible while you work. Stretch your wrists before and after working. Use open fist, elbows or a T-bar to do deep work instead of fingers or thumbs.

If a nodule appears in a finger, try not to use that finger in your work for a week or two; apply pressure with the other fingers of that hand, but raise the finger with the nodule slightly so it is not used. If the nodule persists, work it with transverse friction to break it up. Consult a physician if the nodule will not recede.

Use a paraffin bath for sore hands, ice forearms or use liniment if inflamed.

Vacations and Days Off

Take days off. Success, when it finally comes, can be a shock to your system. If you find yourself very busy, make time to take care of yourself physically and emotionally.

Sometimes it is difficult to switch from the "I need all the clients I can get" consciousness to that of "I need to take time for myself." In the beginning, you do not have enough clients, and you are doing everything you can think of to get more. The time will arrive, however, when the clients will be coming. Allow yourself at that point to step back from your practice and make sure you are not wearing yourself out trying to achieve more "success" than you can stand.

14 Laundry and Linens

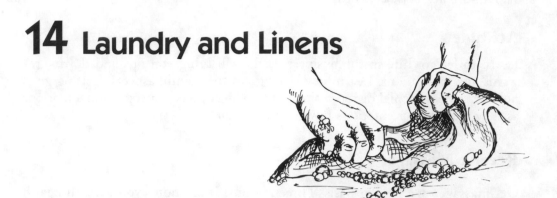

If you do Swedish massage, the issue of laundry is one you will face throughout your career. Unless you work in a setting where your employer takes care of laundry, you will have to make certain decisions about how to supply yourself with fresh linens to practice your trade.

Hire a Laundry Service vs. Do It Yourself

Depending on the laundry service you choose and what type of draping you use, having your laundry done for you can cost between $1 and $2.50 per client. Doing it yourself will bring the cost down dramatically, to between 10 cents and 50 cents per client.

If you hire a service, you will have to choose between furnishing your own linens and using theirs. If you use theirs, the cost will be higher. If you furnish your own, you will need twice as many as if you did your own wash, because at any given time, half your sheets and towels will be at the laundry.

Hiring a service makes the most sense in these situations:

1. You do not have a washer and dryer in your home or office. Trips to the laundromat can be very wearing when you are taking several loads per week.

2. You have a busy massage practice. If you are seeing lots of clients, then you are making enough money to afford paying a service to launder for you. If you have a busy practice, you probably do not have the time or energy to be dealing with the large amount of laundry your practice generates.

Choosing a Laundry Service

If you decide to use a laundry service, shop around. The prices charged by different services will vary quite a bit, as will the quality of their service.

Things to consider in hiring a service:

1. They may require you to use their sheets and towels, or they may be willing to sell you sheets and towels at wholesale prices. If you purchase the sheets and towels, the laundry will charge less to

104

launder them than they would if they supply them. However, any damaged linens will be your responsibility.

2. Be sure that this company can supply sheets and towels that you will like. See and feel samples before making an agreement.

3. Some massage oils can be difficult to remove from linens unless the company has the proper chemicals. Be sure they have experience with massage therapists and understand how to get these linens clean.

4. If you use a service, and they deliver a load of sheets and towels which are unsuitable in some way, you will be stuck with them unless the company is willing to make a special trip to remedy the problem. Find out how willing the company is to make sure problems will be taken care of and your needs will be met.

Finding Suppliers of Sheets and Towels

Buying a few linens at a time

If your practice is a casual one, meaning that you work on just a few clients a week, you will need a relatively small amount of linens, and should therefore purchase sheets and towels in the same way you do for personal use.

One option to consider is buying twin sheet sets. These include one fitted sheet, one flat sheet and one pillowcase, and sometimes can be found on sale for not much more than the cost of a single sheet. The fitted sheet on the table covered by the matching flat sheet creates a pleasant appearance.

Some therapists are quite particular about the linens they use, and this can be a very sensible attitude. The sheets and towels come in contact with a client's body, and you may want to create a luxurious impression by using colorful linens with a lush texture.

Buying in quantity

If you are most interested in presenting a clean (white) image, and keeping your costs to a minimum, consider purchasing sheets and towels through business channels. This is a decision to make when you begin to establish yourself in the field. It is not unlike a carpenter buying a set of tools — think toward the future and invest in a supply of sheets and towels you will be able to use for years to come.

Most companies that sell sheets and towels commercially are in the habit of selling at least 50 dozen at a time. The difficulty lies in finding a vendor who supplies linens commercially and is also willing to sell by the dozen. These are rare, but they do exist.

You will get some help looking in the yellow pages under "laundries." If your community has a Business-to-Business yellow pages, check under "linens." Occasionally, a commercial or institutional laundry will sell you one or two dozen odd or surplus sheets. These companies have large clients, and need to buy sheets by the gross for their own purposes. If they are willing to deal with you, you may be able to get a couple of dozen sheets from them at a discount price.

If you cannot locate any such businesses in your area, consider contacting someone who may have the connections you do not have. Your local hospital may be a wholesale purchaser of sheets and towels, and if you get in touch with the purchasing agent, she or he may be willing to resell a few dozen to you.

Choosing Sheets and Towels

Sheets

Whether you do your own laundry or use a service, you will still need to decide what size and quality sheets and towels to use. The thicker and more luxurious the linens, the more they will cost to buy and the more they will cost to launder.

Composition of sheets. The quality and comfort of sheets is determined by the "thread count." This is the number of threads used in a square inch of the fabric the sheet is made of. A higher thread count means a softer sheet. A thread count of 180 or higher usually signifies a good quality sheet. A thread count of 250 or more signifies a very luxurious sheet.

Also consider the fabric composition. The higher the percentage of cotton, the softer the sheet; the higher the percentage of polyester, the coarser the sheet.

Size of sheets. Keeping the size small helps a great deal in keeping the cost down at laundry time. Sheets come in a great variety of sizes, and the actual size of the sheets you receive may be a few inches different than the stated measurements.

If your goal is to create a luxurious feeling about your therapy room, and you are not being cost-conscious, buy large, thick sheets that will convey a sense of comfort and style. However, if your goal is simply to have a clean and pleasant sheet for your clients to lie on and under, consider the actual measurements of the sheets you need.

The normal size of a massage table is between 72" × 26" and 72" × 30". Two standard sheet sizes to consider are 72" × 42" and 75" × 54".

The actual size of the sheets you buy will be slightly smaller than the size stated on the package. This is partly because the stated size is "before hemming," and partly because it is accepted practice in the industry to have minor variations in sheet sizes. Therefore, a sheet that is called 72" long will actually be a few inches shorter than that, and will not quite cover the length of a massage table.

A 72" × 42" sheet is ideal for a table that has a face hole; it will cover the rest of the table and overlap a bit on all sides. It is also a good size to drape over a client, as it will cover most people from the neck down. A 75" × 54" sheet will cover the entire massage table, and will drape a few inches farther over the sides.

For a better looking image, you can leave a larger sheet draped over the table, concealing the legs, covered by a smaller sheet that you can change for each client.

These smaller sheets are convenient to handle in laundry, and will take up a minimum of space in your washing machine. In fact, well over a dozen 72" × 42" sheets will fit into a normal washing machine at a time.

As you shop for sheets, you may hear a confusing mix of terms used to describe sheets — terms like "draw sheet," "twin sheet," "standard," and other terms. These names have general meanings, but they do not convey accurate information about the size of the sheets you will actually be buying. Keep in mind actual measurements only. Decide what size will be best for your style of draping and the image you want to create, and then shop with these requirements in mind.

Towels

The same considerations apply to towels as apply to sheets. The larger and more luxurious a towel is, the costlier it will be to purchase and launder. Keeping the size down is a big help.

Many standard sizes are available to fit almost any need. The size I find most convenient is 20" × 40". This is the size of a small bath towel. I find it meets my needs for draping very well, while taking up a minimum of space in the cabinet and the washer.

The quality of towels is measured in "pounds per dozen." This means, simply, how much does a dozen of these towels weigh? For a given size towel, the "pounds per dozen" figure will give you an idea of how thick and fluffy the towel is.

For the size I use, 20" × 40", a normal weight might be 6 or 7 pounds per dozen. I use a towel that weighs 8.5 pounds per dozen, because I want a soft and hefty feel to my towels. Towels like these are available for around $2 each, plus shipping, when purchased wholesale. However, it may be difficult to get a wholesale price on orders of less than 16 dozen.

If you are doing comparison shopping, remember that increasing thickness increases "pounds per dozen," and increasing size also increases "pounds per dozen." It helps to decide on the size you want, and then compare the different towels of that size based on the "pounds per dozen" figure. So long as you are comparing towels of same size, the "pounds per dozen" figure will give you a good clue as to the thickness of the towel.

Tips for Do-It-Yourself Launderers

Doing your own laundry has advantages. First, you are in control of how many clean sheets and towels you have, and you know you will not run out unexpectedly, or have to rely on someone else to get your needs met.

Second, it is much cheaper to do your own laundry. Even factoring in the cost of a washer and dryer, in the long run doing your own laundry will probably cost only 10% to 20% as much as hiring a service.

Have the machines at your place

The most important consideration, if you plan to do your own laundry, is to have your own washer and dryer, in your home or in your office — whichever will be most convenient to your practice.

When your washer and dryer are convenient to use, you can throw in a load and be busy working, reading or relaxing. Throwing in a load becomes a routine activity and not a tedious chore, as it is when you have to leave your home or office to go to a laundromat. In addition, if the washer and dryer are for the exclusive use of your business, their cost can be deducted for income tax purposes (see Chapter 18).

Water dispersible oils

Most oil manufacturers now sell water-dispersible oils that are said to put an end to oil buildup in sheets and towels. These oils are a considerable help, and the oil removal process is now needed much less frequently than it was a few years ago. However, you may still find that oil accumulates in your linens, so you may need to purchase a product to remove oil residues.

Beating oil residues

Three products are marketed to massage therapists for removing oil residues from massage linens: Fresh Again, Sunfresh Soap, and Totally Clean and Fresh. You can purchase these products from the following suppliers:

Fresh Again is available from:

> **Biotone**
> 4757 Old Cliffs Rd
> San Diego, CA 92120
> 1-800-445-6457
> (619) 582-0027

> **Golden Ratio Bodyworks**
> P.O. Box 440
> Emigrant, MT 59027
> 1-800-796-0612

Sunfresh Soap is available from:

> **Diamond Light**
> Massage Products
> 14 Las Palomas
> Orinda, CA 94563
> (510) 253-0543

> **The Body Shop**
> 2051 Hilltop Drive #A5
> Redding, CA 96002
> (530) 221-1031

Totally Clean and Fresh is available from:

> **Totally Clean and Fresh SW**
> 91 Taylor Drive
> Fairfax, CA
> Toll free 1-800-458-2411

> **Totally Clean and Fresh SE**
> 612 - 3rd Street NW
> Attalla, AL 35954
> Toll free 1-877-370-3828

> **Totally Clean and Fresh NW**
> 604 Whitman
> Rosalia, WA 99170
> Toll free 1-800-541-8904

Hints for success with Fresh Again

Fresh Again is the oil removal product I tried first. I have been happy with it, so I have stayed with it. Through experience, I have learned the following:

You do not need to use Fresh Again each time you wash. Use it to treat your sheets and towels when you notice a buildup of oil. You will notice either a rough texture, or the odor of cooked oil when the linens get hot in the dryer.

Shake well before pouring to mix the detergent fully. Use the hottest water you can. Use a larger amount of detergent for heavy oil stains. For persistent stains, soak the linens in hot wash water overnight and complete the wash in the morning.

If you have stubborn oil stains, try leaving the linens in a strong concentration of Fresh Again for several days. Another option is to use extreme heat to take the oil out. If your linen will fit into a crock pot, try soaking it for an hour or so on "high" in a concentration of Fresh Again. Otherwise, use an old pan to boil the linen in a solution of Fresh Again on your stove.

Use about 1/3 cup Fresh Again to one or two gallons of water, and boil the linen in this mixture at a low boil for at least five minutes. You will be amazed how much oil comes out of a soiled linen, even if this linen has just been soaked overnight in hot wash water. Although extreme heat can accelerate the wearing out of the stitching and fabric, it can save discarding a sheet or towel that may have a lot of life left in it.

15 Professional Associations
Profiles

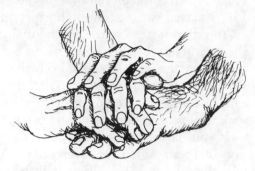

This chapter is divided into two sections; General Membership Organizations and Specialized Membership Organizations.

General Membership Organizations are those for massage practitioners and practitioners of bodywork in general.

Specialized Membership Organizations are those for practitioners of specific types of bodywork. For additional specialized membership organizations see the Bodywork Directory that starts on page 193, as many individual forms of bodywork have guiding organizations.

General Membership Organizations

American Massage Therapy Association (AMTA)

The AMTA is the oldest and largest national professional association for massage. It was founded in Chicago in 1943.

Requirements for membership:

> *Associate Membership* is available to massage students and recent graduates, and to massage therapists who were trained outside the United States. Associates may belong to the organization for up to three years while they pursue the requirements of Professional Active Membership. ($169 per year plus chapter fee of $0 to $30).

> *Professional Active Membership* is available to practitioners certified by NCTMB, or licensed by states that meet AMTA's 500-hour curriculum requirement, or who have graduated from a COMTA-approved school or have previously been Active or Professional AMTA members. ($235 per year plus chapter fee of $0 to $30).

All members receive professional and general liability insurance, optional health, life, business and disability insurance at group rates, member discounts on catalog products, listing in AMTA's *Membership Registry*, voice at AMTA meetings, *Massage Therapy Journal* and *HANDS ON Newsletter*, right to use ATMA logo in promotional materials, right to participate in state chapter and state and national committees.

Professional Active members also receive inclusion in the free therapist locator service, voting privileges at meetings, the right to serve as officer of the organization, and pin and patch.

AMTA's Commission on Massage Therapy Accreditation (COMTA) accredits massage therapy training programs, and as of the publication date, the following schools (identified by their ID number in the State-by-State Directory) were approved or accredited by COMTA: 9, 11, 26, 38, 63, 87, 96, 125, 126, 132, 135, 147, 155, 172, 174, 178, 180, 184, 195, 198, 202, 207, 219, 234, 241, 242, 248, 254, 271, 278, 279, 283, 285, 291, 292, 295, 302, 316, 349, 357, 366, 374, 376, 377, 382, 385, 386, 387, 399, 413, 424, 435, 448, 481, 499, 501, 527, 538, 550, 551, 563, 571.

COMTA can be contacted directly at the mailing address below or at (847) 864-0123.

AMTA has created the AMTA Foundation, a tax-exempt public charity which funds massage therapy related research, community outreach, educational scholarships and conferences (see Chapter 19).

Each year the association sponsors one national conference and one national convention. Chapters exist in all 50 states, the District of Columbia, and the Virgin Islands, and some chapters have regional meetings.

Of the professional associations for massage, AMTA is the most active in the legislative arena. AMTA helps chapters and members to promote legislation which it believes will assist the profession, and it funds selected efforts to keep or change laws governing massage. Some individuals within the AMTA work to have laws passed that require attendance at an AMTA-approved school, and some states have passed laws requiring AMTA-approved schooling (see page 131), but the advocacy of such laws is not official AMTA policy.

> American Massage Therapy Association® (AMTA®)
> 820 Davis St., Suite 100
> Evanston, IL 60201-4444
> (847) 864-0123
> www.amtamassage.org

Associated Bodywork And Massage Professionals (ABMP)

ABMP was founded in 1987. It attempts to be an effective, efficient, non-bureaucratic networking and services organization.

Requirements for membership:

> *Certified* or *Professional* membership requires a practitioner to be licensed by a state that licenses massage, *or* be currently a registered or certified member of an approved association, *or* obtain a passing score on a recognized certification exam, *or* demonstrate at least 50 hours massage training plus a nursing or physical therapy degree. Certified level requires 16 hours continuing education every two years. Cost of membership: *Certified,* $229 per year; *Professional,* $199 per year.

Practitioner level membership is available to those in non-licensed states with at least 100 hours training from an approved program. Cost of *Practitioner* level membership is $199 per year.

Student level ($39 per year)

Supporting level ($60 per year)

Certified, Professional and Practitioner level members all receive professional liability insurance including yoga instruction coverage (Certified has higher liability limit), referral service, regulatory interaction, pin, decal and certificate, subscription to *Massage & Bodywork*, membership newsletter, Massage & Bodywork Yellow Pages, and Successful Business Handbook. Members are also eligible for group rates on business insurance and disability insurance. Members who join for longer than one year receive a discount on the second year's dues.

ABMP sponsors IMSTAC, the International Massage & Somatic Therapies Accrediting Council, which accredits massage schools. IMSTAC can be contacted at the address and phone number printed below. As of publication time, the following schools had been accredited by IMSTAC: 12, 136, 210, 227, 238, 239, 289, 294, 305, 315, 318, 325, 371, 435, 437, 447, 448, 458, 480, 482.

ABMP sponsors research by Touch Research Institute and the Stanford Myofascial Institute.

ABMP attempts to foster a favorable legal climate for its membership, and has worked for and achieved amendments of laws it considered biased, notably in West Virginia and Maine.

For complete information, contact the ABMP:

Associated Bodywork and Massage Professionals
28677 Buffalo Park Road
Evergreen, CO 80439-7347
1-800-458-2267 or (303) 674-8478
www.abmp.com

International Massage Association (IMA Group)

IMA was founded in 1994. Its mission statement includes the goals of taking massage mainstream, uniting all natural health care professionals and gaining respect for their professions, providing members with liability insurance at the lowest possible cost, and giving members marketing tools to help their practices grow.

Requirements for membership: 100 hours of approved training for practicing members.

Practicing membership costs $129 per year and includes liability insurance.
Associate membership costs $79 per year.
Student membership costs $50 per year.

Benefits of membership, in addition to liability insurance for Practicing Members, include free internet referral service, opportunity to establish merchant accounts to accept credit cards, opportunity for mortgage financing for home or office, and debt consolidation loans.

The IMA Group links the International Massage Association to its other divisions for movement therapies, aromatherapy, reflexology, yoga, caricaturists, colonic educators, kinesiology, personal trainers, aerobics instructors, and dance teachers.

In addition, the IMA Group sponsors the IMA Group Education Foundation, which provides massage training to single mothers, and the IMA Group Research Foundation, which benefits Touch Research Institute.

IMA hosts two annual conventions in Washington, D.C.; one for members and one for school owners.

IMA Group, Massage Division
P.O. Box 421 / 92 Main St.
Historic Old Town Warrenton, VA 20186
(540) 349-0775
www.imagroup.com

International Myomassethics Federation (IMF)

IMF is an organization of professionals whose goal is to incorporate a wide range of accepted massage and bodywork techniques to promote health and well-being. It is run by the members, and the officers are volunteers. IMF hires an executive director to run its daily operations. Its motto is: IMF is the "Organization with a Heart".

Requirements for membership:

Myomassologist: Minimum of 500 hours education from a state licensed or approved school of Myomassology or Massage Therapy, or equivalent. Continuing education requirement applies.

Certified Myomassologist: Successful completion of any recognized state, national or international massage or bodywork examination. Continuing education requirement applies.

Student Member: Currently enrolled in a state licensed or approved school or myomassology or massage therapy, or equivalent. Limit: two years.

Cost of membership is $65 per year in states without affiliate organization, and is determined by the affiliate in those states that have affiliates (currently Illinois, Michigan, Wisconsin and Ontario).

Benefits of membership include fellowship and networking, volunteer service recognition, discount on continuing education at conventions and affiliate conferences, product discounts, quarterly newsletter and professional massage journal, listing in IMF's International Directory, discounts on liability insurance through IMA Group or ABMP, available group medical and dental insurance, 800 number for home office resource information, certificate, patch and pin.

International Myomassethics Federation, Inc.
1720 Willow Creek Circle, Suite 517
Eugene, OR 97402
(800) 433-4 IMF
www.imf-inc.org

Specialized Membership Organizations

American Oriental Bodywork Therapy Association (AOBTA)

The AOBTA is a nonprofit membership organization for practitioners of oriental bodywork that was formed in 1989. It maintains a "Council of Schools and Programs" (COSP) which approves curricula that meet AOBTA educational standards. As of publication time, 17 schools and programs had been accepted into the Council.

Requirements for membership:

Certified Practitioner level: 500 hours training, at COSP-approved school or taught by AOBTA-certified instructor. Application fee $30, dues $100 per year.

Associate level: 150 hours training, taught by AOBTA-certified instructor or qualified certified practitioner. Application fee $30, dues $75 per year.

Student level: Must be studying with AOBTA-certified instructor or practitioner. Application fee $10, annual dues $30.

Benefits of membership include the Organization's protection of the interests and rights and professional standards of Oriental Bodywork Therapy, high quality educational opportunities, legislative support and action-oriented representation, *Pulse* quarterly newsletter, member discount for advertising, optional insurance (professional liability, group health, disability), annual membership directory, practitioner referral service.

American Oriental Bodywork Therapy Association
Laurel Oak Corporate Center, Suite 408
1010 Haddonfield-Berlin Rd.
Voorhees, NJ 08043
(609) 782-1616
www.healthy.net/AOBTA

American Polarity Therapy Association (APTA)

Established in 1985, The American Polarity Therapy Association sets standards in Polarity Therapy practice and ethics, promotes public awareness, and cooperates with public agencies and other professional groups.

APTA approves polarity training programs, and as of publication date, there were 29 approved programs in the United States.

The association hosts an annual conference, publishes a membership directory, and produces Energy, a quarterly newsletter.

Membership costs $60 per year. Student membership is $40.

American Polarity Therapy Association
2888 Bluff St., ste. 149
Boulder, CO 80301
(303) 545-2080 or 1-800-359-5620
www.polaritytherapy.org

National Association of Nurse Massage Therapists (NANMT)

The NANMT was formed in 1987. The NANMT is committed to bringing an increased awareness and acceptance of touch therapy to the mainstream medical and hospital community. It supports gaining insurance reimbursement for massage services, and also supports research into the health benefits of massage. Active membership costs $75 per year, senior and student memberships cost $50, corporate membership costs $125, and supporting membership costs $75. Benefits of membership include NANMT's bulletin and quarterly publication, listing in annual directory, copy of directory, discounts, CEU's and use of NANMT seal on promotional material.

For further information, contact:

National Association of Nurse Massage Therapists (NANMT)
P.O. Box 904
Carrboro, NC 27510
1-888-805-7879 voice mailbox 125

Nursing Touch & Massage Therapy Association, International

A recently formed association for nurse-massage therapists. Active membership costs $100 per year, supporting membership costs $80, student and senior memberships cost $70. Contact them at:

Nursing Touch & Massage Therapy Association, International (NTMTA)
1438 Shortcut, Suite E
Slidell, LA 70458
(504) 893-8002
http://members.aol.com/ntmta/

Transformation Oriented Bodywork Network

Transformation Work involves acting as a facilitator for the client's healing process. Massage and bodywork practitioners who participate in the TOB-Network are dedicated to this type of work.

This is a member-driven network that will publicize trainings, provide a forum for therapists to communicate with each other, provide a membership directory and a newsletter. It is open to all graduates of a licensed massage school. Membership is $30 per year, and a packet of two sample newsletters plus information on the network costs $5.50.

For further information, contact:

Transformation Oriented Bodywork Network (TOB-NET)
Mickey McGinnis, Coordinator
P.O. Box 24967
San Jose, CA 95154-4967
(408) 371-6716

State and Local Organizations

Many states and regions have their own massage and bodywork associations. Since these are usually volunteer organizations, the contact information changes frequently as officers serve their terms of office and move on. The best sources of up-to-date information for state and local associations are massage schools and practitioners in the local area.

16 Insurance

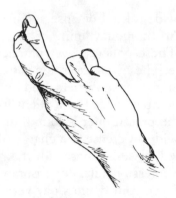

This chapter is about the types of insurance you can buy to protect yourself against certain risks. This chapter does not discuss having your work paid for by your clients' insurance, which is covered in Chapter 20.

Why Buy Insurance?

Insurance is risk protection. If you have no insurance, you bear all the financial risks of life alone.

The kinds of risks that insurance covers are illustrated by the following examples:

- If you are sued by a client and lose, you are responsible to pay the amount awarded to your client by the court.

- If a client slips and falls in your office, you might be required to pay for that injury.

- If you are sued by a client for any reason, you will have to pay your own legal fees for defending the suit.

- If your office burns down or is vandalized, you absorb the loss.

- If you are injured and cannot work for a period of time, you will have no assistance in meeting your financial obligations.

- If you fall ill and need medical attention, you will have to pay the full amount of the medical expenses.

Each of the examples above illustrates one type of risk for which the self-employed bodyworker can purchase insurance. Each kind of insurance is profiled in the next part of this chapter.

Kinds of Insurance Available to the Professional Bodyworker

Professional Liability Insurance

This insurance defends you against claims by clients that you harmed them in the course of performing your professional services. The insurance company will provide a legal defense against a claim, and will pay any judgment against you, up to the policy limit.

These policies cover practically all claims of harm to a client during a massage. The major exception is for allegations of sexual misconduct by a practitioner. The insurance carriers used by ABMP and AMTA provide a legal defense when a member is sued by a client for sexual misconduct, but will not pay a judgment if the practitioner is found guilty. The insurance carrier used by IMA does not provide a defense to a charge of sexual misconduct, nor will they pay a judgment based on sexual misconduct.

Professional liability insurance has become very expensive in other professions. Lawyers and doctors pay very large annual premiums for this type of coverage because of the large number of lawsuits that are filed and the large judgments that result. In massage and bodywork, these suits are very rare, and the insurance is therefore relatively inexpensive.

Professional liability insurance is a benefit of membership in the AMTA, ABMP and IMA. The associations purchase group insurance policies, and their per-member cost is very low. Discounted professional liability insurance is also available at an additional charge to members of the AOBTA, Rolf Institute, American Polarity Therapy Association, Trager Institute and Feldenkrais Guild. Professional liability insurance is also available for $175 per year through Healthcare Providers Services Organization without joining an association. (1-800-982-9491, www.hpso.com)

Two general types of professional liability insurance are sold: "claims-made" insurance and "occurrence form" insurance.

A claims-made policy covers you for claims that are made while the policy is in force. "Claim" refers to the announcement by the client of their complaint against you. With this type of policy, you are covered if it was in force when the claim was filed.

An occurrence form policy covers you for incidents that "occur" while your policy is in force. The act occurs at the moment you allegedly caused harm to the client. With this type of policy, you are covered if it was in force when the alleged misconduct occurred.

The difference between these two types of policy comes up if you discontinue your insurance — for example, if you stop practicing massage. Say you retire from the practice of massage and discontinue coverage effective January 1, 2000. A client comes forth on February 1, 2000 and claims you injured her during a massage you gave her on June 30, 1999.

An occurrence form policy would cover you in this case, because the alleged injury *occurred* while the policy was in force. A claims-made policy would not cover you, because the *claim* was made after your insurance had lapsed. All of the major professional associations offer "occurrence form" policies.

If you plan to have a significant career in the massage or bodywork field, professional liability insurance is virtually a necessity. While you may think you do not need such insurance because you have no significant possessions to lose anyway, consider the broader question of how being uninsured might handcuff your future.

Spa owners, chiropractors and other massage employers will usually not hire an uninsured massage therapist. If the therapist is uninsured, then any client with a claim against the therapist would likely sue the employer, who does have insurance. An uninsured therapist is seen as an unnecessary risk. This is a career disadvantage you do not want to have.

Business Liability Insurance

Business Liability, or premises liability insurance, is "slip and fall" coverage. It protects you against suits that result from injuries people sustain on your business premises. The cause of these injuries might be icy steps, loose carpet, or any other cause of accidental injury.

Legally, you are liable for these injuries only if you do not keep your office in a reasonably safe condition for your clients. The legalities of how safe you need to keep it vary slightly from place to place. However, as a practical matter, any injury to a client is a potential problem, even if you are not ultimately legally responsible for it. If the client sues, you still will have to bear the expense of lawyer's fees to defend the action.

Business liability insurance covers both attorneys' fees to defend an action and any recovery that is ultimately awarded. It is included in the cost of membership in some professional associations (check with the association), and can be purchased on the open market through insurance agents and insurance companies.

If you practice in a home office, you can try to get a rider for your homeowner's policy to cover business liability. Some companies will issue these and others will not. You may need to change insurance carriers after setting up a home office because some companies will discontinue your coverage if they learn you operate a business in a home office. If available, a rider for your home office should cost between $50 and $150 per year.

Business Insurance

Business insurance covers your business equipment and premises against losses such as fire and theft. These policies usually cover the replacement cost of your equipment and supplies, and perhaps even petty cash in the office. Many will also cover lost income while your office is closed and the cost of renting temporary office space if your office is destroyed. Policies are generally available through major insurance companies and independent agents. Prices usually range from $200 to $400 per year.

Disability Insurance or Business Interruption Insurance

In the event you are unable to work due to accident or illness, disability insurance provides you with continued weekly income. You usually must be disabled for several weeks (or several months) before the policy will pay you a weekly income, and you can usually collect payments under the policy up to a maximum of one year.

Disability insurance is not cheap; a policy to provide you with $300 to $400 per week in the event of disability may cost around $1,000 per year to purchase.

It has also become increasingly difficult to find a company willing to write a disability insurance policy, especially for women. Decide whether or not to buy such insurance based on how strong your need is to be sure of continued income.

Medical Insurance / Group Medical Insurance

Policies for medical insurance are available in many forms, from bare-bones to deluxe. The costs of such insurance range from high to exorbitant.

The least expensive coverage is referred to as "catastrophic illness insurance." This insurance will pay for most of the expense of a hospital stay, after a deductible of, for example, $2,000. This is protection against being turned away from a hospital when you need care, and against being placed into bankruptcy by an illness. Such insurance may cost $500 to $2,000 per year, depending on your age and place of residence. It is not available in all states.

The most expensive coverage is major medical, which will cover a wide range of treatments, procedures and medications. The cost of this type of coverage seems to be going up weekly, and no one can tell where it will stop.

In between are a wide range of compromise plans with varying price tags. AMTA and ABMP offer members opportunities to purchase discounted group health policies. Many other groups offer their members group health insurance of one sort or another. One good source is the local chamber of commerce or other nonprofit civic group. You can also check with National Association for the Self-Employed (1-800-232-6273) and the Home Office Association of America (1-800-809-4622). Other options are Costco (1-800-974-0500), farmers' cooperative organizations, and any organization that bands together large numbers of consumers to improve their bargaining power.

17 Laws You Should Know About and State Regulation of Massage

Many laws have some effect on bodyworkers. The first section of this chapter summarizes basic laws you should know about and legal principles you should understand.

The second section details state laws regulating massage, and also describes legislative activity in states that have not yet adopted laws regulating the practice of massage. A chart summarizing all state laws regulating massage appears on page 131.

Laws you should know about

Federal, State, County and Local Governments. Most Americans live under the authority of four different governments. Each one has its own areas of major influence, in terms of what it offers you and what it requires of you.

The *Federal* government requires you to pay federal taxes on all the money you earn. The federal government also authorizes certain organizations to accredit massage schools, paving the way for the granting of financial aid for massage education. (Financial aid information is noted in schools' listing in the State-by-State Directory.)

State governments sometimes enact laws regulating the practice of massage in the state. These laws are described in the second part of this chapter, and summarized on page 131. State governments sometimes require the payment of income taxes on the money you earn.

County governments occasionally pass laws concerning the practice of massage in the county. Such laws apply only in unincorporated areas of the county — that is, in areas which are not within the borders of a town or city that has a municipal government. The county government may also take over zoning and health requirements in unincorporated areas within the county, and has the power to levy some taxes.

County governments also keep track of business names ("assumed names" or "fictitious names") and issue certificates to businesses allowing them to use a business name.

City (or township or village) governments, also called *municipal* governments, regulate zoning, parking, health concerns, and the operation of businesses within the city limits. They have the power to decide what businesses can and cannot operate in the city, and what locations within the city are permissible locations for different types of businesses. Some cities have regulations for the practice of massage within the city limits. Some cities prohibit the practice of massage within city limits. Many cities have some form of municipal taxation.

If there is ever a conflict between the laws of different governments, the power structure works as follows: Federal law always has priority; state laws have priority over county and local laws; municipal laws control within the borders of the city, town or village; in unincorporated areas of the county, county law applies unless it is in conflict with state or Federal law.

County and Municipal Professional Licensing Laws. As mentioned above, laws specifically regulating the practice of massage can be enacted by state, county or local governments. In many areas, no regulatory law applies to the practice of massage, as neither the state, county nor city has enacted one.

Many local laws regulating the practice of massage require the applicant for a massage license to submit items like fingerprints, recent photo, recent employment history, references, and physician's certificate that he or she has no communicable disease. In addition, some have educational requirements.

Some representative municipal educational requirements are listed below:

Ames, IA 750 hours at AMTA-approved school; Cedar Rapids, IA 500 hours; Colorado Springs, CO 1,000 hours; Davenport, IA 500 hours over a period of at least one year; Des Moines, IA 1,000 hours; Las Vegas, NV 500 hours; Pueblo, CO 70 hours; St. Louis, MO 70 hours; St. Paul, MN, 40 hours; Tempe, AZ 600 hours; Tucson, AZ 1,000 hours (500 in-class hours).

As you can see, the range of 40 hours to 1,000 hours is quite a broad one, and this reflects the situation within the nation as a whole concerning massage licensing.

Other Local Requirements. If your local government has a law regulating massage establishments, the law may have requirements for bathrooms, lighting, signs and other specifics concerning the office. If there is no such law, consider contacting the health department, fire department and the police department to see if there are any requirements you should know about before committing to a particular office space.

Business License. Business licenses are usually required by city governments. Occasionally a county requires a business license, and the state of Alaska requires such a license. It is used by the city government to keep track of who is performing what business activity, to generate money for the municipal treasury, and to make sure that zoning laws are being followed.

Zoning Laws. Most cities have a special map of the city that divides every location into one of several zones. (See Sample Zoning Map, page 59.) A key explains the meaning of each zone. The zones create different kinds of neighborhoods — business areas, residential areas, industrial areas, and areas of mixed usage.

When you open a massage or bodywork practice, you will need to be sure you are locating your office in an area that is zoned for your type of business. You may find there is a dispute about the type of business you have — some zoning agencies classify massage as a profession, others consider it a health service, others call it a personal service, and others classify it as adult entertainment. The zoning board's classification decision can affect permissible locations for your office.

Local Taxes. Some local governments charge businesses a tax on business property. That means that they decide the value of the business property you own, and tax you a fixed percentage of that value each year. Some local governments also charge a sewer tax, which may be based on water usage or number of plumbing units.

Fictitious Name (or Assumed Name) Statement. If you use a made-up name for your business that does not include your own name, you should register that name with the county government. There is a fee, usually around $20, and you may be required to search through the county's record books to make sure that no one has already taken the name you are choosing. You may also be required to advertise the name in the legal classifieds of your local newspaper. Registering your fictitious name is a requirement for opening a checking account in the name of the business.

Taxpayer Identification Number. If you are a sole proprietor (see below) and do not have any employees, you can use your social security number on all tax documents. If you have employees, or if you incorporate or form a partnership, you will need to apply for a taxpayer identification number. Obtain form SS-4 from the Internal Revenue Service. For information on how to get the form, see the end of Chapter 18.

Business Identity. In the eyes of the law, there are several possible "identities" for your business. The main ones are corporation, partnership and sole proprietor.

Corporations have a separate legal identity apart from the shareholders and employees. They can have tax advantages in some sophisticated situations, but if you are a self-employed bodyworker, it is not an advantage to incorporate.

Partnership is a special legal relationship in which the two or more partners can speak and act for each other. A promise by one binds the other, so if your partner makes a business deal and then fails to follow through, you can be held responsible for it. Partners usually share the partnership income, without regard to who actually did the work that generated the money.

Sole Proprietor means you, and you alone, run your business. In legal terms, there is no difference between you and your business. Your business income and personal income are simply added together to determine what your income is. Your business is treated legally just as it is in fact — as an extension of your life and a part of yourself.

Practically every bodyworker operates as a sole proprietor, and unless you have some good reason not to, you should too. Becoming a corporation or a partnership will not benefit you unless you are involved in some complicated or sophisticated business dealings. If you become involved in a group practice, the group may choose to incorporate. This is something the group will decide in consultation with a lawyer or accountant.

Contractual relationship. A contract can be oral or written. It is simply an exchange of promises in which each party agrees to do or give something of value to the other party. Once made, a contract is legally enforceable until it is ended by the parties who made it.

Written contracts are easier to enforce, because the exact terms of the agreement are on paper for all to see. Oral contracts can also be enforced, but the specifics must be proven by testimony about the agreement.

Simply opening a checking account involves making a contract. The bank agrees to hold your money and give it to you or the people you write checks to, according to certain rules the bank establishes. You agree to pay a set fee per check written, or keep a minimum monthly balance, and to pay prescribed penalties for writing checks that your account cannot cover.

As a massage therapist, contracts you are likely to enter into include agreements to work for others or to have others work for you, rental agreements for office space, contracts with the phone company for business phone service, and contracts for performance of services like printing, laundry and cleaning.

State Laws Regulating Massage

The following is an index to state regulation of massage as of July, 1998. In states that have governmental regulation of massage, this index lists their educational requirements, notes states that have adopted the National Certification Exam as their written exam, and gives the address and phone number for the licensing body. Additional requirements, such as health certificate, required fees, and continuing education requirements are not listed.

For states that do not regulate massage but have had recent legislative activity, a summary is given of the action that has taken place in the legislative arena.

Information of this nature necessarily goes out of date, since legislation regarding massage is changing rapidly. Fortunately, there are sources you can turn to that will provide periodic updates to this information.

For current information on massage laws that have been enacted, one resource is *Massage* Magazine, which prints a summary of current

licensing laws toward the back of each issue. Another source of current licensing information is any of the massage schools located in a state. In addition, most professional associations keep abreast of licensing laws nationwide and can provide current information. The information in this chapter is also updated at the publisher's website, www.CareerAtYourFingertips.com. From the home page, click on the link to "State Laws Regulating Massage."

In states that require or accept the National Certification Exam as their written exam, passing that exam in any location will satisfy the written test requirement. However, other licensing requirements must also be met to qualify for a license, such as specific educational requirements.

The current state licensing laws are summarized in a chart on page 131. The information in this section is meant to give fuller information about what is happening in individual states than can be contained in a one-page explanatory chart.

Alabama

State licensing, 650 hours until 1/1/00, 1,000 hours thereafter, from an institution approved by the Board.

Applicants must pass either state-administered exam or *National Certification Exam*

Alabama Massage Licensing Board
660 Adams Ave., Suite 301
Montgomery, AL 36104
(334) 269-9990

A bill to exempt reflexology practitioners from the operation of the massage licensing law was introduced in 1998 but did not pass. It will likely be resubmitted in the 1999 legislative session. There is also a plan to submit legislation which would do away with the state-administered written test and require the National Certification Test for all applicants, but as of press time this had not been introduced in the legislature.

Arkansas

State licensing, 500 hours required
Reciprocity is on a case-by-case basis and requires education in an accredited school

Arkansas Massage Board
P.O. Box 20739
Hot Springs, AR 71903
(501) 623-0444

California

California does not have statewide massage regulation. Licensing of massage practitioners in California is done only by city and county governments. A State of California law (Chapter 6, sections 51030 through 51034) gives authority to cities and counties to regulate massage. The law states what aspects of the practice may and may not be regulated. Section 51034 states that local laws may not restrict massage to same-sex massage only.

Some southern California jurisdictions exempt Holistic Health Practitioners from their massage laws. This is usually defined as someone with demonstrable training and experience in massage.

The following table of municipal and county licensing requirements was compiled in 1991, and has been only partially updated since then. While most of this information is still accurate, it is the nature of such information that it slowly goes out of date. Nonetheless, this table provides a useful picture of the diverse state of massage licensing in California.

Aside from the educational requirements listed below, most cities have some practical requirements for a person who wants to practice massage. For example, some towns prohibit "outcall" massage, or house calls, and some regulate it separately and require a special outcall massage license.

The amount charged for business or professional licenses varies tremendously from place to place, from a few dollars to over two thousand dollars. Some towns require a business license but no professional credentials. Some regulate massage as "adult entertainment." Some prohibit the practice of massage altogether.

For updated information about local laws, inquire at the city hall or county government building in the county seat. If you cannot locate a city government, contact the League of California Cities, 1400 K Street, Sacramento, CA 95814.

1,000 HOURS: Orange, San Clemente, Santa Paula, Thousand Oaks, Tustin, Vista

600 HOURS: Fontana, Rialto, San Bernardino

500 HOURS: Alameda County (NCE), Brea, Cupertino, Palm Desert, Seal Beach

300 HOURS: Newport Beach

225 HOURS: Marina

200 HOURS: Alhambra, Auburn, Bakersfield, Big Bear Lake, Camarillo, Carlsbad, Carson, Chula Vista, Covina, Cudahy, Cypress, El Segundo, Fairfield, Glendale, Grover City, Hayward, Hercules, Highland, Imperial, Imperial Beach, Kern County, Laguna Beach, Loma Linda, Los Alamitos, Huntington Park, Marysville, Montebello, Ontario, Orange County, Placentia, Ridgecrest, San Bernardino County, San Buenaventura, Santa Barbara, Signal Hill, Solano Beach, Torrance, Twentynine Palms, Union City, Ventura County, West Sacramento, Yuba County.

180 HOURS: Atwater, Ceres, Dublin, Livingston, Merced, Modesto, Turlock

100 HOURS: Corona, Desert Hot Springs, Dublin, El Dorado County, Escondido, Fresno, Gardena, Hollister, La Mesa, Livermore, Merced County, Monterey, Monterey County, Novato, Palm Springs, Redlands, San Francisco, San Leandro, San Luis Obispo, Santa Monica.

70 HOURS: Alameda, Burlingame, Colma, Contra Costa County, Daly City, Half Moon Bay, Lakewood, Livermore, Manteca, Milpitas, Pacifica, Palo Alto, Portola Valley, Richmond, San Mateo County, San Pablo, San Ramon, Santa Clara, Santa Clara County, Saratoga, Selma.

Any approved or recognized school: Adelanto, Arroyo Grande, Azuza, Beaumont, Belmont, Beverly Hills, Cloverdale, Encinitas, Eureka, Foster City, Fullerton, Glendora, Healdsburg, Imperial County, Lemon Grove, Millbrae, Napa, Oceanside, Oxnard, Pacific Grove, Pleasanton, Poway, Rancho Mirage, Sacramento County, San Bruno, San Diego County, San Marcos, San Mateo, Santa Rosa, Santee, Simi Valley, South Lake Tahoe, Stockton, West Covina, West Hollywood, Westmoreland, Whittier.

No educational requirement but other requirements: Anaheim, Bell Gardens, Burbank, Commerce, Culver City, Hemet, Long Beach, Los Angeles, Manhattan Beach, Riverside, Riverside County, San Ramon, Santa Fe Springs.

Colorado

In 1989, representatives of AMTA and ABMP, school owners, and several unaffiliated massage therapists came together to form a coalition to represent massage practitioners on licensing issues. These efforts resulted in a law defining "Massage Therapist" as a graduate of a state-approved school with at least 500 hours of education. One who meets this definition is exempted from the "massage parlor" law.

Massage regulation in Colorado is done by city and county governments, and approximately 15 county and municipal governments have laws regulating the practice of massage. At present, there is no plan to pursue state regulation of massage or bodywork.

Connecticut

State licensing, 500 hours at a school approved by COMTA *and* by an accrediting agency recognized by the U.S. Department of Education
Reciprocity is available if school is on CT's approved list - contact the department.
National Certification Exam

> Ct. Dept. of Public Health
> Massage Therapy Licensure
> 410 Capitol Ave. MS #12, APP
> P.O. Box 340308
> Hartford, CT 06134
> (860) 509-7570

Delaware

Massage and Bodywork Therapist, 500 hours (300 hours massage modalities, 100 A&P, 100 contraindications) *National Certification Exam*
> or
Certified Technician, 100 hours (curriculum not specified)

Delaware Committee of Massage Practice
Cannon Building, suite 203
861 Silver Lake Blvd.
Dover, DE 19904
(302) 739-4522, ext. 205

Only licensed massage and bodywork therapists may work by prescription of physicians. Certified technicians may work in any other massage setting. To practice massage in Delaware, one must be either licensed or certified. As of 1998, Delaware had 200 certified technicians and 48 licensed massage and bodywork therapists.

District of Columbia

A bill for licensure of massage therapists was enacted in 1995, but as of press time for this edition (late 1998), it still had not been implemented by the government. The law requires 500 hours of education, which can be waived through a grandfathering provision to be in effect for two years. (Grandfathering means those already practicing can become licensed without meeting all the requirements of the new law)

Implementation of the law seems to have been caught up in a political tussle about the large number of professional regulation boards in D.C. There is a movement under way to reduce the number of regulatory boards, and massage licensing has been held up by that political issue. As of press time, the D.C. Control Board had issued its final regulations, clearing the way for the Board of Massage Therapy to begin the process of licensing massage therapists.

For updated information, contact one of the massage schools in the D.C., or call the Licensing Board at (202) 727-7823, or check for updates on our website at: www.CareerAtYourFingertips.com.

Florida

State licensing, 500 hours required
Reciprocity (called Endorsement in Florida) for graduates of a school or apprenticeship approved by the Board.
National Certification Exam

> Division of Medical Quality Assurance
> Board of Massage Therapy
> Northwood Centre
> 1940 N. Monroe St.
> Tallahassee, FL 32399
> (850) 488-6021

Georgia

Bills to regulate the practice of massage have been introduced in Georgia in 1992, 1995, and 1997. None of these passed the legislature. The process of attempting to create massage legislation has brought out varying opinions from practitioners within the state. The state AMTA chapter's president wrote in 1998 that he believed the process of voicing conflicting concerns and ideas would result in eventually enacting a unified law representing the different modalities of the massage therapy profession.

Hawaii

State licensing, 570 hours required; or apprenticeship of 150 in-class hours and 420 hours practical.

Educational institution must be approved or licensed by a state department of education *or* approved by an accredited community college, college or university *or* approved by the AMTA *or* approved by the Rolf Institute.

> Hawaii Department of Commerce and Consumer Affairs
> Professional and Vocational Licensing Division
> P.O. Box 3469
> Honolulu, HI 96801
> (808) 586-3000

Iowa

State licensing, 500 hours
National Certification Exam

> Iowa Massage Therapy Board
> 321 E. 12th St.
> Lucas State Office Building
> Des Moines, IA 50319
> (515) 281-6959

Louisiana

State licensing, 500 hours
National Certification Exam (optional)

> Louisiana Board of Massage Therapy
> P.O. Box 1279
> Zachary, LA 70791
> (504) 658-8941

National Certification Exam may be used to substitute for the written portion of State Exam.

Maine

State Licensing, 500 hours from a school approved by the Department of Professional and Financial Regulation, *or*
National Certification Exam

> Maine Department of Professional and Financial Regulation
> Division of Licensing and Enforcement — Massage Therapists
> State House Station #35

> Augusta, ME 04333
> (207) 624-8624

Maine recently upgraded its regulatory requirement from "registration" to "licensure". During the transition phase, until 12/31/01, registered practitioners may upgrade to licensure if they have 1) completed 250 hours of formal massage education and have five years of active practice or 2) have 10 years of active practice.

Maine's law does not prohibit the practice of massage by non-licensed persons, but it prohibits the use of the terms "massage therapist" or "massage practitioner" by unlicensed persons.

Maryland

State Certification, 500 hours until 1/1/02, 60 college credit hours thereafter
National Certification Exam (tentative)

> Maryland Board of Chiropractic Examiners
> (410) 764-4726

Maryland has been a battleground between the professions of Physical Therapy and Massage. The Physical Therapy Board made a serious attempt to prohibit the practice of massage by anyone except physical therapists. This battle raged in Maryland for about a decade, and it has finally (almost) ended with the enactment of massage licensing legislation.

As of press time for this edition, near the end of 1988, Maryland's newly-enacted massage law had not yet been implemented. Massage will be regulated by the Chiropractic Board. In devising the final regulations, the Chiropractic Board is advised by an Advisory Committee composed of two chiropractors and four massage therapists. Disputes between the Advisory Committee and the Chiropractic Board were holding up implementation of the law at press time.

Some provisions have been agreed on: Current practitioners will be grandfathered in — they can be certified without meeting the requirements of the new law. The Board also may offer an alternative to the National Certification Exam. Practitioners who are certified before 1/1/02 and maintain active certification status will not need to satisfy the requirement for 60 hours of college credit.

Michigan

A statewide massage licensure law was adopted in 1974 and modified in 1980, but it is legally defective and has never been implemented. Even though there is a licensing law "on the books," there is no license available in Michigan to those who practice massage or bodywork.

Minnesota

Proposed legislation was introduced in 1998 but did not pass. The group sponsoring the bill planned to refine it for reintroduction in the 1999 legislative session

Mississippi

Proposals to regulate massage have been introduced in Mississippi in 1993, 1994, 1997 and 1998. The latest bill was approved by the House Public Health and Welfare Committee, but it failed to pass the House of Representatives.

Missouri

State licensing, 500 hours

Missouri's law was enacted in July of 1998, and as of press time, the regulations to implement the law had not been drafted. One provision of the law is that the only written test required for licensure is the testing done at the state-certified massage school.

Nebraska

State licensing, 1000 hours
National Certification Exam
Reciprocity for those attending a school approved by the Board, or upon review of school transcript.

Department of Health
Credentialing Division
301 Centennial Mall South
P.O. Box 94986
Lincoln, NE 68509
(402) 471-2117

New Hampshire

State licensing, 750 hours
National Certification Exam

NH Dept. of Health and Human Services
Bureau of Health Facilities Administration
6 Hazen Drive
Concord, NH 03301
(603) 271-4594

New Jersey

In 1993, New Jersey's bodywork community formed a coalition to work toward the creation of a law regulating massage. Legislation was introduced in 1997 that did not succeed. Bills were introduced in the House and Senate during 1998, and both received hearings. At press time, both measures were still before the legislature.

New Mexico

State licensing, 650 hours (may be 300 hours plus 350 hours Alternative Qualifying Experience)
National Certification Exam plus Jurisprudence Exam
Reciprocity on a case-by-case basis (referred to as "by credentials")

New Mexico Board of Massage Therapy
P.O. Box 25101
Santa Fe, NM 87504
(505) 476-7090

New York

State licensing, 605 hours until 1/1/00, 1,000 hours thereafter
Reciprocity is case-by-case and requires proof of practice for two years

New York State Education Department
State Board for Massage Therapy
Cultural Education Center, Room 3041
Albany, NY 12230
(518) 474-3817 (general info)
(518) 474-3866 (practice issues and applications)

North Carolina

Bills to regulate the massage profession in North Carolina were introduced in 1993, 1995 and 1997, and none succeeded. Sponsors of the legislation intend to try to have a bill introduced in 1998, or failing that, in 1999.

North Dakota

State certificate of registration, 500 hours
Requires attendance at COMTA-approved school

North Dakota Massage Board
P.O. Box 701
Dickinson, ND 58601
(701) 225-3906 (Phil Reisenauer)

Ohio

State licensing, 600 hours (during at least 12 months)
Reciprocity is on a case-by-case basis, but an exam is still required.

Ohio State Medical Board
77 South High St., 17th floor
Columbus, OH 43266
(614) 466-3934

In Ohio, a massage license is required for use of the title "licensed massage therapist." A massage license is required to practice therapeutic massage, but is not required to practice relaxation massage. Unlicensed practitioners probably cannot receive reimbursement from insurance companies.

Oklahoma

A bill to regulate massage was introduced in 1997 and carried over into the 1998 legislative session, but it did not pass the legislature.

Oregon

State licensing, 330 hours until 1/1/99, 500 hours thereafter
No Reciprocity

> Oregon Board of Massage Technicians
> 3218 Pringle Rd. SE, Suite 250
> Salem, OR 97302
> (503) 378-2070

Pennsylvania

A coalition of 16 organization worked for more than five years to develop a legislative proposal to regulate massage, reflexology, and healing arts. Legislation was introduced in 1997. As of press time for this edition, the bill was under consideration by the legislature but no action had been taken on it.

Rhode Island

State licensing, 500 hours at a COMTA-approved school or an equivalent academic and training program of 1000 hours
National Certification Exam

> Rhode Island Department of Health
> Room 104, Cannon Building
> Three Capitol Hill
> Providence, RI 02908
> (401) 222-2827 ext. 112

A bill was introduced in the legislature in 1998 that would give every city and town in RI authority to adopt ordinances and license and regulate massage establishments (massage parlors) and massage therapists. The state would still retain licensing authority. The measure was still before the legislature at press time.

South Carolina

State licensing, 500 hours
National Certification Exam

> Department of LLR
> Massage Therapy Board
> P.O. Box 11329
> Columbia, SC 29211
> (803) 896-4830

Tennessee

State Licensing, 500 hours from State-accredited school, *or*
National Certification Exam
Reciprocity is on a case-by-case basis

> Board of Massage Therapy
> First Floor, Cordell Hull Building
> 425 5th Ave North,
> Nashville, TN 37247-1010
> (615) 532-5083

Students who attend a school on the state's list of accredited schools do not need to take a written test. Anyone who has passed the National Certification Exam and submits proof of passing may be licensed, regardless of what school they attended. In addition, those licensed in states with equivalent educational requirements may be admitted by reciprocity.

Texas

State registration, 250 hours plus 50 hours internship

> Texas Massage Therapy Registration
> Texas Department of Health
> 1100 W. 49th St.
> Austin, TX 78756
> (512) 834-6616

Registration is required to legally practice massage in Texas.

Utah

State licensing, 600 hours at COMTA-approved school, *or*
apprenticeship of 1000 hours
Theory Exam and Laws & Rules Exam
Reciprocity is available to licensed out-of-state therapists whether or not their training was at COMTA-approved school. For purposes of reciprocity, *National Certification Exam* can substitute for Theory Exam.

> Utah Department of Commerce
> Division of Occupational and Professional Licensing
> Herbert M. Wells Building
> 160 East 300 South
> P.O. Box 45805
> Salt Lake City, UT 84145
> (801) 530-6551

Virginia

State certification, 500 hours
National Certification Exam

> Virginia Board of Nursing
> 6606 West Broad St., 4th floor
> Richmond, VA 23230
> (804) 662-9909

Washington

State licensing, 500 hours
National Certification Exam

> Washington Department of Health
> Massage Licensing Program
> P.O. Box 47867
> Olympia, WA 98504
> (360) 586-6351

West Virginia

State licensing, 500 hours from a massage therapy school approved in its home state, *or*
National Certification Exam, or
grandfathering for those in practice before Dec. 1, 1994

> Massage Therapy Licensure Board
> P.O. Box 8038
> South Charleston, WV 25303
> (304) 736-0621 (Chairwoman Anna Pekar)

As originally enacted, the law required attendance at a COMTA-approved school (even though there were none in the state). Before long, a coalition of members of all the major massage associations worked together to amend the law to its current form.

Wisconsin

State licensing, 500 to 600 (to be determined)
Exam to be determined

> Department of Regulation and Licensing
> Secretary Marlene Cummings
> 1400 E. Washington Ave./P.O. Box 8935
> Madison, WI 53708
> (608) 266-8609

Wisconsin's law is newly-enacted, and as of press time, the regulations to implement the law had not been formulated. One provision built into the statute is that practitioners can be "grandfathered" in if they have at least 100 hours of education and adequate practical experience. The board implementing the statute can choose to have a written test or not, and if they choose to have a written test, they may choose the National Certification Exam or may use another test.

State Licensing Chart as of July, 1998

State	Type of Regulation	Education Required	NCE	Number licensed
Alabama[1]	License	650 / 1000	yes[4]	325
Arkansas	License	500 hours	no	1,413
Connecticut	License	500 hours COMTA	yes	1,740
Delaware	Certification	500 (therapist) 100 (technician)	yes	48 (therapist) 200 (technician)
Dist. of Columbia	License	500 hours	yes	(not implemented)
Florida	License	500 hours	yes	16,250
Hawaii	License	570 hours or 150 plus 420 apprenticeship	no	2,903
Iowa	License	500 hours	yes	1,112
Louisiana	License	500 hours	yes[4]	925
Maine	License	500 hours	yes	775
Maryland[2]	Certification	500 hours / 60 credits	?	(not implemented)
Missouri	License	500 hours	no	(not implemented)
Nebraska	License	1000 hours	yes	472
New Hampshire	License	750 hours	yes	878
New Mexico	License	650 hours or 300 plus 350 experience	yes	2,535
New York[3]	License	605 / 1,000	no	9,000
North Dakota	Registration	500 hours COMTA	no	188
Ohio	License	600 hours	no	3,247
Oregon	License	500	no	2,900
Rhode Island	License	500 hours COMTA or 1000 hours	yes	396
South Carolina	License	500 hours	yes	550
Tennessee	License	500 hours or NCE	yes	872
Texas	Registration	300	no	11,914
Utah	License	600 COMTA or 1,000 apprenticeship	yes[4]	2,100
Virginia	Certification	500 hours	yes	1,007
Washington	License	500 hours	yes	7,000
West Virginia	License	500 hours	yes	(not implemented)
Wisconsin	License	500 to 600 (tentative)	?	(not implemented)[5]

1. Alabama's educational requirement is 650 hours until 1/1/02, 1,000 hours thereafter.
2. Maryland's law requires 500 hours until 1/1/02, and 60 accredited college hours thereafter.
3. New York requires 605 until 1/1/00, 1,000 hours thereafter.
4. In Alabama, Louisiana and Utah, NCE may be used in place of all or part of the state's written exam.
5. Wisconsin's regulations had not yet been formulated as of July, 1998.

18 Income Taxes

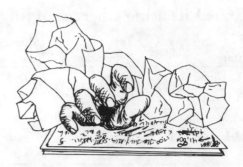

This chapter cannot give you all the information and advice you will need to prepare your income tax return. Instead, this chapter will:

1. Familiarize you with all of the key facts and ideas you need to understand about Federal income tax;

2. Explain what records you should keep for tax purposes, why you need them and how to keep them;

3. Guide you to all the resources you will need to do your own taxes, or to hire a professional to do your taxes for you.

The Big Picture

The following discussion gives you the basis of the federal tax laws that determine how much money you give the government at the end of the year.

This information is presented in condensed form, and on the first reading it may seem difficult to understand. This is only because the words are strange, not because the ideas are difficult.

Really try to "get" this big picture in your mind. Everything else in this chapter relates to this overall picture.

Some of the statements in this "big picture" would need additional explanation to be 100% accurate, so just use this information to understand the concepts at this point.

1. Employment income only

If you are an employee, and have no income from self-employment, your taxes will be very simple. You employer will give you a W-2 form showing income and withholding, and the forms the IRS sends you to fill out your taxes should be sufficient.

2. Self-employment income

Almost all massage therapists and bodyworkers, however, are completely or partially self-employed. When you are self-employed, your business activity is reported on a separate IRS form, called Schedule C (see page 136). In reporting your business activity on your Schedule C, you add up all of the money you received during the year in your business, and you subtract your business deductions. (What you can subtract as business deductions will be discussed later).

If the money you *received* is a larger amount than your allowable *deductions*, you have a *profit*. We will call this your "business profit." You have to pay a percentage of your business profit as self-employment tax, and you also have to pay a percentage of your business profit as income tax.

3. Self-employment tax

Business profit is subject to a self-employment tax (which includes a Medicare tax). This is the self-employed person's equivalent of Social Security Tax. The amount of the self-employment tax for tax year 1997 was 18.2% on business profits up to $65,400, and 2.9% of amounts over $65,400.

4. Income tax

Business profit is also subject to income tax, which is separate from self-employment tax. In 1997, Income tax was approximately 15% for those who did not make large incomes. If your income rises to around $60,000, you will pay a higher tax on the excess income.

Your income from non-business sources is called "Personal Income". Examples are interest and dividend income. Personal income is subject to the income tax only, *not* the self-employment tax.

If you have been following along this far, see if the following chart makes it a little clearer for you:

Business earnings	Personal income
minus	*minus*
Business deductions	Personal deductions
equals	*equals*
Business profit	Personal profit

Pay self-employment tax	Pay income tax
on business profit	on personal profit
(approximately 18%)	(approximately 15%)
and	
Pay Income tax	
on business profit	
(approximately 15%)	

Notice that you pay both self-employment tax and income tax on your business profit. Personal (non-business) profit is subject only to the income tax.

Deductions are beautiful

Once you grasp the overall picture of how taxes are figured, it becomes apparent that business deductions and personal deductions are money in your pocket.

Since they reduce the total amount subject to taxes, they reduce the total taxes you have to pay.

Business deductions are especially helpful, since they reduce both the self-employment tax and the income tax. Personal deductions reduce only the income tax. Personal deductions include items such as charitable contributions, medical expenses, and the like.

Business deductions are discussed in some detail below. Become familiar with this information so that you have a clear understanding of what is deductible, and what records you need to keep to support your deductions.

Deductions are listed on "Schedule C" which is the form all self-employed persons file with their income tax returns. If your gross business receipts were under $25,000, you may be able to use Schedule C-EZ (see page 137). Otherwise, you must use the slightly more complicated Schedule C.

What Can I Deduct?

In general, if it's a business expense, it's deductible. The expense must be for something "appropriate and helpful in developing and maintaining your trade or business" and the cost must be reasonable. This allows for a broad range of business deductions.

The following list demonstrates the most common deductible items.

- Business use of your automobile
- Office rental fees
- Painting or repair costs for office
- Your appointment book
- Business cards and any other business printing jobs
- Advertising
- Business phone and long-distance business phone calls (but not the base monthly service charge for the first residential line)
- Business travel expenses (cost of lodging plus 80% of cost of meals)
- Entertainment expenses
- Gifts to clients (up to $25 per client per year)
- Professional convention fees (and travel expenses)
- Continuing education expenses, including books
- Professional association dues
- Licensing fees
- Laundry expenses
- Costs of oil and other supplies
- Massage table and other equipment for treatment room (up to $10,000 in one year)
- Cassette player or disc player for treatment room
- Music for use in treatment room

Education

You can deduct the cost of education, plus travel and meals expenses, if the education maintains or improves your professional skills, or is required by law for keeping your professional status.

Educational expenses are *not* deductible for training in a new field, or to meet minimum professional requirements, because that is considered a "start-up" cost, and start-up costs are not deductible. So once you are a practicing massage therapist, the expenses of continuing education are deductible, but the costs involved in becoming a massage therapist are not deductible.

Since expenses are deductible even if they are for education that "improves" your professional skills, you can probably deduct a major educational expense, as long as you are already a practicing massage therapist.

This is one advantage of taking a small amount of training and practicing massage on the side (in states where this is permissible) before making a commitment to a more serious educational program.

Gifts

You can deduct the cost of gifts you give as part of doing business, up to a maximum of $25 worth of gifts to any one individual in one year. If there is a question whether something is a gift or entertainment (like football tickets) it will be considered entertainment.

Home office expenses

Rent and other costs for an office in your home are deductible if you use a part of your home "regularly and exclusively" as:

1. Your principal place of business, *or*

2. A place to meet and deal with clients in the normal course of your practice, *or*

3. If you use a separate building regularly and exclusively for your business, such as a cottage or detached garage.

The home office deduction used to be allowed *only* if your home office was your main place of business. The rules have been eased up and the "principal place of business" has been relaxed.

Now, to qualify as a home office, the room or part of your house only needs to be used "regularly" and "exclusively" in your practice. That means you have to use it for your business on a regular basis — not just on rare occasions. It also means you cannot use it for any other purpose, such as a den or guest bedroom.

Second, your home office must qualify under number 1, number 2 or number 3, above. Most home offices for massage therapists qualify under number 2. You give massages to clients there, so obviously, you meet and deal with clients there in the normal course of your practice. You qualify for the home office deduction.

The same applies if your office is in a separate building on your property. (An office in a separate building is deductible even if you only do your bookwork

SCHEDULE C (Form 1040)
Department of the Treasury
Internal Revenue Service (99)

Profit or Loss From Business
(Sole Proprietorship)
▶ Partnerships, joint ventures, etc., must file Form 1065.
▶ Attach to Form 1040 or Form 1041. ▶ See Instructions for Schedule C (Form 1040).

OMB No. 1545-0074
1997
Attachment Sequence No. 09

Name of proprietor | Social security number (SSN)

A Principal business or profession, including product or service (see page C-1)
B Enter principal business code (see page C-6) ▶
C Business name. If no separate business name, leave blank.
D Employer ID number (EIN), if any
E Business address (including suite or room no.) ▶
City, town or post office, state, and ZIP code
F Accounting method: (1) ☐ Cash (2) ☐ Accrual (3) ☐ Other (specify) ▶
G Did you "materially participate" in the operation of this business during 1997? If "No," see page C-2 for limit on losses . . ☐ Yes ☐ No
H If you started or acquired this business during 1997, check here . . . . ▶ ☐

Part I Income

1 Gross receipts or sales. **Caution:** *If this income was reported to you on Form W-2 and the "Statutory employee" box on that form was checked, see page C-2 and check here* . . . . . . ▶ ☐ | 1
2 Returns and allowances . . . . | 2
3 Subtract line 2 from line 1 . . . . | 3
4 Cost of goods sold (from line 42 on page 2) . . . . | 4
5 **Gross profit.** Subtract line 4 from line 3 . . . . | 5
6 Other income, including Federal and state gasoline or fuel tax credit or refund (see page C-2) . . | 6
7 **Gross income.** Add lines 5 and 6 . . . . ▶ | 7

Part II Expenses. Enter expenses for business use of your home **only** on line 30.

8 Advertising . . . . . | 8
9 Bad debts from sales or services (see page C-3) . . | 9
10 Car and truck expenses (see page C-3) . . . . | 10
11 Commissions and fees . . | 11
12 Depletion . . . . . | 12
13 Depreciation and section 179 expense deduction (not included in Part III) (see page C-3) . . | 13
14 Employee benefit programs (other than on line 19) . . | 14
15 Insurance (other than health) . | 15
16 Interest:
a Mortgage (paid to banks, etc.) . | 16a
b Other . . . . . . | 16b
17 Legal and professional services . . . . . | 17
18 Office expense . . . . | 18

19 Pension and profit-sharing plans | 19
20 Rent or lease (see page C-4):
a Vehicles, machinery, and equipment . | 20a
b Other business property . . | 20b
21 Repairs and maintenance . . | 21
22 Supplies (not included in Part III) . | 22
23 Taxes and licenses . . . | 23
24 Travel, meals, and entertainment:
a Travel . . . . | 24a
b Meals and entertainment . .
c Enter 50% of line 24b subject to limitations (see page C-4) .
d Subtract line 24c from line 24b | 24d
25 Utilities . . . . . . | 25
26 Wages (less employment credits) . | 26
27 Other expenses (from line 48 on page 2) . . . . | 27

28 **Total expenses** before expenses for business use of home. Add lines 8 through 27 in columns . ▶ | 28
29 Tentative profit (loss). Subtract line 28 from line 7 . . . | 29
30 Expenses for business use of your home. Attach **Form 8829** .
31 **Net profit or (loss).** Subtract line 30 from line 29.
• If a profit, enter on **Form 1040, line 12,** and ALSO on Sched[...], see page C-5). Estates and trusts, enter on Form 1041, line 3.
• If a loss, you MUST go on to line 32.
32 If you have a loss, check the box that describes your investment [...]
• If you checked 32a, enter the loss on **Form 1040, line 12,** [...] (statutory employees, see page C-5). Estates and trusts, enter [...]
• If you checked 32b, you MUST attach **Form 6198.**

For Paperwork Reduction Act Notice, see Form 1040 instructions.

IRS form 1040 Schedule C, page 1

Schedule C (Form 1040) 1997 | Page **2**

Part III Cost of Goods Sold (see page C-5)

33 Method(s) used to value closing inventory: a ☐ Cost b ☐ Lower of cost or market c ☐ Other (attach explanation)
34 Was there any change in determining quantities, costs, or valuations between opening and closing inventory? If "Yes," attach explanation . . . . ☐ Yes ☐ No
35 Inventory at beginning of year. If different from last year's closing inventory, attach explanation . . | 35
36 Purchases less cost of items withdrawn for personal use . . | 36
37 Cost of labor. Do not include salary paid to yourself . . | 37
38 Materials and supplies . . . . | 38
39 Other costs . . . . | 39
40 Add lines 35 through 39 . . . . | 40
41 Inventory at end of year . . . . | 41
42 **Cost of goods sold.** Subtract line 41 from line 40. Enter the result here and on page 1, line 4 ▶ | 42

Part IV Information on Your Vehicle. Complete this part ONLY if you are claiming car or truck expenses on line 10 and are not required to file Form 4562 for this business. See the instructions for line 13 on page C-3 to find out if you must file.

43 When did you place your vehicle in service for business purposes? (month, day, year) ▶ . . . / . . . / . . .
44 Of the total number of miles you drove your vehicle during 1997, enter the number of miles you used your vehicle for:
a Business . . . . b Commuting . . . . c Other . . . .
45 Do you (or your spouse) have another vehicle available for personal use? . . . . ☐ Yes ☐ No
46 Was your vehicle available for use during off-duty hours? . . . . ☐ Yes ☐ No
47a Do you have evidence to support your deduction? . . . . ☐ Yes ☐ No
b If "Yes," is the evidence written? . . . . ☐ Yes ☐ No

Part V Other Expenses. List below business expenses not included on lines 8-26 or line 30.

48 Total other expenses. Enter here and on page 1, line 27 . . . . | 48

IRS form 1040 Schedule C, page 2

SCHEDULE C-EZ
(Form 1040)

Department of the Treasury
Internal Revenue Service   (99)

Net Profit From Business
(Sole Proprietorship)

▶ Partnerships, joint ventures, etc., must file Form 1065.
▶ Attach to Form 1040 or Form 1041.   ▶ See instructions on back.

OMB No. 1545-0074

19 97

Attachment
Sequence No. **09A**

Name of proprietor | Social security number (SSN)

Part I   **General Information**

**You May Use
This Schedule
Only If You:** ▶

- Had business expenses of $2,500 or less.
- Use the cash method of accounting.
- Did not have an inventory at any time during the year.
- Did not have a net loss from your business.
- Had only one business as a sole proprietor.

And You: ▶

- Had no employees during the year.
- Are not required to file **Form 4562**, Depreciation and Amortization, for this business. See the instructions for Schedule C, line 13, on page C-3 to find out if you must file.
- Do not deduct expenses for business use of your home.
- Do not have prior year unallowed passive activity losses from this business.

A   Principal business or profession, including product or service

B   Enter principal business code
(see page C-6) ▶

C   Business name. If no separate business name, leave blank.

D   Employer ID number (EIN), if any

E   Business address (including suite or room no.). Address not required if same as on Form 1040, page 1.

City, town or post office, state, and ZIP code

Part II   **Figure Your Net Profit**

1	**Gross receipts. Caution:** If this income was reported to you on Form W-2 and the "Statutory employee" box on that form was checked, see **Statutory Employees** in the instructions for Schedule C, line 1, on page C-2 and check here . . . . ▶ ☐	**1**
2	**Total expenses.** If more than $2,500, you **must** use Schedule C. See instructions	**2**
3	**Net profit.** Subtract line 2 from line 1. If less than zero, you **must** use Schedule C. Enter on **Form 1040, line 12**, and ALSO on **Schedule SE, line 2.** (Statutory employees **do not** report this amount on Schedule SE, line 2. Estates and trusts, enter on Form 1041, line 3.)	**3**

Part III   **Information on Your Vehicle.** Complete this part **ONLY** if you are claiming car or truck expenses on line 2.

4   When did you place your vehicle in service for business purposes? (month, day, year) ▶ ...... / ...... / ....

5   Of the total number of miles you drove your vehicle during 1997, enter the number of miles you used your vehicle for:

a Business ....   **b** Commuting ....   **c** Other ....

6   Do you (or your spouse) have another vehicle available for personal use? . . . .   ☐ Yes   ☐ No

7   Was your vehicle available for use during off-duty hours? . . . .   ☐ Yes   ☐ No

8a Do you have evidence to support your deduction? . . . .   ☐ Yes   ☐ No

b If "Yes," is the evidence written? . . . .   ☐ Yes   ☐ No

For Paperwork Reduction Act Notice, see Form 1040 instructions.   Cat. No. 14374D   Schedule C-EZ (Form 1040) 1997

IRS form 1040 Schedule C–EZ

there, as long as you use it only for business). And if you have another business, such as selling products to your clients, the room where you store your inventory or where you do your bookkeeping for that business also qualifies as a home office under number 1, as long as you use it exclusively for business.

If you qualify for a home office deduction, you can deduct a proportionate share of all household expenses from your taxable income. Such expenses include real estate taxes, mortgage interest, rent, utility bills, insurance, repairs, security systems and depreciation. *Not* included are repairs or improvements that increase the value of a home you own.

To determine the percentage of your home expenses that is deductible as a business expense, calculate the total square footage of your home, and the square footage of your home office. Divide the square footage of the office by the total square footage of the home, and you will get a decimal, for example .23. You then multiply your home expenses (or your rent if you are a renter) by .23 (or whatever number applies) to find the amount of your deduction for your home office.

If the rooms in your home are roughly the same size, and you use one room as an office, you can use a fraction instead of doing the square-foot computation. For example, if you have six equal-sized rooms and use one as an office, deduct one sixth of your household expenses (or rent) as your home office expense.

The home office deduction cannot be larger than the amount of business income generated in the home office. In other words, the deduction cannot be used to create a business loss, only to offset income that you actually earned using that office.

Meal and Entertainment Expense

If you purchase meals or entertainment as a means of conducting business, you can deduct 80% of the cost of the meals and entertainment, including 80% of tips (as long as the costs are reasonable). You can also deduct 100% of your automobile costs for driving to the meal or entertainment. An example of meal and entertainment expense would be taking a chiropractor to lunch to discuss the possibility of cross-referrals.

Rent and other office expenses

Rental payments for your business office are fully deductible, as are other costs such as heat, electricity, insurance and the like.

Self-employed health insurance

In 1998, you could deduct 45% of the premiums you paid for health insurance if you were self-employed.

Self-employment tax

You can deduct one-half of your self-employment tax from your gross income when you figure your income tax.

Start–up costs

If you are already a practicing massage therapist, and open a new office, or expand an existing office, the costs involved in doing so are ordinary and necessary business expenses, and are fully deductible.

However, when you first begin your business as a massage therapist, the costs involved in starting your business are "start-up costs" and these are *not* deductible.

This issue generally will not arise for a massage therapist or bodyworker, since opening an office without prior professional experience is not usually a realistic approach. It does, however, become an issue when you want to deduct education expenses. Continuing education is deductible, but your initial educational expense is a nondeductible "start-up" cost.

Travel

When you travel away from home for business, most of your expenses are deductible. Travel away from home means going for more than just a day's work, and must include going away long enough to need sleep or rest before coming home.

Deductible items

When traveling away from home on business, your deductible expenses include airplane, rail or bus tickets, automobile expenses, taxi fares, baggage costs, meals, lodging costs, cleaning and laundry expenses, telephone, telegraph, fax, tips, and other similar expenses related to travel.

Travel receipts

Keep receipts during your trip. If you travel by car, keep an envelope in the glove compartment, and put all receipts in the envelope. When you get home, staple them together and put them in the place where you collect all business receipts. At the end of the year, they will be together and easy to handle when you are totaling your deductions.

Optional methods for deducting meal costs when traveling

Meals can be deducted two ways — you may either deduct 50% of the amount you actually spend (so long as the amount is not lavish), or you may deduct the "standard meal allowance" which varies between $30 and $42 per day, depending on location (tax year 1997). For detailed information on the standard meal allowance, request Publication 463, free from the IRS. (see end of chapter)

When using the standard meal allowance, you do not need to produce receipts for your meals. For all other expenses, however, you need to have receipts to document your travel expenditures.

Mixed business and personal travel

If a trip is mainly business but partly personal, you can deduct the round trip travel expenses to get to your business destination, and the meals, lodging and incidental expenses that relate to the business portion of your trip. Any personal side trips, or expenses on days that were vacation days, are not tax-deductible.

If your trip was primarily for vacation and partly for business, no part of the expense is tax-deductible.

Business use vs. Personal use

If a particular expense has aspects of business and personal activity mixed together, remember that the test is whether it is "appropriate and helpful in promoting your business." If it meets this test, the fact that it also helps you personally is irrelevant; it is still deductible.

Some activities are personal and not business-related. For example, if you go to a bar on Saturday night hoping to meet someone who will become a bodywork client, you will not convince the IRS that your expenses are business-related.

However, if you go to the hardware store to get a wing nut to repair your massage table, that is a business trip, and it remains a business trip even if you also pick up a surge protector for your VCR while you are there.

If you pay attention to all the things you do for your business, you will see that much of your lifestyle actually is deductible. The cost of professional books, business phone calls, entertainment, uniforms, and business laundry are all deductible expenses. You can also deduct the cost of traveling to shop for items for the business and to do errands for the business. You are entitled to proper business deductions, so plan for them, document them and take them.

Documenting deductions

The key to documenting deductions is keeping receipts, canceled checks, and in the case of automobile mileage, a log of business miles driven in your car.

What is documentation?

The IRS needs a paper record of any transaction you are claiming as a deduction. If you pay a bill for a business expense, keep the bill. When you get your canceled checks from your bank, save the ones that relate to business expenses.

Where to keep your documents

Create a space, in your office or your home, where you regularly keep a whole year's bills, receipts and canceled checks. It can be a drawer, a filing cabinet, a sturdy box, or any space that you can regularly keep these records. At the end of the year, you will take them out and organize them so they can be totaled and included in your tax return.

What to document

Keep all records of money spent on goods or services that relate to your business. These are items listed above under the heading "What Can I Deduct?", and any other items which are related to the operation of your business.

At the end of the year

When you go through your year's receipts and canceled checks, gather them into categories of deductions. This will make it easier for you or your accountant to make a final presentation of your business activity on your Schedule C.

Schedule C contains a partial list of business deductions. These include: advertising, bad debts, car and truck expenses, depreciation, insurance, legal and professional services, office expenses, supplies, travel, meals, and entertainment. In addition, the form provides space for other expenses than the ones listed.

Use this list as a basis for organizing your receipts. Other categories you might use for organization purposes are printing and photocopying, telephone expense and gifts to clients. Receipts which do not fit into any other category can be labeled "miscellaneous."

Business use of your car

Are you a commuter?

Business use of your car is deductible, with one important exception: Commuting expense is not deductible. For tax purposes, commuting means traveling between your home and your main or regular place of work. The trip to your work and the trip home again are both considered nondeductible commuting. The IRS enforces this prohibition against deducting commuting expenses strongly and completely.

Perhaps you have no regular place of work; you may do house calls, or you may work in several different locations doing massage. In such a case, you are not a commuter. However, if you work principally in one office, that is your main or regular place of work, and the miles you drive to and from that place are not deductible... unless you have a valid home office.

If you have a home office, then travel between your home office and your workplace is not commuting, but business travel. The idea is that going from office to office is business travel, but going from home to office is commuting. With a home office, you get to decide whether it is your home or your office you are leaving from.

To qualify as a home office, your space in your home must be used exclusively for business. However, you can work at other locations and still have your home office qualify so long as you see most of your clients at home. If you use a garage or outbuilding, the rules are more lax. (See page 135.)

If you have a home office, step into your home office just before you leave on any other business trip. Then you are going from one place of business to another. When you return, step into your home office before doing anything else. Thus your return trip is from one office to another. In this way, none of your business driving is considered commuting. While this may sound a little shady, it is apparently entirely within the law, at least at the present moment.

It is possible the IRS would question this deduction if you were audited. If you wish to be more conservative, then deduct mileage expenses only on days when you see clients in your home office. If you are actually working in your home office on a particular day, there can be no legitimate question that travel from that office to some other business destination is business travel.

Two methods of computing automobile deduction

You may choose either of two methods to compute your deduction for business use of your car.

The methods are to use the standard deduction (31.5 cents in tax year 1997) for each mile driven for business, or to calculate actual expenses of operating your car for the year and to figure mathematically the amount of your deduction.

If you have a car that is not very expensive and costs little to operate, such as a Toyota Tercel, you will come out ahead using the 31.5 cents per mile computation. If you have an expensive new car or one that required lots of expensive repairs this year, you may come out ahead using the actual computation method.

The standard per-mile method is quite simple to use, and the actual cost method can become quite involved. I use the per-mile rate on my tax return, because I don't enjoy keeping all the records necessary to use the actual cost method. Even if I am paying a little extra in taxes, for me it is worth it to simplify my record-keeping.

A brief explanation of both methods follows.

Standard deduction method — 31.5 cents per mile (tax year 1997)

Keep a daily log of the use of your car. You should record business and personal use.

The best kind of record to keep lists the starting and ending odometer mileage for each business trip. This type of record shows each business trip individually, and also shows how many miles were personal use. It is also acceptable to list only the destination and the miles driven for each trip.

At the end of the year, total all the business miles and multiply the total by .315 to get the deduction for business use of your car.

Example: Your total business miles turn out to be 3,000.

$$\begin{array}{r} 3000 \\ \times\ .315 \\ \hline \$\ 945.00 \end{array}$$

Your deduction for business use of your car is $945. This figure is included on your Schedule C as your mileage deduction.

Actual cost method

Keep itemized records of all expenses related to operating your car. These include gasoline, oil, tires, lubrication, repairs and maintenance, insurance, license and registration fees and automobile club membership dues.

These actual costs will be added up at the end of the year. Another actual cost that can be included is the depreciation in value of your car during the year. The IRS has guidelines for computing depreciation.

Keep a log of business and personal miles, since you will need to figure the percentage of business use. At the end of the year, divide the year's total business miles by the year's total miles to arrive at the percentage of business use. Multiply the total of actual expenses by percentage of business use to determine your deduction.

For example, assume that your total costs of operating your car for the year were $1,758. In addition, your depreciation allowance was $2,500. The total of these figures is $4,258.

If your business use of the car was 20% of the year's total use, your calculation would be:

$$\begin{array}{r} 4258 \\ \times\, .20 \\ \hline \$851.60 \end{array}$$

Your deduction for business use of your car is $851.60. This figure is included on your Schedule C as your mileage deduction.

Depreciation

Depreciation is one of the most complex concepts facing someone trying to understand income taxes. Fortunately, you can get along just fine without ever conquering this particular challenge.

Depreciation refers to spreading out the cost of a large expense over a period of years, and deducting part of the expense each year. This usually applies to heavy equipment which costs a great deal and lasts for many years. During each tax year, the owner takes a portion of the total cost as a deduction. The idea is simple enough, but the rules for putting it into practice can get confusing.

The government has given small businesses the option of avoiding the whole problem, by enacting a rule that any business expense up to $10,000 per year may be taken as a *deduction* entirely during that year.

Therefore, even if you purchase ten massage tables this year, you can take the whole deduction as a business expense during the year in which you spend the money.

In some cases, there can be tax advantages to using depreciation instead of taking the whole deduction. For example, if you make a large expenditure this year, and earn very little, the expenditure would be "wasted" if you took the whole deduction this year, because you would pay no taxes whether or not you take the deduction. Next year, when you have more income, you would like to be able to use part of the deduction to reduce you income taxes.

If you think that using depreciation could help you, send for IRS publication 534, Depreciation, or buy *Small-Time Operator*. See the end of this chapter for information on obtaining these items.

Estimated tax payments

If you expect to owe at least $1,000 in tax next year, you are required to pay estimated tax payments four times a year, on April 15, June 15, September 15 and January 15. You can also be penalized if you make your estimated tax payments late.

Estimated taxes are paid on IRS form #1040-ES, and the form includes a worksheet for you to use to calculate the amount of your estimated tax payments. It is based on last year's income, and if you follow the instructions in the worksheet, you are guaranteed not to be assessed a penalty for underpayment.

Consider this: Your estimated tax payments are based on last year's income. If you make exactly the same income this year, your estimated payments will exactly pay your tax bill. However, what if you make more this year than last year? Your estimated tax payments cover the amount you earned last year, but on April 15, you will owe tax on any amount more than that. If you had a really good year, this additional amount could be several thousand dollars.

Consider also that April 15 is the date you must pay your first estimated tax payment for the coming year. In addition to paying the excess tax for last year, you must now make the first installment on next year's taxes. This "double whammy" can make April 15 a very expensive day for the self-employed bodyworker. Remember this if your practice is increasing, and find the discipline to put some money away in a safe place so you will have it to pay your taxes in April.

Hiring an accountant

Accountants are not cheap, but often they can pay for themselves in tax savings they find that you might miss. If you are motivated to do your own taxes, there is no reason you cannot do so. The resources listed below will give you all the information you need. With some time and study, you can learn what you need to know.

However, it can get complex, and unless you enjoy this sort of thing, consider hiring professional help. The non-CPA tax preparers may know just as much as an accountant, and may charge a little less.

Ask other therapists for recommendations for an accountant. When they recommend someone, ask why they like him (or her), or why they think he is a good accountant. If the reasons they give refer to things that matter to you in an accountant, consider using him.

Consider finding an accountant who will trade accounting services for massage. Use the yellow pages, and call accountants. Explain that you are just getting established, have a simple return, and would like to find an accountant who appreciates massage. You may catch someone in the proper mood to make an arrangement to trade services.

Consider, also, hiring an accountant to get you started with bookkeeping and tax systems you can understand, so that you can do your own taxes in future years. An accountant may be able to explain everything you need to know, and set you up with forms you will be able to use in future years.

Even if you use an accountant or tax preparer, keep your records clear and organized. If possible, keep them in categories that will make it easy to sort out at tax time. This will make the accountant's job easier, and may encourage him to keep his fees reasonable.

Getting further information

If you want help doing your own taxes, there are several good resources you can turn to.

1. One is a book, written by an accountant, for the purpose of helping small business owners take care of bookkeeping and taxes. It is well-organized, well written and inexpensive. It goes into more detail about depreciation, and a few other minor subjects, than this chapter, and has practical advice about bookkeeping. The book is called *Small-Time Operator* and is available from:

   Bell Springs Publishing
   Box 640 Bell Springs Road
   Laytonville, CA 95454
   (707) 984-6746

2. Check out your local bookstore as tax season comes around. All major bookstores will carry a selection of Do-It-Yourself tax guides. One good one is by Consumer Reports, but there are several to choose from. They are usually several hundred pages, and cost around $12.00. They cover in detail any subject you would need to know about in order to do your tax return. When April 15 rolls around and you are up against a deadline, book like this can be a comforting resource to have with you.

3. The final source of information is the IRS, and its information is available at no charge. The IRS will send you booklets explaining various aspects of your taxes, and is also available to answer questions by phone.

   IRS publications can be ordered by calling:
   1-800-829-3676 (1-800-TAX-FORM)

The first publication to order is Tax Guide for Small Businesses, Publication 334. This contains the basics of record-keeping and taxes for small businesses, including filled-in forms.

The second publication to order is "Guide to Free Tax Services." This lists all the other IRS publications. Once you have this booklet, you can leaf through it to see what else is available and what you need.

Some of the subjects covered in these IRS publications are listed below. The IRS publication number is listed after each name. These can be ordered from the toll-free number listed above.

Travel, Entertainment and Gift Expense 463
Tax Withholding and Estimated Tax 505
Educational Expenses 508
Moving Expenses 521
Reporting Income from Tips 531
Self-Employment Tax 533
Depreciation 534
Business Expense 535
Retirement Plans for the Self-employed 560
Taxpayers Starting a Business 583
Business Use of Your Home 587
Alternative Minimum Tax for Individuals 909
Business Use of a Car 917

All of these publications provide good detail, and are written in clear and readable fashion. However, they are written by the IRS, and will not necessarily tip you off to the best ways of getting the most out of your deductions.

To reach an IRS representative by phone, check your local phone book blue pages under Federal Government, Internal Revenue Service. Major cities have local offices. In other locations, call the IRS toll-free at: 1-800-829-1040.

19 Scientific Research on the Benefits of Massage

Although massage has been practiced for thousands of years, helping millions, perhaps billions of people, little scientific documentation of the health benefits of massage has existed until very recently. The massage field has been seeking to be taken seriously by the health care establishment without adequate scientific evidence of its value.

All that is changing now. Scientific research is producing hard data showing the efficacy of massage for a large variety of health problems. This documentation will be useful in promoting hospital-based massage, in securing reimbursement for massage from insurance companies, in gaining physician referrals and collaborations, and in convincing the general population of the benefits of massage as a health modality.

Three organizations currently involved in massage and bodywork research are the AMTA Foundation, the National Institutes of Health, and Touch Research Institute.

AMTA Foundation

The AMTA Foundation was created by AMTA in 1990. The Foundation awards grants to individuals or teams which promise to advance our understanding of specific therapeutic applications of massage, public perceptions of massage or attitudes toward massage, and the role of massage therapy in health care delivery. At publication time, eight research grants had been awarded, and two of those had resulted in completed studies. These studies are summarized below:

Reduced Anxiety During Periods of Stress

Massage given to medical students one day prior to exams resulted in decreased anxiety and decreased respiratory rate.

Massage in Spinal Injury Cases

Massage was tested as a treatment for spasticity in spinal cord injury cases. It was shown to depress H-reflexes for all subjects tested, showing it holds promise as a non-invasive, non-drug treatment of spasticity in spinal cord injured persons.

Other ongoing studies funded by AMTA Foundation are examining the effect of Trager Psychophysical Integration on mothers whose children have died, the efficacy of massage as a treatment for sickle cell anemia, the effects of connective tissue massage on migraine, the effect of work-site massage and acupressure on job stress, the ability of massage to reduce chronic pain, and the use of massage on cancer pain and anxiety.

AMTA Foundation can be reached at:

> AMTA Foundation
> 820 Davis Street, Suite 100
> Evanston, IL 60201
> (847) 864-0123

Information about the foundation may also be available on the AMTA's website at www.amtamassage.org.

National Institutes of Health

Also sponsoring research in massage and bodywork is National Institutes of Health (NIH), a federal agency. NIH's research in massage is coordinated by their Office of Alternative Medicine (OAM). Using federal grant money, the OAM requests proposals for research, and then funds the projects they believe are the most promising.

Projects currently being conducted under grants from NIH/OAM are studying the effects of massage on bone marrow transplant patients, on HIV-1 patients, on post-surgical outcomes, on HIV-exposed infants, on manual palpation of the lumbar spine, and on the immune response to stress.

For information about NIH/OAM visit http://altmed.od.nih.gov

For basic information about OAM, contact:

> Office of Alternative Medicine Clearinghouse
> P.O. Box 8218, Silver Spring, MD 20907
> (888) 644-6226, fax (301) 495-4957

You can contact the Office of Alternative Medicine directly at:

> National Institute of Health
> Office of Alternative Medicine
> 9000 Rockville Pike, building 31, Room 5B-38
> Bethesda, MD 20892
> (301) 402-2466

Touch Research Institute

Of the three groups sponsoring or conducting massage research, by far the most studies are being conducted by Touch Research Institute, which was established in 1992 at the University of Miami School of Medicine. Under the direction of Tiffany Field, Ph.D., the institute has been conducting numerous studies to document the health benefits of massage. Some of their studies use licensed massage therapists, and others use college students or parents or grandparents who are given some training in how to give a massage.

The rest of this chapter is devoted to summarizing the results of their research efforts to date.

Adolescent and Child Psychiatric Patients

Adolescents and children who had been hospitalized for depression or adjustment disorder were given a 30-minute back massage each day for five days. Depression and anxiety were reduced and sleep increased compared to a control group who viewed relaxing videotapes.

72 children and adolescents aged 7 to 18 were studied. 52 received daily massage from psychology students who had massage training. The control group of 20 watched relaxing videotapes of pleasant sounds and images with psychology students while the subject group received massage. Observations, questionnaires, and measurements of pulse and saliva samples showed decreases in depression, anxiety, fidgeting and stress hormones (cortisol) immediately after treatment sessions. At the end of 5 days, depression levels were lower (though not in the control group) and nurses noted improved affect and cooperation. Massaged subjects also spent more of their bedtime sleeping and less time awake. The benefits of massage were greater for those subjects who were depressed.

Field, T.; Morrow, C.; Valdeon, C.; Larson, S.; Kuhn, C. & Schanberg, S. (1992). Massage therapy reduces anxiety in child and adolescent psychiatric patients, *Journal of the American Academy of Child and Adolescent Psychiatry*, 31(1), 125

Anorexia

Massage therapy reduced anxiety and stress, and resulted in decreased body dissatisfaction associated with anorexia.

Hart, S.; Field, T.; & Hernandez-Reif, M. (1988) Adolescents with Anorexia Show Improved Body Image with Massage Therapy. *Women's Health*. In Press.

Asthma

Asthmatic children were massaged by their parents and showed improvement.

The study compared massage with relaxation therapy, in both cases administered by parents who were taught the technique and performed it for 20 minutes at bedtime each day for 30 days. The 4 to 8 year-olds showed an immediate decrease in anxiety and stress hormones, and their peak air flow and other pulmonary functions improved over the course of the study. The 9 to 14 year-olds showed decreased anxiety and their attitude toward asthma improved during the study, but only one measure of pulmonary function improved.

Field, T.; Henteleff, T.; Hernandez-Reif, M.; Marting, E.; Mavunda, K.; Kuhn, C. & Schanberg, S. (1997). Asthmatic Children Have Improved Pulmonary Function After Massage Therapy. *Journal of Pediatrics*. In Press.

Attention Deficit Hyperactivity Disorder

Adolescents with ADHD rated themselves as happier and were observed to fidget less after massage sessions. Also, teachers rated children receiving massage as less hyperactive and as spending more time on-task.

Field, T.; Quintino, O. & Hernandez-Reif, M. (1997). Attention deficit hyperactivity disorder adolescents benefit from massage therapy. *Adolescence.*

Autistic Children

After exposure to massage therapy, relatedness to teachers increased, and touch sensitivity, attention to sounds and off-task classroom behavior decreased.

Field, T.; Lasko, D.; Mundy, P. & Henteleff, T.; Talpins, S.; Dowling, M. (1996). Autistic children's attentiveness and responsivity improved after touch therapy. *Journal of Autism & Developmental Disorder* 27(3), 329-334.

Bulimic Adolescents

Massage decreased anxiety, depression and stress hormone levels in bulimic adolescent females, and improved body image and attitudes about their eating disorder.

Field, T.; Shanberg, S.; Kuhn, C.; Fierro, K.; Henteleff, T.; Mueller, C.; Yando, R. & Burman, I. (1997). Bulimic adolescents benefit from massage therapy. *Adolescence.* In Press.

Burn Patients

Massage with cocoa butter reduced anxiety, depression, pain and itching.

Burn patients were either massaged with cocoa butter for 30 minutes, two times per week for five weeks, or given standard medical treatment for burns. The massaged group reported less anxiety, depression, pain and itching immediately after the first and last therapy session, and their ratings on these measures improved over the five-week period.

Field, T.; Peck, M.; Krugman, S.; Tuchel, T.; Schanberg, S.; Kuhn, C. & Burman, I. (1997). Massage therapy effects on burn patients. *Burn Care and Rehabilitation.* In Press.

Chair Massage enhances alertness & math computations, reduces depressed mood and job stress

Subjects were given chair massage for 15 minutes, twice a week for five weeks. The control group were asked to relax in the massage chair during the same period. Both groups had increased relaxation and reduced depression. The massaged group, however, also exhibited enhanced alertness (as shown by altered EEG levels), greater speed and accuracy on math computations, reduced anxiety levels, lower salivary cortisol levels, and lower job stress.

Field, T.; Ironson, G.; Scafidi, F.; Nawrocki, T.; Goncalves, A.; Burman, I.; Pickens, J.; Fox, N.; Schanberg, S. and Kuhn, C. (1996). Massage therapy reduces anxiety and enhances EEG pattern of alertness and math computations. *International Journal of Neuroscience* 86(3-4). 197-205.

Children with Diabetes

Massage helped children with diabetes and their parents who gave the massages.

Parents of children with diabetes were taught massage or relaxation techniques. Children were massaged for 20 minutes at bedtime for 30 consecutive nights. Giving massage was found to decrease anxiety and depression in the parents, and receiving massage was found to reduce anxiety, fidgeting and depressed affect in the children. Over the course of the 30-day study, compliance for insulin and food regulation improved and blood glucose levels decreased from 159 to 118 (within the normal range).

Field, T.; Hernandez-Reif, M.; LaGreca, A.; Shaw, K.; Schanberg, S. and Kuhn, C. (1997). Massage therapy lowers blood glucose levels in children with Diabetes Mellitus. *Diabetes Spectrum* 10, 237-239.

Chronic Fatigue Syndrome

Immediately following massage therapy, depression, anxiety and stress hormones decreased. Following 10 days of massage, fatigue-related symptoms, particularly emotional stress and somatic symptoms, were reduced, as were depression, difficulty sleeping, and pain.

Field, T.; Sunshine, W.; Hernandez-Reif, M.; Quintino, O.; Schanberg, S.; Kuhn, C. and Burman, I. (1997). Chronic fatigue syndrome: massage therapy effects on depression and somatic symptoms in chronic fatigue syndrome. *Journal of Chronic Fatigue Syndrome* 3, 43-51.

Cocaine-Exposed Premature Infants

Cocaine-exposed preterm neonates who received massage averaged 28% better weight gain than the control group and had better motor and stress scores on the Brazelton scale.

Babies were stroked and given passive movements for 15 minutes at a time, three times a day for ten days and were then compared to control group who were not massaged.

Scafidi, F.; Field, T.; Wheeden, A.; Schanberg, S.; Kuhn, C.; Symanski, R.; Zimmerman, E. and Bandstra, E. S. (1996). Cocaine exposed preterm neonates show behavioral and hormonal differences. *Pediatrics* 97, 851-855.

Fibromyalgia Patients

Fibromyalgia patients who received two 30-minute massages per week for five weeks had reduced anxiety and depression, less stiffness and fatigue, and fewer nights of difficult sleep.

One group received massage, one group received TENS (transcutaneous electrical stimulation) and one group received sham TENS (TENS equipment attached to subject but not activated). Massage therapy was most effective of the three, TENS was the next most effective, and even the sham TENS group had some improvement.

Sunshine, W.; Field, T.; Schanberg, S.; Quintino, O.; Kilmer, T.; Fierro, K.; Burman, I.; Hashimoto, M.; McBride, C. and Henteleff, T. (1996). Massage therapy and transcutaneous electrical stimulation effects on fibromyalgia. *Journal of Clinical Rheumatology* 2, 18-22.

HIV-Positive Gay Men

Massage resulted in improvement of immune function for HIV-positive subjects.

Daily massage was given for one month. Significant increases in relaxation were noted, and significant decreases in anxiety. Also, significant increases were noted for Natural Killer Cell number, Natural Killer Cell Cytotoxicity, soluble CD8, and the cytotoxic subset of CD8 cells.

Ironson, G.; Field, T.; Scafidi, F.; Hashimoto, M.; Kumar, M.; Kumar, A.; Price, A.; Goncalves, A.; Burman, I.; Tetenman, C.; Patarca, R. and Fletcher, M. A. (1996). Massage therapy is associated with enhancement of the immune system's cytotoxic capacity. *International Journal of Neuroscience* 84(1-4), 205-217.

Infants Born to HIV-Positive Mothers

Neonates who received massage had greater weight gain and higher Brazelton scores than the control group.

Babies born to HIV-positive mothers were given three 15-minute massages per day for 10 days. The control group did not receive massage. The massaged group showed superior performance on almost every Brazelton newborn cluster score and had greater daily weight gain at the end of the treatment period, unlike the control group who showed declining performance.

Scafidi, F. and Field, T. (1996). Massage therapy improves behavior in neonates born to HIV-positive mothers. *Journal of Pediatric Psychology* 21(6), 889-897.

Infants of Depressed Mothers

Massage was more effective than rocking to reduce stress, improve weight gain, promote sleep, and increase sociability and soothability.

Full-term 1 to 3 month old infants were either massaged or rocked for 15 minutes, two days per week for six weeks. Their mothers were all single adolescents of low socioeconomic status who suffered from depression. The massaged infants cried less, spent more time in active alert and active awake states, and had lower stress levels and lower stress hormone levels and their serotonin levels increased.

Field, T.; Grizzle, N.; Scafidi, F.; Abrams, S.; and Richardson, S. (1996). Massage therapy for infants of depressed mothers. *Infant Behavior and Development* 19, 109-114.

Infant Massage With Oil vs. Without Oil

Massage with oil was more effective than massage without oil.

Infants were separated into two groups, one which received massage with oil and one which received massage without oil. Both groups benefited, but the group massaged with oil were less active, showed fewer stress behaviors and head averting, and their stress hormone levels decreased more. Vagal activity also increased more with oil massage.

Field, T.; Schanberg, S.; Davalos, M. & Malphurs (1996). Massage with oil has more positive effects of neonatal infants. *Pre and Perinatal Psychology Journal* 11, 73-78.

Infants sleep better after massage

Massage was more effective than reading to children to promote sleep.

Parents in one group massaged infants and toddlers with sleeping problems for 15 minutes; parents in another group read bedtime stories to infants and toddlers with sleeping problems. The massaged infants showed fewer sleep delay behaviors and fell asleep more quickly by the end of the study.

Field, T.; Kilmer, T.; Hernandez-Rief, M.; Burman, 1. (1997). Preschool Children's Sleep and Wake Behavior Improve After Massage Therapy. *Early Child Development & Care*. In Press.

Job Stress

A 10-minute massage was as effective to reduce job stress as were 10-minute sessions of music relaxation, muscle relaxation with guided imagery, or social support group interaction.

Hospital workers were given one of the above brief treatments. Each group showed reduction in job stress as a result, and the reductions were approximately the same for all the methods tested.

Field, T.; Quintino, O.; Henteleff, T.; Wells-Keife, L. and Delvecchio-Feinberg, G. (1997). Job stress reduction therapies. *Alternative Therapies in Health and Medicine* 3(4), 54-56.

Massage During Labor

Massage therapy during childbirth decreased anxiety and pain, and decreased the length of labor.

Field, T.; Hernandez-Rief, M.; Taylor, S. & Quintino, O. (1997). Labor pain is reduced by massage therapy. *Journal of Psychosomatic Obstetrics and Gynecology*. In Press.

Pediatric Dermatitis (eczema)

Massage produced improvement in children's affect and activity levels, as well as measurements of skin condition including less redness, lichenification, excoriatis and pruritis. Parents' anxiety levels also decreased.

Schachner, L.; Field, T.; Hernandez-Reif, M.; Duarte, A.; Krasnegor, J. (1997). Atopic Dermatitis Symptoms Decrease in Children Following Massage Therapy. *Pediatric Development*. In Press.

Post-Traumatic Stress Disorder

Children who survived Hurricane Andrew received massage therapy, resulting in decreased anxiety, depression and stress hormone levels. In addition, their drawings became less depressed.

Field, T.; Seligman, S.; Scafidy, F. and Schanberg, S. (1996). Alleviating post-traumatic stress in children following Hurricane Andrew. *Journal of Applied Developmental Psychology* 17(1), 37-50.

Premature Infants

Preterm neonates who received massage averaged 47% better weight gain and averaged six days shorter hospital stay than the control group, resulting in savings of approximately $3,000.00 per infant.

Babies were stroked and given passive movement for 15 minutes at a time, three times per day for 10 days. The massaged infants were more alert, more mature, had better motor activity, and ranked higher on the Brazelton scale than the control group. These findings were replicated in a subsequent study which showed 21% greater weight gain, and discharge five days earlier than the control group.

Field, T.; Schanberg, S. M.; Scafidi, F.; Bauer, C. R.; Vega-Lahr, N.; Garcia, R.; Nystrom, J. & Kuhn, C. M. (1986). Tactile/ kinesthetic stimulation effects on preterm neonates. *Pediatrics*, 77(5), 654-658.

Scafidi, F.; Field, T.; Schanberg, S.; Bauer, C; Tucci, K.; Roberts, J.; Morrow, C. & Kuhn, C. M. (1990). Massage stimulates growth in preterm infants: A replication. *Infant Behavior and Development* 13,167-188

Rape and Spouse Abuse

Massage therapy reduced aversion to touch and decreased anxiety, depression and stress hormone levels for victims of rape and spouse abuse.

Field, T.; Hernandez-Reif, M.; Hart, S.; Quintino, O.; Drose, L.; Field, T.; Kuhn, C. & Schanberg, S (1997). Sexual abuse effects are lessened by massage therapy. *Journal of Bodywork and Movement Therapies* 1, 65-69

Senior Citizens

Grandparent volunteers massaged infants for a 3-week period, and then received massages during a 3-week period. While giving massage, anxiety, depression and stress levels were decreased, and lifestyle, self-esteem and health improved. These effects were not as strong while receiving massage, possibly because of awkward feelings about being massaged.

Field, T.; Hernandez-Reif, M.; Quintino, O.; Schanberg, S. & Kuhn, C. (1997). Giving massage helps "grandparent" volunteers. *Journal of Applied Gerontology*. In Press.

Women who have experienced sexual abuse

Massage was more effective than relaxation therapy for women who had experienced sexual abuse.

Massage was given by licensed massage therapists for 30 minutes twice a week for one month. A control group received relaxation therapy at the same time. Both groups experienced decreased anxiety and slightly decreased depression. The massage group also had decreased stress hormones (salivary cortisol) and less life event stress. The massage group did not experience a changed attitude toward touch, but the control group reported an increasingly negative attitude toward touch. The study suggests that a longer-term massage experience may be necessary to achieve change in attitude toward touch and significant change in depression.

Ongoing Research

Additional ongoing studies at the time of publication included work with abused and neglected children, aggressive adolescents, aromatherapy, back pain, breast therapy, children with severe burns, carpal tunnel syndrome, infants with cerebral palsy, colic, coma, couples therapy, massage for dancers, cystic fibrosis, Down syndrome, HIV in adolescents, hypertension, irritable bowel syndrome, migraine headaches, multiple sclerosis, pediatric oncology (children with cancer), pregnancy, premenstrual symptoms, preterm physiology, sickle cell anemia, spinal cord injuries, sports massage, and sudden infant death syndrome risk.

Because returning telephone calls depletes the limited resources of TRI, they request that persons wanting further information visit their website. It is routinely updated with new publications and studies, and it also includes information on studies conducted by other labs: www.miami.edu/touch-research

TRI publishes Touchpoints, a quarterly update on their research. Ordering information is on page 189.

Those needing to establish contact with the Institute can write to them at the following address:

> Touch Research Institute
> Department of Pediatrics
> P.O. Box 016820 (D-820)
> 1601 NW 12th Avenue
> Miami, FL 33101
> fax (305) 243-6488

For those wishing to do serious research into existing studies on massage and bodywork, the following are resources that may help.

Richard Van Why has compiled a large library of research papers from around the world on touch therapy. A bibliography is $40, and his 1,000-page research collection is $350. To view his database, you can visit his website at www.erols.com/fibrosym. He can be contacted at Bodywork Research Institute, 123 E. 8th St., #121, Frederick, MD 21701, (301) 698-0932.

National Library of Medicine (NLM) manages MEDLARS, the Medical Literature Analysis and Retrieval System, which includes more than 40 on-line databases and databanks. An overview can be obtained at www.nlm.nih.gov, and they can be contacted at National Library of Medicine, 9000 Rockville Pike, Bethesda, MD 20894, 1-888-FIND-NLM or (301) 496-6308. To contact the MEDLARS management section, call 1-800-638-8480.

20 Reimbursement For Your Service by Insurance Companies

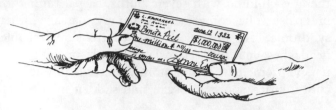

This chapter is written with the assistance of David Dolan, L.M.T., author of *Insurance Reimbursement and Specialty Physician Referrals*. Information about this book, and about his teaching and consulting can be found on page 187.

The Current Status of Insurance Reimbursement for Massage

The issue of insurance reimbursement is a source of confusion for many in the massage industry. The question "is your work covered by insurance" sounds like a simple question, but when you try to answer it, it can become quite complicated.

Consider, for example:

- Some health insurance policies cover massage, some do not.

- Some cover massage only if it is performed in a doctor's office.

- Some states license massage, and being in a non-licensed state may affect reimbursement.

- Automobile accident victims are under auto insurance, which has a different set of rules than health insurance.

- Within the automobile insurance industry, there are different rules in different states.

The variations in insurance policies, in types of insurance cases, and in state laws, combine to make the subject of insurance reimbursement for massage a difficult one to explain. However, it is not so difficult that it cannot be understood, and this chapter will give you the basics for understanding the insurance reimbursement system as it applies to massage therapy.

How big a part of the profession are we talking about?

In 1990, the AMTA surveyed its members about insurance reimbursement. Of those who answered the survey, 27% never participate in insurance billing. 9% have tried without success for insurance reimbursement. 34% report that they sometimes receive insurance reimbursement, and 20% receive reimbursement whenever they submit a claim. This survey was conducted among AMTA members, who are probably more oriented toward medical massage than the average massage therapist. The national averages for the entire massage community would probably show a smaller percentage of the total pursuing insurance reimbursement than is reflected by that study.

Some massage therapists do exclusively medical massage, and have mastered the skills required for insurance billing. These therapists routinely receive compensation for their services from insurance companies. Others, who may not do much insurance billing, and may not understand the correct procedures, become frustrated by what they perceive as roadblocks or red tape in the insurance billing field. They tend to shy away from insurance reimbursement clients. Still other therapists decline to undertake the extra work involved in charting each client's progress, reporting to insurance companies, obtaining pre-approval, tracking billings and payments, and following up on unpaid cases. These therapists choose not to participate at all in insurance billing.

Some of the political issues discussed in Chapter 3 have their effect in the insurance billing field. The issues of credentialing, certification, and standardization of educational requirements all have relevance in this field. However, even with the national picture unsettled at this time, you as a practitioner can still learn what is necessary to successfully do insurance billing and make this a successful part of your practice if you choose to do so.

Before exploring "how to" do insurance billing, we will consider the advantages and disadvantages of this type of practice.

Advantages and disadvantages

Insurance reimbursement for massage is a two-edged sword. On one side, people who could not otherwise afford massage, or who otherwise would not choose to pay for massage, become clients, often repeat clients over a period of time. On the other side, your control over what you do as a massage therapist can be compromised, and each massage session you bill to insurance companies brings added paperwork for you.

These are the days of managed care. Doctors complain that managed care has ruined the practice of medicine. Insurance companies, eager to keep costs to a minimum, have become aggressive in telling doctors, psychotherapists and chiropractors what treatments will be paid for, at what rate, and under what conditions. Professionals who rely on insurance reimbursement are losing much of their freedom to practice as they see fit because they must conform to insurance company guidelines.

Massage therapists are not primary providers of health-care like physicians are. Massage therapists are "adjunct" therapists who work by prescription from a primary provider. As such, we are not quite so closely controlled by managed care as are doctors. However, there is definitely a set of procedures that must be adhered to, and a set of rules that must be followed, and not following proper procedures can result in your not being paid for your work.

Another question to consider is what kind of massage work you will do if you practice insurance reimbursement massage. The kind of work you do may vary depending on which doctor is referring, what skills you have, and how you have structured your practice. Some massage therapists have a clear vision of what kinds of work they do, they do the work they feel needs to be done, and they make the system work for them. Others work in a practice that can cast them more in the role of a technician, being told to work certain muscles only, or to warm up an area for chiropractic adjustment. The kind of therapy you specialize in and your level of professional experience can make a large difference in this regard.

Another consideration is that you should expect at least some resistance by insurance companies to which you submit your claims for reimbursement. Insurance companies, like any other companies, make a profit by paying out less money than they take in. Most companies will pay legitimate claims, but they may require substantial paperwork to demonstrate that the claims are legitimate. Some companies resist even legitimate claims, requiring duplicative or excessive paperwork from the therapist.

The big advantages of working for insurance compensation are higher compensation and a stable client base. The billable hourly rate for clinical massage is usually between $60 and $100. (It is often closer to the high end in licensed states and closer to the low end in non-licensed states). The possibility of insurance compensation will also bring you clients who otherwise could not afford to use your services. These are very substantial advantages to an individual who is committed to the full-time practice of massage therapy.

It is up to you to decide whether the advantages to you outweigh the disadvantages, and you may not really know until you try it.

Your Role in the Health Care System

As a massage or bodywork practitioner working by doctor's prescription, your therapy is a part of the treatment plan of the referring doctor. He or she prescribes your services much the same as prescribing physical therapy or psychiatric care.

The doctor must provide a diagnosis in order to initiate the process. Diagnosis means identification of the patient's medical problem. The problem can be a general one, indicating a need for relaxation massage, or a specific one, indicating a need for specific therapeutic techniques.

Relaxation Massage

Occasionally, a doctor will prescribe massage solely for its benefits in relaxing the client. Relaxation massage may or may not be reimbursable, depending on the patient's diagnosis and treatment plan.

Some chiropractors prescribe massage for patients who are too rigid to adjust, in hopes that the massage therapist will be able to help the patient release muscle tension, thus facilitating chiropractic care. A few medical doctors also prescribe massage for patients who are overly tense, as relaxation can help with a variety of medical problems that result from anxiety.

Medical Massage

Most prescriptions, however, are of a different sort, and involve what is commonly called "medical massage" or "clinical massage." This includes understanding of certain pathologies and knowledge of specific techniques that will be helpful in recovery from specific conditions and injuries. Certain schools specialize in medical massage, and other schools offer limited training in medical massage as part of their curriculum. You can find a list of all the schools teaching medical massage on page 204.

No *legal* requirement exists that you take a training in medical massage before working from a doctor's prescription. However, to attempt to do medical massage without proper training would be ill-advised, and would lead to frustration for you and for the doctor. Unless you have substantial training, you will not be able to understand the doctor's orders, and you will not know what to do to carry them out. Most doctors do not understand what massage therapists know and don't know, and therefore the responsibility to keep communication clear rests with you. Unless you are familiar with the terminology and procedures to be used in medical massage, problems will arise.

There is still no industry standard for training in medical massage. Courses in pathology, medical terminology, neuromuscular therapy or trigger point therapy, cranio-sacral therapy, myofascial release, postural evaluation and deep tissue massage are useful. Also consider programs that include rehabilitative exercises and treatments for specific injuries and conditions. The medical massage component of your education could easily take 500 classroom hours, plus clinical practice.

Professional arrangements

A variety of professional arrangements are available to a massage therapist or bodyworker who wants to work with clients for insurance reimbursement.

1. The client pays the therapist at the time of service, and the client then submits the therapist's bill to the insurance company for reimbursement.

2. The therapist works by prescription of a physician, and the therapist deals directly with the insurance company for reimbursement.

3. The therapist works closely with the prescribing physician (or physical therapist) and the physician's office handles insurance reimbursement. The physician or physical therapist may pay therapist by the hour or by subcontract. This arrangement is most common in non-licensed states, and is especially common when massage therapists work in chiropractors' offices.

No matter which of these three arrangements you participate in, you should have a good understanding of insurance guidelines and the billing process. Even if the doctor's office does your billing, you should be able to supervise and assist the process, since the doctor's office person may not understand how to classify and bill for your services.

Procedures for Insurance Reimbursement

Assuming you have made the choice to work for insurance reimbursement, what follows is a nuts-and-bolts approach to the procedures you should follow. Note that there are entire manuals devoted to this topic, and the brief discussion in this chapter is meant to get you started, but cannot answer every question and cover every issue.

Step One — Preapproval

When a new client comes to you for insurance reimbursed work, your first task is to make sure they have a doctor's referral or prescription. If they do, then you can proceed with the preapproval process.

Obtain the following information:
Patient's name
Date of birth
Social Security Number
Address
Phone Numbers
Date of Injury
Insurance Company's Name
Policy Number and Name of Insured Party

From the physician's referral or prescription, note the following information:
Diagnosis codes
Frequency of Treatments
Total Number of Treatments
Name and UPIN# (Doctor's ID#) of Referring Physician
Statement That Massage Therapy is Medically Necessary

A sample Physician's Prescription Letter of Referral is on page 165. You should create your own Letter of Referral on your own letterhead. In the space titled "Treatment to include" create a list of the treatments you are able to do so the physician can check them off. Use accepted orthopedic language in this section so the physician will be comfortable with it.

Have a physician complete a Letter of Referral for each client you will be working with. It establishes medical necessity, and it also lets the physician know what you do. By educating the physician about your practice, you are doing a form of direct marketing of your service to the medical community.

Once you have the above information, contact the client's insurance company and ask for preapproval. State that you are a massage therapist, and that the treatment has been declared "medically necessary" by a physician. You may want to seek preapproval for "soft tissue mobilization" or "myofascial release" rather than "massage." Find out how many visits will be paid for, how much the company will pay per visit or what CPT code procedures are acceptable, and whether there are any restrictions on who performs the service or where it is performed.

Write down the name of the person you spoke with and the date. Make note of the answers to all of the above questions, and make sure you have the correct phone number and extension in case you need to reach this person again to follow up. Place the note in the client's file for future reference.

Step Two — Documentation

The first session should be documented in a separate report titled "Report of First Massage Therapy". Detail your objective findings, the client's symptoms, and any postural or range of motion measurements you made. This report will serve as a baseline from which you can measure future progress.

Each session should be individually documented. The customary format is the SOAP format. This stands for Subjective, Objective, Assessment, Plan/Prognosis.

Subjective refers to the complaints and symptoms as the client expresses them. What pain is she having, and how often?

Objective refers to postural distortions, gait pattern, and range of motion evaluation, and all measurable limitations.

Assessment refers to the improvement resulting from this session. Did pain levels drop? Are there structural improvements? What aspects of the treatment plan are working ?

Plan/Prognosis refers to the future treatment plans. Note goals for this client, including which muscles or regions of the body need treatment and what techniques are to be used.

Some therapists have modified the SOAP format to SOTAP format. The added "T" is for *Treatment,* and in this category they list the therapeutic procedures used in the session, such as massage (Mass), neuromuscular therapy (NMT), myofascial release (MFR), therapeutic exercise (Ther-X) for example. These prefixes are matched with insurance CPT codes for use on the HCFA insurance form used nationally by all health care providers.

After several visits, a "Progress Report" may be required to show the status of the client's progress. This report compares all the objective client information to date with the measurements made at the initial visit, and reports on the change (if any) in the client's conditions and any circumstances that may be interfering with the client's progress.

Step Three — Billing the Company

You will submit your bill for insurance reimbursement on HCFA Form 1500. This form must include the CPT codes used by practitioners of physical medicine, and should be filled out in the language used by health care providers nationally. The CPT code book is available from the American Medical Association. The 1997 edition identified the following codes that are commonly used by massage therapists and bodyworkers:

97530 Therapeutic Activities—Direct (one on one) patient contact by the provider (use of dynamic activities to improve functional performance), each fifteen minutes
[Most massage or bodywork techniques could fit under this code in 15 minute units]

97250 Myofascial Release—Myofascial release/soft tissue mobilization, one or more regions
[This code could apply to bodywork techniques that focus on elongation, manipulation and treatment of fascia]

97122 Manual Traction (no CPT definition)
[This refers to continued manual force used to decompress joints and elongate soft tissue, such as continuous pulling]

97110 Therapeutic Exercises—Therapeutic procedure, one or more areas, each fifteen minutes; therapeutic exercises to develop strength and endurance, range of motion, and flexibility.
[This procedure is used when exercises or movement therapies are performed in the presence of the therapist. Typically, these are taught for home use]

97112 Neuromuscular Re-Education—Neuromuscular re-education of movement, balance, coordination, kinesthetic sense, posture and prorioception
[This refers to techniques that focus on improving the client's sense of balance or coordination, body awareness, posture or skeletal alignment, or awareness of biomechanical movement.]

On the HCFA form, the diagnostic codes given by the physician in the Letter of Referral are matched with the CPT codes and the reasonable and customary fees. Most insurance companies base their allowable fees on a national or regional average, and will furnish you with their schedule of fees upon request. Note that if you are providing services under a Worker's Compensation claim, lower fees are paid, different CPT codes are used, and different rules apply to insurance billing. An explanation of how to do Worker's compensation billing is beyond the scope of this chapter.

Step Four — Follow-up

If you do not receive payment within 45 days after you submit your bill, contact the representative at the insurance company (see the note you made when you called for preapproval). Make sure the bill has been received, and find out if there is any reason it has not been paid, or when you can expect payment. If forms have been incorrectly completed, your claim could be substantially delayed. Finding out about the error can help you clear it up. Other times, simply drawing attention to your claim can help the wheels of bureaucracy turn a little faster; sometimes the "squeaky wheel" gets the oil.

Kinds of Insurance

One complicating aspect of this field is that there are different kinds of insurance carriers you may be submitting to. What follows is a brief discussion of the kinds of insurance you may encounter in this field, and how they differ.

Workers' Compensation. Generally a reliable payer; stay strictly within the authorized number of treatments, and work only on the regions of the body that are diagnosed and approved by the adjuster.

Automobile Insurance. Each policy will have a PIP (Personal Injury Protection) limit. This is the total amount available to pay all health care claims. Inquire at the time of preapproval as to the amount of PIP coverage, and whether the remaining balance is sufficient to pay for your treatment. Generally a reliable payer; when benefits expire, client will be responsible for balance if Financial Responsibility Form has been signed (see below).

Liability Insurance. In rare cases, liability insurance will be responsible for payment for massage, such as a slip-and-fall in a grocery store. When preapproved, these carriers are usually reliable in paying for treatment. Sometimes payment is withheld until the end of treatment.

Group Health Insurance/Indemnity Policies. These policies usually have an annual deductible that must be met before benefits are paid to the insured, as well as a client co-pay amount, such as 20% of your fee. You would then bill 80% of your fee to the insurance company, and if the deductible is not yet satisfied, your fee would go toward the deductible. Billing this type of insurance carrier involves more details and restrictions than the types described above. These carriers are usually reliable payers after proper preapproval.

Managed Care/HMO/PPO. This type of insurance billing is not for the novice. Unless you have expertise in the field of insurance billing, have this type of client pay for your service and provide the client with a bill that she can submit to her carrier for reimbursement.

Financial Responsibility Form

Except as to Workers' Compensation, all clients may be made responsible to pay fees that insurance will not reimburse. This form should be signed at the first office visit. Many clients have never considered that they might be responsible for fees insurance will not pay, and some therapists choose not to use a Financial Responsibility Form, choosing instead to waive their fee if insurance will not pay. A sample form is in *Insurance Reimbursement and Specialty Physician Referrals*, or you can draw up your own if you have a basic understanding of drafting legally binding documents.

States With Licensure vs. States Without Licensure

When all the proper procedures are followed, insurance reimbursement for massage should definitely be received in states with massage licensure (see page 131 for State Licensing Chart). As a practicing therapist, you should know your own state's law concerning scope of practice, and any variations there may be in procedures in your state.

In states without massage licensure, it is risky to directly bill insurance carriers. The least risky form of insurance to bill to is automobile insurance. If you are in an unlicensed state, the safest approach is to work in an establishment where a licensed provider bills under her or his provider number, for example a physical therapist or physician.

When working with a licensed provider, you must consider whether you are an independent contractor or an employee (see page 35). You can agree on a fixed payment per session, or an hourly rate. You may create a situation where you pay rent for a room and receive a fixed amount per session or per hour worked.

A Note about Objective Findings

Objective measurements of the skeletal system and of range of motion are widely accepted as valid documentation in all branches of physical medicine — orthopedics, osteopathy, chiropractic, and physical therapy. Your work is more likely to be accepted as corrective and restorative if you are able to document your results in the common language of objective measurements of structure and function. "Speaking the same language" as doctors and physical therapists is helpful in increasing your credibility, and thus in promoting referrals.

Litigation and the "Letter of Protection"

In a personal injury case, you may be asked to wait until the conclusion of the lawsuit to be paid for your work. Your client's attorney may offer you a Letter of Protection that guarantees you will be paid out of the settlement or judgment.

Be aware, however, that there is not always enough money available to pay everyone. Claims may be paid in the order they are received, and if the funds are exhausted before yours is paid, you can lose out. Some litigation cases guarantee 100% payment, but usually you must wait until massage therapy treatment is completed.

Most of these claims are paid eventually, and if you can do without the money at present, it can be a welcome surprise to finally receive a large check for work long since completed.

Documentation is Direct Marketing

If you are feeling like all the documentation involved in working for insurance reimbursement is tedious and time-consuming, take heart. It may be those things, but it is also an effective marketing tool. Your notes, reports, phone calls and updates communicate your results directly to the gate-keepers of health care. These reports and contacts educate all involved about your work, your understanding of the body and health, and the effectiveness of your treatment. It is much cheaper than advertising and is targeted at those who can send you clients or pay you for your work.

This chapter has provided you with "the basics." You may feel comfortable taking this information and beginning to bill insurance companies, or you may feel that you need additional information and guidance. See the resources on pages 187-188 and consider also people in your community who have expertise in insurance billing who could give you some help or instruction as you get started.

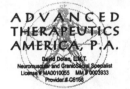

Specializing in Neuromuscular & CranioSacral Therapy Injury Rehabilitation

ADVANCED
THERAPEUTICS
AMERICA, P.A.
David Dolan, L.M.T.
Neuromuscular and CranioSacral Specialist
License # MA0010055   MM # 0003933
Provider # C6168

PRESCRIPTION/LETTER OF REFERRAL

Patient's Name	Address
John Doe	123 Any Street

	City	State	Zip
	Jacksonville	FL	32216

Date of Birth	Date of Accident	Sex: Male ☒ Female ☐	S.S. #
6/30/52	6/30/97		123-45-6789

ICD-9-CM Principal Diagnosis	Date
Myofascial Pain Syndrome	Present Date

Treatment to include: Neuromuscular Therapy which includes the following: Soft Tissue Mobilization, Neuromuscular Re-Education, Postural Evaluation, CranioSacral Evaluation, Hot/cold packs (as needed), Movement Therapy, Assisted Flexibility, Myofascial Release, Manual Traction, Palpation findings, Postural Education, Ergonomic Education, and self-care skills to enhance self-responsibility.

Treatment for the following area(s)/Diagnosis Codes

_X_ 784.0 Headaches ____847.0 Cervical Strain/Sprain _X_ 840.0 Shoulder Strain/Sprain ____840.9 Unspecified Upper Extremities: R____ L____ B____ 842.0 Wrist Strain/Sprain: R____ L____ B____ 847.1 Thoracic Strain/Sprain ____847.2 Lumbar Strain/Sprain ____846.0 Lumbosacral Strain/Sprain _X_724.3 Sciatica (pain in leg, no back pain) _X_844.9 Unspecified site of knee and leg (strain/sprain): R _X_ L____ 848.5 Pelvic Strain/Sprain ____723.4 Cervical Radiculitis ____354.0 Carpal Tunnel Syndrome
____Other:_____
Safety Measures: No manipulation of cervical spine-fusion C4-C5

Orders of Discipline and Treatment Plan

Duration: ____8 weeks _X_6 weeks ____4 weeks ____Other_____
Frequency: ____Daily ____3x/weekly _X_2x/weekly ____Weekly ____Biweekly ____Monthly

Medically Necessary: _X_Yes ____No
Start of Care: present date

Physician's Name, Address, and Telepohne

Dr. John Smith
555 Medical Park East
Olney, MD 21222

Physician's Signature	Date
John Smith, M.D.	Date of Dr.'s signature

Physician's U.P.I.N.

Physician's Identification Number

4237 Salisbury Road • Suite 106 • Salisbury Lakes Medical Park • Jacksonville, Florida 32216
t. (904) 296-7566 • f. (904) 296-1657

21 Keeping Client and Financial Records

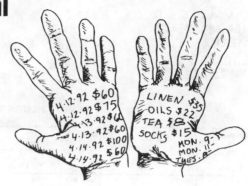

There are three basic kinds of records to keep, and they are all important.

Tax records

These are your records of all the money you earn and all the money you spend on deductible items. If you should be called on one day to demonstrate to the IRS the truth of all the entries in your tax return, you will need to produce accurate records of your income and deductions. These records should be kept at least three years after your return is filed, as your return can be audited up to three years after you file it.

Business records

These are the records you keep to give you a better understanding of your own practice. Different practices have different slow and busy times. Your practice may slow down for three weeks every August, which would make that a perfect time for your vacation in the Colorado Rockies. If you don't keep accurate records, you probably would never see that pattern, and might wind up staying in town during your slow season and leaving when clients will miss you more.

Client records

Client records allow you to better know and serve each client. Your records will let you know basic personal and medical information about each client, and will show you their history of receiving treatments from you. When appropriate, your records will give you an at-a-glance view of how your treatments affected specific problems or situations in your clients' lives.

This chapter discusses how to keep each of these three kinds of records, and suggests some ways to design your own record-keeping system that will make the whole process easier and more efficient. Sample forms appear at the end of the chapter. You may copy and use these forms, modify them to suit you, or create your own.

Record-keeping For Tax-Time

The records you need to keep are those proving your income and your deductions. Chapter Eighteen explains income and deductions.

The main things you should do to support proper tax record-keeping are (1) write down every payment you receive for your work in some type of ledger, (2) keep track of your automobile business mileage in a ledger, and (3) keep bills, receipts and canceled checks in one container until the end of the year, when you can sort them out and tally them up.

SHOE by Jeff MacNelly

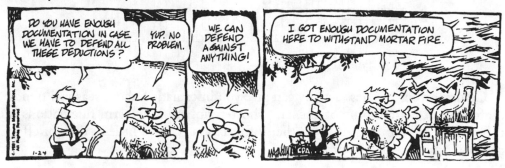

Recording income and business mileage

There is no required form for these records. The only requirement is that they be accurate and complete. If your car has a trip odometer, you can easily compute miles for each business trip by resetting the trip odometer to zero when you begin, and reading the trip odometer when you finish. Keep your log in the car, and record the mileage when you finish each business trip.

No matter what system you decide to use, take the time each day to record all of the day's business activity. Record the day's business mileage, and all income you receive each day. Get in the habit of recording each day's business activity before you go to sleep.

Records of Business Activity

Your records should show you your business activity for each day, each week, each month, and each year. It takes a minimum amount of effort to keep your records in good order, and the rewards can be substantial.

Charting your business activity not only gives you information about when you can expect seasonal ups and downs, but it also tells you whether your overall business activity is going up, going down, or staying about the same.

During some slow weeks, I could have become depressed or pessimistic about the progress of my practice. Instead, I glanced at my business activity chart, and I saw that last month I had a slow week and it was in-between two better weeks. Instead of thinking my practice was going sour, I realized I was experiencing a normal fluctuation and nothing was going wrong. That insight did a lot for my emotional health.

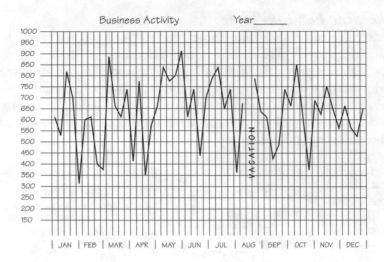

Business Activity   Year_____

| JAN | FEB | MAR | APR | MAY | JUN | JUL | AUG | SEP | OCT | NOV | DEC |

Charting your business activity can give you information about seasonal trends, usefulness of certain promotions, and short-term and long-term fluctuations in the volume of your practice. No other information costs so little in time or effort compared to the value it produces.

Keeping Client Records

If you or your clients are going to bill insurance companies for your services, you need to keep detailed records for each treatment you perform. See Chapter 20 dealing with billing insurance companies, and see page 187 for resources to help with record-keeping for insurance clients.

Even if you are not dealing with insurance billing, you should keep accurate records. For each client, you should have a completed intake form that includes the following basic information:

- Date of first treatment

- Client's name, address, and date of birth

- Phone number

- Medical history (as much as you feel is necessary)

- Previous experience with massage or bodywork

- Current symptoms or problems

- Reason for seeking treatment

Date of first treatment will be useful to you later as you review your records on a particular client.

The address is necessary if you ever want to mail something to the client (such as a Christmas card, birthday card, promotional flyer, or bill) or do a house call.

The phone number is necessary in the event of cancellation or change of plans on short notice.

Medical history gives you a better sense of how your treatment can fit into this person's whole picture, and can be useful in discovering contraindications for part or all of the treatment you will give.

Whether the person has previously had bodywork helps you to know how to approach this session.

Current symptoms or problems, and reason for seeking treatment give you information about what this client wants from you. Failure to get this information can result in doing a session that does not satisfy a client. They will not usually spontaneously tell you what they expect from your work.

The sample intake form on page 170 is one you can modify to suit your own needs. If you do remedial work, you may want substantially more medical information. Keep in mind that the intake form has two basic purposes. First, it provides you with contact information and essential data about your clients. Second, it serves to open a dialogue between you and your client, and thereby begin the therapeutic relationship. It is a tool for communication.

If the client's care does not involve insurance billing, you may not need to keep further records for this client, except those necessary for business activity and tax purposes. If you do need to keep further records, you can use the back of the client's intake form, or create a separate file for records about continuing care clients.

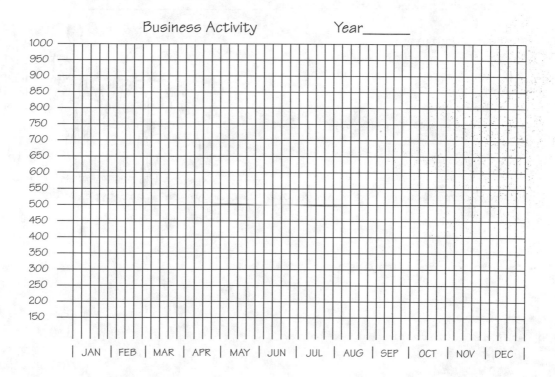

Client _____ Date of birth _____

Address _____

_____ Phone (_____) _____

Date of first treatment _____

Occupation _____

Medical History:
Previous major Illnesses:

Previous broken bones or other injuries:

Are you currently under a physician's care?

    Physician_____

    For what condition?_____

    Are you taking any medications? _____

Current Condition:
Areas of pain or discomfort:

Reasons for seeking massage:

Have you previously had massage or other bodywork? What type?

What do you do to manage your stress?

What is your routine of exercise?

Weekly Business Log

Week of _____

Date	Client	fee	miles

22 Managing Your Money
Some Ideas On Financial Planning

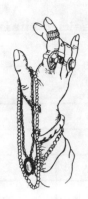

In the early years of your massage career, you will not have much money to manage. Spare dollars will go to necessities, and to improvements in your professional equipment.

In time, however, success will bring with it prosperity, and when it does, you will need to give at least a little thought to how to manage your money.

Savings

One of the hardest things for a self-employed person to do is to put money into a savings account. However, it is a very important habit to get into. Consider the following expenses you will have:

1. Quarterly estimated tax payments

2. Health insurance, auto insurance

3. Professional association dues

These expenses come quarterly, semiannually, or annually. They can put a strain on your budget if you are living from month to month. Having a reserve in your savings (or checking) account makes life easier when these expenses come due.

Open a savings account at your bank. Start it with at least $100, and add whatever amounts you can. Avoid making withdrawals unless absolutely necessary. The fact that you have a few hundred dollars, or a couple of thousand dollars, can be very comforting when the mechanic tells you you need a transmission overhaul.

Beyond this issue of emergency reserves to meet unforeseen expenses, you will also want to consider the larger financial reserves you will need to meet the major expenses you can expect sooner or later:

4. Buying a new car

5. Buying a home

6. Rearing children

7. Retirement

These are the expenses that require you to make, and save, substantial sums of money, and to manage that money in a way that gives you the most advantage out of it.

Long-range planning

As a rule of thumb, there are two critical points in the careers of many would-be massage therapists — two years into a career and five years into a career.

Many practitioners give up somewhere near the two-year mark. Either they failed to pursue any organized marketing approach, or they gave up before getting the benefit of the approach they were using.

Those who survive the two-year mark usually find some degree of success in the field. Another point often comes at the five-year mark, when the physical nature of the work may begin to take its toll, or the practitioner may decide to branch off into another kind of work.

Practitioners who stay with the work longer than five years can usually keep doing the work practically indefinitely. Some keep working into their seventies. If you are staying in the field longer than five years, you will do well to take up the study of estate planning and investment.

You can't live on Social Security

Consider what you will have to live on when you retire.

Social security may be enough to keep a roof over your head, and three very low-budget meals on the table, but it is not enough money to live on. Before you reach retirement age, you should have put aside enough to create your own retirement plan. The earlier you start, the easier it will be.

Kinds of Savings Plans

Savings plans can take many forms.

1. You can stockpile cash, but if you do so you earn no interest, and can lose everything in a theft or fire.

2. You can keep your money in a savings account, certificate of deposit, or money market account. These will earn interest, and your money will be basically safe.

3. You can choose a "tax shelter" keyed to retirement. While you must still pay self-employment tax on the money you put into your retirement plan, you do not pay federal income tax on this money. You pay income tax on the retirement money only when you receive it, at retirement. Tax breaks available to retired persons may help you pay lower taxes on your money at retirement time than you would now.

Tax Shelter Retirement Plans

In a nutshell, the great thing about tax shelter retirement plans is that they force you to keep your money invested until you retire. Because of high penalties for withdrawing money prior to age 59½, you are forced to keep your "nest egg" safe for your future.

This is both the advantage and the disadvantage of these plans — you lose the flexibility to deal with your money on a whim; you have fewer options now, but more security later.

The government makes this appealing by giving you a slightly better tax treatment if you put your money into a retirement plan. Consider the following example:

It is April 14th, and you are preparing your tax return for the previous year. You do all your computations, find out you owe $2,104 in income tax (we are ignoring self-employment tax in this example, because retirement plans do not change your self-employment tax).

If you use some money you have saved to make a contribution of $2,000 to a qualified retirement plan, your income tax bill will be reduced to $1,804. You therefore reduce your tax by $300 by placing $2,000 in a retirement plan. As long as you make this contribution by April 15, it counts as a deduction for the preceding year's taxes.

Save now, Save later

To take the example a step further, consider the long-term effects of this decision. If you *do not* make the contribution to your retirement plan, you must spend $300 of the $2,000 on taxes. This leaves you with $1,700.

Assume that you keep this $1,700 invested at "average" interest rates for thirty years. Interest rates are always changing, but as a rule of thumb, you can figure that money well-invested will double itself every ten years. Therefore, in 30 years, an investment should grow to eight times the original amount. (After 10 years, the original investment will double; after 20 years it will double again, or be four times the original amount; after 30 years it will double a third time, and be eight times the original amount).

This rule of thumb tells us that $1,700 today will be $13,600 in 30 years.

Now consider the alternative where you put $2,000 in a retirement account. The same rule of thumb tells us that the $2,000 today will turn into $16,000 in 30 years. However, this $16,000 will be subject to income tax when you receive it at retirement. Current rates of income tax, 15%, would reduce that $16,000 to $13,600 — exactly the same amount as if you had paid your $300 tax in the first place and left the $1,700 invested.

However, unless you are a person of incredible will power, you will not leave that $1,700 alone for 30 years to gain interest. What you will wind up with will be somewhat less than the $13,600 you know you can count on if you sock the money away in a retirement plan where you cannot reach it without substantial penalties.

In addition, tax breaks available to retired persons may make it possible for you to pay less than 15% tax on the money when you receive it at retirement. Any such breaks you get make it definitely advantageous to have your money in a retirement account.

Kinds of Retirement Plans

The Tax Relief Act of 1997 created new retirement plans and modified some traditional ones. It is beyond the scope of this chapter to discuss all of these fully, but the information below highlights their provisions.

With the exception of the Education IRA, all of the plans described below require you to keep the money in the account until retirement (usually age 59½), and have penalties for early withdrawal. The plans described below are all available to self-employed persons.

IRA (Individual Retirement Account)

Easy to set up and widely available, an IRA allows you to shelter up to a maximum of $2,000 per year. The amount you put in is a tax-deduction in the year you make the contribution, so you receive a tax advantage for putting money into an IRA. However, you must pay tax on the money, and on accumulated interest, when you withdraw it, usually after age 59½.

Roth IRA

Your contributions to a "Roth IRA" are not deductible from your current year's taxes. However, you will not have to pay taxes on the accumulated investment earnings when you receive the proceeds after age 59½. This can give you a better overall result that a regular IRA.

Education IRA

This is a fund for your children's education. You can contribute up to $500 per child per year, to be used for their educational expenses. Distributions are tax-free if used for educational purposes.

Simple IRA

Contributions are allowed up to $6,000 per year, no matter what your income.

Simple 401(K)

Contributions are limited to 25% of income, up to maximum of $6,000 per year.

SEP (Simplified Employee Pension)

Easy to set up and widely available, the SEP allows you to shelter up to 13.04% of your self-employed annual earnings (to a maximum contribution of $24,000 in any one year).

Keogh

Keogh's are more complicated to set up, and can be more expensive to create and maintain than the other plans described.

If you are interested in establishing one of these accounts, start with your local bank, savings and loan, accountant, financial advisor, or insurance advisor. Chances are, they can consult with you about the various kinds of accounts and set up an account for you, often at no charge.

Once established, these accounts cannot be modified, so be very careful that you understand how your account will fit into your future plans.

V

Equipment and Other Professional Resources

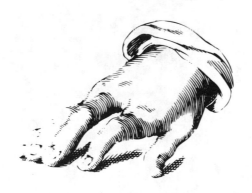

Massage Tables and Chairs

All of the following companies ship their products nationwide. They will all send you brochures or information packets about their massage tables and other products at your request.

American Bodycrafters, Inc.
21602 Surveyor Circle
Huntington Beach, CA 92646
1-888-822-5328 (1-888-TABLE 2 U)

Portable massage table with face hole, lightweight on-site massage chair.

Astra Lite Tables
120 Manfree Rd.
Watsonville, CA 95076
1-800-368-5483 or (408) 763-0397

Extremely lightweight, portable table; stationary table; fixed or push-button adjustable height, with recessed legs & cables and built-in face cradles; bolsters, carrying cases.

Blue Ridge Tables
Rt. 6 Box 490
South Industrial Park
Corinth, MS 38834
1-800-447-2723 or (601) 286-7007

Full line of massage equipment; portable, stationary and electric tables, on-site chairs.

Care-Tech Research Corp
4337 River Road W.
Delta, BC., V4K 1R9, Canada
(604) 946-1574

Transportable, height-adjusting massage table.

Colorado Healing Arts
P.O. Box 2247
Boulder, CO 80306
1-800-728-2426

Portable and non-portable tables, oils, linens, bolsters, massage tools, charts, professional office forms and other items. Free brochure includes "How to select a massage table."

Comfort Craft Bodywork Tables
P.O. Box 520638
Longwood, FL 32752-0638
www.comfortcraft.com
(407) 830-7332

Height-adjusting and position adjusting table; adjustable gas-lift stool.

Creative Touch
1713 G Street #1
Sacramento, CA 95814
1-800-441-6759

Lightweight, adjustable height, oval massage tables and accessories

Custom Craftworks
P.O. Box 24621
Eugene, OR 97402
(541) 345-2712
1-800-627-2387
www.customcraftworks.com

A selection of stationary and adjustable height portable tables; on-site chair, electric lift table, desktop portable support, bolsters, carrying cases, and accessories. Lifetime warranty on all wood tables.

Cyan Massage Products, Inc.
8853-63 Avenue
Edmonton, Alberta, T6E 0E9 Canada
(403) 944-9690
www.compusmart.ab.ca/cyan/cyanhome.htm

Portable massage tables and on-site chairs. Cyan also offers to refurbish and recondition existing equipment instead of replacing it.

Earthlite
2750 La Mirada Dr.
Vista, CA 92083
1-800-872-0560

Full line of portable, stationary and electric lift massage tables; bolsters fleece pads, table skate, carry case, stools, headrest covers, flannel sheets

G & A Manufacturers
1004 E. Fairview Blvd.
Inglewood, CA 90302
(213) 207-0023 or 1-800-TABLES-2

Stationary and portable tables, wooden or aluminum legs; very lightweight inexpensive portable, reiki/facial table, on-site chair, bolsters and carrying cases

Galaxy Enterprises, Inc.
5411 Sheila St.
Los Angeles, CA 90040
(213) 728-3980 or 1-800-876-4599

Lightweight, portable, adjustable-height massage table

Golden Ratio Woodworks
P.O Box 297
Emigrant, MT 59027
1-800-796-0612

Full line of stationary and portable tables, spa tables, on-site chair, 14-pound on-site chair, covers, oils, bolsters, charts, books and other accessories.

Integrated Medical, Inc.
8100 S. Akron, ste. 320
Englewood, CO 80112
1-800-333-7617

Stationary massage table with electric motor for height adjustment during treatment.

Living Earth Crafts
600 East Todd Road
Santa Rosa, CA 95407
1-800-358-8292

Complete line of stationary and portable tables, including very inexpensive portable, on-site chair, desk-top face cradle, oils, linens, books, charts, music, videos, and more.

New Generation Products
Montgomery Woods
6721 E. Akron St.
Mesa, AZ 85205
1-800-850-5552

Basic and deluxe lightweight adjustable height massage tables; carry case, fitted face cradle covers, oil pouch belt (lifetime guarantee except for vinyl).

Oakworks, Inc.
34 Main Street
P.O. Box 99
Glen Rock, PA 17327-0099
(717) 235-6807 or 1-800-558-8850

Complete line of stationary and portable tables, on-site chair, carrying cases, bolsters and sheets.

Pisces Productions
380 Morris St., Suite A
Sebastopol, CA 95472
1-800-TABLE-33

Vertical to horizontal, adjusting on-site chair, portable tables and accessories.

Robert Hunter Bodywork Tables
910 SE Stark St.
Portland, OR 97214
(503) 238-6345 or 1-800-284-3988
www.RobertHunter.com

Stationary and portable adjustable height tables, sheets, massage oil, carrying cases, customization available.

Somatron Corp.
8503 N. 29th St.
Tampa, FL 33604
(813) 960-2183 or 1-800-544-4294

Vibro-acoustic massage table that directs vibrations through the client's body during the massage.

Stronglite Massage Table Kits
255 Davidson St.
Cottage Grove, OR 97424
(541) 942-0130
1-800-BUY-KITS (289-5487)
www.stronglite.com

Portable, lightweight adjustable height, inexpensive tables, on-site partially assembled tables and kits at substantially lower cost. Stronglite also makes the ComforTable line of massage tables.

Tatum's Custom Woodworks
1631 SW 170ᵗʰ St.
Newberry, FL 32669
1-800-382-8530

Portable, adjustable height massage table, on-site chair, accessories.

Touch America
P.O. Box 1304
Hillsborough, NC 27278
(919) 732-6968
1-800-678-6824

Complete line of stationary and portable tables, spa products, acoustic music table, on-site chair, stool, sheets, miscellaneous items workshop series, spa therapies.

Tree of Life Bodyworks
1-800-281-4145

Inexpensive on-site massage chair, lightweight portable massage table

Ultra-Light Inc.
3140 Roy Messer Hwy.
White Pine, TN 37890
(423) 674-8111 or 1-800-999-1971

Extremely light portable table, adjustable legs available

Massage Oils

The following companies either manufacture or distribute massage oils. Most of these companies also sell other beauty, body-care, health-related or aromatherapy products. All companies listed below will send a catalogue on request.

The price listed next to the company name is the approximate price of a gallon of their least expensive massage oil including shipping charges (unless otherwise noted). Prices reflect a professional discount, if any applies. Some companies require a wholesale order, usually a four-gallon minimum.

Aroma de Terra
401 Euclid Ave., suite 155
Cleveland, OH 44114
(216) 566-8234

Supplies of a variety of massage oils

Avalon Skin Care Products, Inc.
P.O. Box 150681
Lakewood, CO 80215
1-888-295-OILS (6457)

Massage oil, lotions and cream and essential oils. (Gal. $25.00 plus s/h)

Barclay Labs ($27.50 plus s/h)
4780-A Caterpillar Rd.
Redding, CA 96003
1-800-845-4460

A light massage oil that will not go rancid, is stain resistant, coconut oil based, derived solely from plants; cruelty free, color and fragrance free.

Biotone ($40)
4757 Old Cliffs Rd.
San Diego, CA 92120
1-800-445-6457
In CA: (619) 582-0027

Unscented, and scented massage oils, dual-purpose massage creme, deep tissue lotion, sports therapy creme and gel, pumps, Fresh Again detergent, essential oils, face cradle covers, cruelty-free

Charlie Sunshine's Secret Formula ($40 plus s/h)
88 Santa Marina
San Francisco, CA 94110
(415) 647-3973

Massage oil with a creamy texture like a lotion; 100% oil, will not disappear into the skin; recommended for deep tissue work.

Credo ($30 plus s/h)
4940 E. 73rd St.
Tulsa, OK 74136
1-800-714-9272

Massage and aromatherapy oils

Diamond Light Massage Products
14 Las Palomas
Orinda, CA 94563
(510) 253-0543

Sunfresh soap, valley of the sun natural massage oil (10% discount on orders over $110)

Dr. Hauschka Cosmetics
59C North Street
Hatfield, MA 01038
1-800-247-9907

Dr. Hauschka massage oils are made with specially prepared organic and whole plant ingredients (3.4 ounce bottle $11 to $14; min. order $200)

Duane Karr & Assoc.
Massage Clinic & Store ($85.45)
441 N. Main, rear/P.O. Box 400
Milford, MI 48381
(248) 685-3628

Cold-processed sesame oil, unscented or blended with essential oils; aromatherapy supplies (also distributes massage tables)

Elements Plus
21327 Hilltop
Southfield, MI 48034
1-800-995-6404
(248) 208-1655

Activating massage oil, scented or unscented, replenishing massage lotion, restructuring creme, herbal formula

Effleurage ($19.95 plus s/h)
45054 Palo Vista Dr.
Lancaster, CA 93535
1-888-333-5563

Base is a blend of seven oils; comes in unscented, sports blend, exotic blend and soothing blend.

Everybody, Ltd.
1738 Pearl St.
Boulder, CO 80302
1-800-748-5675 or (303)440-0188

Massage and aromatherapy oils, not tested on animals; skin trip, mother's special blend, custom blending.

Genesis Nail and Skin Care Systems
5987 Park Blvd., Suite 2
Pinellas Park, FL 33781
1-800-406-2457
www.GenesisNailCare.com

Totally Natural - Total Body Therapy oil made from 14 oils including kukui nut, macadamia, avocado and the key oil, copaiba balsam, imported from the Brazilian rainforest.

The Heritage Store ($36)
P.O. Box 444
Virginia Beach, VA 23458-0444
1-800-726-2232
1-800-862-2923

Aura glow massage oil, from a formula prescribed by Edgar Cayce, available in 8 aromatherapeutic scents and unscented; also lotion, liniment and pure oils. Call for free catalogue, professional discounts.

Jacki's Magic Lotion
($59.40 plus s/h)
258 "A" St., #7-A
Ashland, OR 97520
1-800-355-8428 or (541) 488-1388

A 100% natural oil-based massage lotion with a creamy texture. Comes in unscented, lavender, rose-mint, orange-vanilla and almond. Free samples, 10% discount with first order.

Janca's Jojoba Oil & Seed Co.
456 E. Juanita #7
Mesa, AZ 85204
(602) 497-9494

Massage oils, specialty oils, creams, lotions, aromatherapy supplies

Liberty Massage Products ($22)
8120 SE Stark St.
Portland, OR 97215
1-800-289-8427
www.libertynatural.com

Almond oil, coconut, over 400 pure and natural essential oils and botanicals. Order by phone, fax, or on-line.

Pure Pro Massage Oils ($31.90)
955 Massachusetts Ave. #232
Cambridge, MA 02139
1-800-900-PURE (7873)

Showroom: 325 New Boston St., Unit A-B 10 18 massage oils, natural products, water washable, many accessories. Free catalogue and sample, 10% of first order—mention this book.

Pure Touch Therapeutic Body Care
P.O. Box 1281
Nevada City, CA 95959
1-800-442-PURE (7873)

Watersperse massage oil, massage lotion, apricare massage oil, ice ch'i.
Not tested on animals.

Rainbow Research Corp. ($42)
170 Wilbur Place
Bohemia, NY 11716
In NY: (516) 589-5563
Outside NY: 1-800-722-9595

Sports or moisturizing blend; contains almond, olive and peanut oil, plus Vitamin E, lanolin and paba.

**Reign Dance Hawaiian
Massage Oils** (9 oz. $10 to $22)
219 First Ave. South, Ste 405
Seattle, WA 98104
(206) 789-6429 or 1-800-221-1309

Hawaiian flower oils and combination oils for all types of bodywork, deep tissue work and healing work, plus ceremonial oils.

Sunshine Oils
($31.45, min. order $150.00)
12737 28th NE
Seattle, WA 98125
1-800-659-2077

Massage oils, lotions, perfumed oils, essential oils and body-care oils.

**Third Millenium/Body
Care** ($35 plus s/h)
712 Rocio St.
Carlsbad, CA 92008
(760) 431-7181 or 1-800-776-6525

7 water washable formulations of oils and lotions, pain relieving massage lotions, hand and body lotion (discounts for orders of 4 or more gallons).

Total Sensations ($48 plus s/h)
Private Label Cosmetics
85D Mahan St.
West Babylon, NY 11704
1-800-446-4704 or (516) 491-9010

Massage oil with gentle aromatic fragrance.

Uncommon Scents ($29.95 plus s/h)
380 W. First Ave.
Eugene, OR 97401
(503) 345-0952
1-800-426-4336

Massage oil blend, massage lotion, apricot oil, almond oil, coconut oil, cocoa butter, essential balm, tiger balm; customized scents available.

Weleda, Inc. ($119)
P.O. Box 249
Congers, NY 10920
(914) 268-8572

Arnica massage oil, citrus massage oil, Calendula baby oil, essential oils.

Massage Supply Stores and Catalogue Services

Alternative Essentials
P.O. Box 54
Coopers Mills, ME 04341
(207) 623-4551

books, charts, music, gift certificates, accessories, massage tables and chairs, aromatherapy supplies.

Banner Therapy Products
524 Hendersonville Rd.
Asheville, NC 28803
1-888-277-1188
www.BannerTherapy.com

Aromatherapy, massage tools, oils, gels, lotions vibrators, hot and cold packs, hydrocollators, pack chillers, paraffin baths, charts, supports, pillows, desktop portal, 30-day money back guarantee.

Best of Nature
176 Broadway
Long Branch, NJ 07740
1-800-228-6457

Massage tables and chairs, oils, creams, lotions, liniments, essential oils, linens, self-massage tools, incense, books, videos, music, bottles and pillows.

BML (Basic Massage Lines)
1207 W. Kingshighway
Paragould, AR 72450
1-800-643-4751

Oils, lotions, hydrocollators, vibrators, paraffin baths, hot and cold packs, massage tables and chairs, linens, bolsters, pillows, stools, other accessories.

The Body Shop
2051 Hilltop Dr., suite A-5
Redding, CA 96002
(530) 221-1031
1-800-736-6897

Massage Holster, aqua-relief pad, sunfresh soap, stronglite tables, aromatherapy supplies, oils, lotions, charts.

Body Therapy Assoc.
4442 Main St.
Philadelphia, PA 19127
1-800-677-9830
www.gotyourback.com

Massage tables and on-site chairs, accessories, oils & lotions. Large inventory, same-day shipping.

Body Tools
16 Camaron Way, Suite C
Novato, CA 94949
(415) 382-1355 or 1-800-845-6202

Self-massage tools, charts, skin brushes, cocoa butter, ayurvedic massage oils, incense, smudge sticks.

Bodywork Central
5519 College Avenue
Oakland, CA 94618
(510) 547-4313
orders: 1-888-226-8500

Variety of massage tables and on-site chairs, bolsters, Biotone oil & lotions, carrycase, table skate, table carrier, spa supplies, body support cushion, table selection assistance.

Bodywork Emporium (7 locations):

338 North Highway 101
Leucadia, CA 92024
(760) 942-9565

1451 Morena Blvd.
San Diego, CA 92110
(619) 276-2608

414 Broadway
Santa Monica, CA 90401
(310) 394-4475

1804C Newport Blvd.
Costa Mesa, CA 92627
(714) 548-0220

4529 Sepulveda Blvd.
Sherman Oaks, CA 91403
(818) 990-6155

2427 G Street
Bakersfield, CA 93301
(805) 631-1966

1329 State Street
Santa Barbara, CA 93101
(805) 965-5546

Large selection of massage tables and on-site chairs, massage oils and lotions, videos, books, charts, music and other supplies.

Edcat Enterprises
P.O. Box 168
Daytona Beach, FL 32115
(904) 253-2385 or 1-800-274-3566

Large selection of anatomical and other charts, self-massage tools.

Educating Hands School of Massage Bookstore Catalogue
120 Southwest 8th Street
Miami, FL 33130
1-800-999-6991
(in Miami (305) 285-6991)

Books, massage tables, massage oils and Chinese liniments, charts, audio cassettes, videos, hot and cold application equipment, self-massage tools, linen and hand cleaners, crystals, miscellaneous items.

HANDSON BOOKSTORE™
QWL Services
POB 20795
NY, NY 10025
Tel: 212-222-4240

Located at www.qwl.com/mtwc/handson/, this is a virtual bookstore specializing in books for the massage and bodywork professional. Large selection, On-line ordering.

Hands on Health Care Catalog Acupressure Institute
1533 Shattuck Ave.
Berkeley, CA 94709
1-800-442-2232 or (510) 845-1059

Books, reference charts, flash cards, videos, audio tapes, massage and self-massage tools, magnet devices, acupressure model, aroma-therapy supplies, music, massage tables, on-site chair, on-site desktop support.

The Health Touch
261 Main St.
Royersford, PA 19468
1-800-890-6195

Oils, lotions, creams, aromatherapy supplies, massage products, massage tools, massage tables. Free catalogue.

Massage Central
12235 Santa Monica Blvd.
Los Angeles, CA 90025
(310) 826-2209

Large display of massage tables and on-site chairs, and other supplies.

Massage Products West
641 Avilar Court
San Marcos, CA 92069
1-800-747-4802 or (760) 598-1460

Massage tables, chairs, linens, oils and accessories. Catalogue available.

Massage Mart
12217 Santa Monica Blvd., Suite 202
Los Angeles, CA 90025
(310) 207-7013 or 1-888-822-5370

Offering a selection of stationary and adjustable massage tables.

New England Massage Tables and Chairs
20 Bridge St.
Manchester, NH 03101
1-800-545-8497
(603) 641-5928

Massage tables, massage chairs, oils, lotions, gels, essential oils, charts, books, self-massage tools, bolsters, hot and cold applications products, flash cards, other accessories.

Oak Lawn Myotherapy
2728 Oak Lawn
Dallas, TX 75219
(214) 528-2390 or 1-800-775-5685

Over 1,800 products. Extensive catalogue $5.00 Mini-catalogue free upon request or may be downloaded from website at www.bodyworker.com.

Professional Development Catalog Sohnen-Moe Associates, Inc.
3906 West Ina Road, suite 200-367
Tucson, AZ 85741
1-800-786-4774 or (520) 743-3936

Books and other material with an emphasis on marketing, practice building, practice management and self-care.

**Rosenthal Clinic Massage
Tables & Chairs**
141 N. Meramec
St. Louis, MO 63105
1-800-833-3603 or (314) 727-7278

Distributor of most brands of massage tables
and chairs; table selection service
http://1stpage.com/1/rctables.

Sunset Park Massage Supply
2302 S. Hubert Ave.
Tampa, FL 33629
1-800-344-7677 or (813) 251-0320

Massage tables and chairs from 12 companies,
accessories, charts, books, aromatherapy supplies, videos, hydrocollators, paraffin baths,
lotions, oils, massage machines.

Zenith Supplies
6300 Roosevelt Way NE
Seattle, WA 98115
(206) 525-7997 or 1-800-735-7217

Stationary massage table, portable tables, on-
site chair, curtain screen, step-stool, Hydro-
collator, hot and cold packs, charts, pillows
and back supports, massage oils and lotions,
bolsters, paraffin bath.

Miscellaneous Massage Items

Table covers, sheets and related items:

Innerpeace
P.O. Box 940
Walpole, NH 03608
1-800-949-7650

100% cotton flannel sheets, face cradle covers,
bolster slip covers and more.

Daffodil's Associates
12 Shelby Rd.
East Northport, L.I., NY 11731
(516) 368-1197

Disposable 40" x 90" massage sheets in
cartons of 50; electro-stimulator for
pain relief sold only to LMT's.

Printed items such as brochures about massage and gift certificates:

Hemingway Publications
P.O. Box 4575
Rockford, IL 61110
(815) 877-5590

(brochures, gift certificates)

Information for people
P.O. Box 1876
Olympia, WA 98507
1-800-754-9790 or (360) 754-9799

(brochures (English, French and Spanish), selection of books and compassionate touch videos, display cases, gift certificates, greeting cards, post cards)

Touch, Ink. MicroPublishing
225 Harrison
Oak Park, IL 60304
1-800-296-3968

(Touch, Ink. is a promotional newsletter aimed at massage clients. It is personalized with the
name of the massage therapist on the front page, and contains informative articles about
massage and related topics)

Assorted products and services:

Khepra Foot Balm—A preparation for use in massaging the feet, that creates a skin texture with a subtle resistance for better massage, eliminates foot odor, and conditions and refreshes the feet:

Khepra Skin Care, Inc.
3939 IDS Center
80 South Eighth Street
Minneapolis, MN 55402
1-800-367-9799

BodyCushion™ — a contoured system of support that positions the body comfortably, prone, supine or laterally; useful for pregnancy, geriatric, disabled, on-site and seated massage:

Body Support Systems, Inc.
P.O. Box 337
Ashland, OR 97520
1-800-448-2400
(541) 488-1172

Massage Table and on-site chair Selection Service (Service is free, and tables can be ordered at discount from retail):

Tablechoices
Mary Lou Clairmont
(718) 339-9163

Record-Keeping and Insurance Billing Assistance

Insurance Billing Service

Guides and coordinates your process of billing massage services to insurance providers:

CompuMed Billing
16172 Parkside Dr., Suite 101
Parker, CO 80134
(303) 840-7500

Massage Billing Services, David Dolan, LMT
3960 Coastal Hwy, Suite C
St. Augustine, FL 32905
(904) 826-1641

Books for the clinical bodyworker:

Insurance Reimbursement and Physician Referral by David Dolan, LMT, includes perforated forms you can customize with your letterhead. Available from David Dolan, c/o Southeastern School, (904) 448-9499 or (904) 826-1641

The Insurance Reimbursement Manual by Christine Rosche, M.P.H. The author is also available for telephone consultations. 1-800-888-1516

Hands Heal: Documentation for Massage Therapy: A Guide to SOAP Charting by Diana L. Thompson, LMP. $21.95 postpaid from Diana L. Thompson, Healing Arts Studio, 916 N.E. 64th St., Seattle, WA 98115 1-800-989-4743 extension 7 (Forms pack and teacher's manual also available)

Forms for Insurance Billing:

Carol Alfrey, LMT, Bodyworker Business Forms
P.O. Box 1016
Gainesville, GA 30503
1-800-295-7085

Chart notes, insurance billing information, HCFA #1500 claim forms

Computer programs that organize client and financial records and generate and track insurance billing:

The Therapist
L.G. Duffy Violante
297 Hull Ave.
Clintondale, NY 12515
(914) 883-7500 or 1-888-GO DUFFY (1-888-463-8339)

Magazines, Journals, Newsletters and Books

Magazines

Massage Magazine covers a broad range of news and features of general interest to massage practitioners. Each issue also contains up-to-date nationwide licensing information. Published six times a year. Subscriptions 1-800-533-4263

AMTA's *Massage Therapy Journal*, available by subscription to non-members, contains articles of interest to the general massage community, and items of special interest to AMTA members. Published four times a year. Subscriptions (847) 864-0123

ABMP's *Massage & Bodywork* Magazine, available by subscription to non-members, contains articles of interest to the general massage community, and items of special interest to ABMP members. Published four times a year. Subscriptions (303) 674-8478

Journals

The Journal of Soft Tissue Manipulation This is an international, multidisciplinary journal highlighting research, clinical change, aspects of the client/practitioner relationship, precautions and contraindications, and philosophical issues concerning massage and related disciplines. It is a publication of the Ontario (Canada) Massage Therapist Association. Subscriptions (416) 968-6487

Newsletters

Hands-On Digest is a quarterly resource of continuing education nationwide for massage therapists and bodyworkers. It also plans to feature educator profiles, class reviews, and book and product reviews. HandsOn Digest, 143 Tiernan Avenue, Warwick, RI 02886, (401) 739-0685.

The Portable Practitioner A worldwide resource and networking guide for health and healing arts professionals, this is a quarterly newsletter that emphasizes travel, work and study overseas and in the US. Subscribers are able to place free classifieds and also have access to a job hotline. Subscriptions 1-800-968-2877 or (616) 347-8591, P.O. Box 2095, Petosky, MI 49770, www.cybersytes.com/portprac.

The Professional Bodyworker Newsletter is aimed at the clinical bodywork practitioner. It focuses on changes in state laws, insurance policies and practitioner interviews. Published twice a year. Subscriptions 1-800-888-1516

The Rub is a newsletter advocating against licensure or certification of massage and bodywork. Free sample issue. The Rub, P.O. Box 459, Berkeley, CA 94701.

Touchpoints This is the quarterly publication of the Touch Research Institute, Tiffany M. Field, Ph.D., director. The publication reports on the work of the Touch Research Institute in scientifically documenting the health benefits of touch, and also provides information on programs sponsored by the Institute. Subscriptions are $10.00 per year. Touchpoints/Touch Research Institute, Department of Pediatrics (D820), University of Miami School of Medicine, P.O. Box 016820, Miami, FL 33101, (305) 243-6781.

Books for Bodyworkers

The library of books for massage and bodywork seems to grow by the day. The books in the following list were selected because they can assist you with the *career* of massage.

Self-Care Books

Save Your Hands! by Lauriann Greene. This book covers reasons for injury, common injuries, how to use your body, techniques to use or avoid, exercises, stretching and treatment. It retails for $17.95. Published by Infinity Press, P.O. Box 17883, Seattle, WA 98107, 1-800-313-9716.

The Ultimate Hand Book by Maja Evans, CMT, DH. This book focuses on self-care for the massage therapist or bodyworker, offering guidance on such subjects as physical, psychological and psychic self-care, burnout, abundance and success. Available from Laughing Duck Press (415) 221-5530

National Certification Review Books:

The Book by Cal Cooley, L.M.T. This book aims to coach you through passing national or local certification tests. Spiral-bound, 150 pages plus appendix, also available in two-videotape format. Available from Southwest Myotherapies 1-800-263-9646

Complete Review Guide for National & State Certification Examinations by Dr. Patrick Barron. This book is designed as a review to use in preparation for exams. Spiral bound, 178 pages plus Appendix. For information contact Oviedo Physical Medicine & Rehab., Inc., 27 Tomoka Dr., Oviedo, FL, 32765, (407) 672-1140.

Pathology for Massage and Bodywork

Recognizing Health and Illness, Pathology for Massage Therapists and Bodyworkers by Sharon Burch. This oversize textbook is well-organized, with each chapter covering a physiological system. It contains illustrations, study questions, references and chapter reviews. It is available from Health Positive! Publishing, 1510 E. 1584 Road, Lawrence, KS 66046, fax (785) 841-1761.

Pathology A to Z, a Handbook for Massage Therapists by Kalyani Premkumar, M.D. This book is arranged alphabetically. For each pathology, it discusses the cause, signs & symptoms, risk factors, cautions & recommendations, and notes. Published by VanPub Books, 2132 Crowchild Trail, N.W., Calgary, AB, T2M 3Y7, Canada, (403) 220-0632.

Networking, Marketing and Promotional Services

The Quiet Touch International Massage Network
1-800-946-2772
4421 121 Terrace North
Royal Palm Beach, FL 33411
www.massageinc.com

Accepts: Licensed Massage Therapists with current membership in AMTA, ABMP, IMA or you can get corporate discounts through The Quiet Touch from ABMP.

Service Provided: The company markets massage and makes agreements to provide massage services to clients in hotels, offices, health spas, the company's own massage offices and clients' homes. The company started in New York, spread quickly to New Jersey, Connecticut and Florida, and now has clients in all 50 states, and in foreign countries.

Clients schedule appointments through the company's 800 number and participating massage therapists are told where and when to report to fill these appointments. The therapist receives up to 70% of the fee paid by the client. Therapists need not have their own office to participate. Therapists are charged a $250.00 annual fee to participate.

ASSOCIATED MTs℠
Bruria Ginton, LicMT
212-222-4240
www.amts.org

Membership Categories: Active, Student and Supportive.

Service Provided: This is a co-operative promotional, mentoring and advocacy network, created in NYC, 1992, to enhance the reputation, professional status and economic opportunities for licensed massage therapists. The organization maintains a website and places advertisements in national publications. Active members are included in the online global directory, MTs NEAR YOU™. They can use the company logo and other promotional materials. In addition, members may also participate in online and offline co-operative promotions in which several massage therapists share the cost of a specific promotional effort.

Active Membership dues: $120.00 first year, $65.00 per year renewal
Student Membership: $25 per year, upgrade to Active Membership at renewal rate.

1-888-MASSAGE
As of the publication date for this edition, this marketing company was in the formation stages. The company expects to market massage nationwide through this toll-free number and to employ a network of massage practitioners to provide massage services.

VI

Bodywork
Organizations
and
Trainings

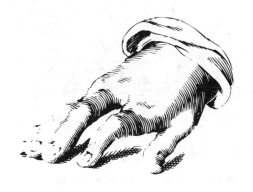

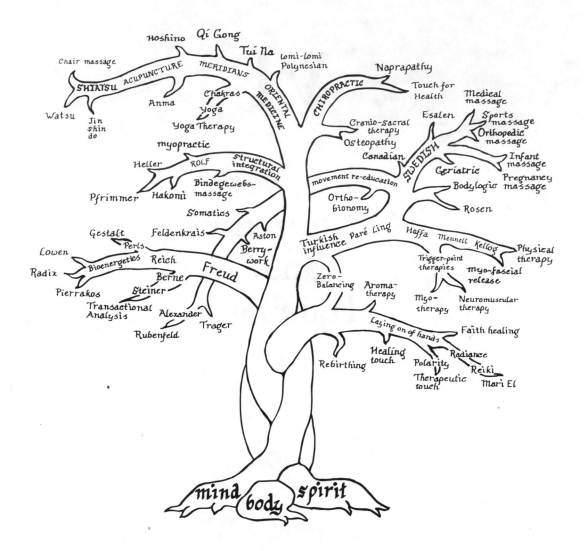

The Bodywork Tree © 1999

Based on a concept by David Linton

Bodywork Systems, Organizations and Trainings

For purposes of this Directory, "bodywork" refers to a body-centered therapy that is different from Swedish massage.

Some of the forms listed below are very similar to Swedish massage—for example, sports massage, Esalen, pregnancy massage. Some are entirely different from Swedish massage—for example, Alexander Technique, Reiki, Somatics Psychology.

For each form of bodywork, the listing includes a brief explanation of the nature of the work, the name and address of an official organization representing the form (if any) and a list of schools that offer instruction in that form of bodywork. Massage schools are listed by their code numbers in the State-by-State directory. Schools may teach these forms of bodywork as part of their massage training program, or as continuing education, or as an advanced training. Contact individual schools for more specific information.

New forms of bodywork are continually created as imaginative and dedicated bodyworkers explore their own unique gifts and systematize their work. Factors that go into the decision to include a form in this directory include how long the form has been in existence, how widely it is practiced, and whether it is taught in mainstream massage schools.

Forms appearing for the first time in this edition are: Berrywork, Bowen Technique, Canadian Deep Muscle Massage, Colon Hydrotherapy, Facial Rejuvenation, Geriatric Massage, Healing Touch, Jin Shin Jyutsu, Myopractic, Orthopedic Massage, Qi Gong, Spa Treatments, Thai Massage, Tui Na, Vibrational Healing Massage Therapy, and Yoga Therapy.

Acupressure

See Shiatsu

Alexander Technique

The Alexander technique is an educational method for improving coordination, and for developing awareness of unnecessary tensions in the body.

F. M. Alexander was an actor who had a problem with losing his voice. By studying his habitual movements in a mirror, he discovered ways he was using his body that created his vocal problem and was able to resolve the difficulty. He went on to create a system for enhancing balance, posture and the use of the body, which is called the Alexander Technique. Practitioners refer to themselves as teachers of the Alexander method and refer to sessions as lessons.

The following schools offer some training in Alexander: 62, 113, 125, 145, 149, 155, 255, 336, 386, 409, 449, 452, 458, 536, 537, 538, 546, 572

AMMA® Therapy (or ANMA)

AMMA therapy is a method of restoring the flow of life energy in the body, and is used to treat a wide range of medical conditions. It combines Oriental medical principles with a Western approach to organ dysfunction. AMMA Therapy may include dietary plans, detoxification, herbs and vitamins, and therapeutic exercises.

AMMA or AMNA is taught at schools 13, 69, 136, 145, 193, 203, 222, 263, 338, 351, 374, 382, 402, 421, 543, 544, 552.

Applied Kinesiology (see also Touch for Health)

Applied Kinesiology is a technique used mainly by chiropractors to gain diagnostic information through muscle testing and to strengthen muscles to aid in structural correction. Muscles are related to specific organs or systems through the acupuncture meridian network.

The following schools offer training in applied kinesiology: 3, 4, 12, 20, 29, 30, 37, 39, 50, 67, 79, 86, 106, 108, 110, 117, 120, 125, 126, 129, 131, 132, 136, 142, 145, 149, 159, 160, 175, 179, 181, 191, 192, 193, 196, 203, 207, 210, 216, 219, 221, 230, 232, 246, 249, 255, 257, 263, 266, 271, 272, 273, 303, 304, 316, 320, 321, 347, 357, 362, 367, 369, 378, 379, 380, 384, 393, 394, 402, 422, 435, 436, 437, 442, 452, 465, 469, 473, 476, 524, 525, 529, 531, 533, 536, 540, 542, 544, 546, 569.

Aromatherapy

Aromatherapy involves working with aroma as a healing modality by using pure essential oils, each distilled from a single botanical source. Aromatherapy is often done in conjunction with massage, but not always.

Professional Associations—Aromatherapy

**The American Alliance
of Aromatherapy**
P.O. Box 309
Depoe Bay, OR 97341
1-800-809-9850
www.aaoa.org

**National Association for
Holistic Aromatherapy (NAHA)**
P.O. Box 17622
Boulder, CO 80308-7622
1-888-ASK-NAHA (1-888-275-6242)
www.naha.org

Journals—Aromatherapy

**The International Journal
of Aromatherapy**
P.O. Box 309
Depoe Bay, OR 97341
1-800-809-9850

Aromatherapy Quarterly
P.O. Box 421
Inverness, CA 94937-0421
(415) 663-9519

The Aromatic Thymes
18-4 E. Dundee Road, Suite 200
Barrington, IL 60010
(847) 526-0456

Aromatherapy World
c/o ISPA, ISPA House
82 Ashby Road
Hinckley, Leics. LE10 1SN, England
Tel: 011-44-1455-637987

Aromatherapy Times
Stamford House
2-4 Chiswick High Road
London W4 1TH, England
Tel: 011-44-181-742-2605

The Aromatherapist
Essentia House
Upper Bond Street
Hinckley, Leics. LE10 1RS, England
Tel: 011-44-1455-615466

Suppliers of essential oils

There are many suppliers of essential oils. Some of the massage oil companies listed on pages 181-183 also supply essential oils. The companies listed below have been recommended by practitioners as having a good reputation in the industry and supplying good quality oils:

Amrita Aromatherapy Inc.
1900 W. Stone
Fairfield, IA 52556
(515) 472-9136

Changes Within
P.O. Box 326
Freeburg PA 17827
(717) 374-6735
www.sunlink.net/~changes/

Elizabeth Van Buren, Inc.
P.O. Box 7542
Santa Cruz, CA 95061
(Showroom: 303 Potrero St., #33)
1-800-710-7759 or (408) 425-8218

Leydet Aromatics
PO Box 2345
Fair Oaks, CA 95628
(916) 965-7546
http://leydet.com

Nature's Gifts Custom Aromatherapy
1040 Cheyenne Blvd.
Madison, TN 37115
(615) 612-4270
www.naturesgift.com

Prima Fleur
1525 E. Francisco Blvd., Suite 16
San Rafael, CA 94901
(415) 455-0957

Snow Lotus Inc.
P.O. Box 1824
Boulder, CO 80306
(303) 443-9289

Warren Botanicals
75-1027 Henry St., #111A
Kailua-Kona, HI 96740 (808) 325-7900
Distributor: Kathy Ziola, 708 Ivy Place
Grand Junction, CO 81506
(970) 245-7172 (9:00 to 6:00 Mountain time)

Fragrant Earth
2000 Second Ave., Ste. 206
Seattle, WA 98121
(206) 374-8773 or 1-800-260-7401
www.fragrantearth.com

Natura & Isha Essentials
27134A Paseo Espada, Suite 323
San Juan Capistrano, CA 92675
1-800-933-1008

Original Swiss Aromatics
P.O. Box 6842
San Rafael, CA 94903
(415) 459-3998

Samara Botane
300 Queen Anne Ave. N, Ste 378
Seattle, WA 98109
(206) 282-4532

Time Laboratories
P.O. Box 3243
South Pasadena, CA 91031
(208) 232-5250

Aromatherapy trainings

The following schools offer training in aromatherapy: 3, 4, 8, 10, 12, 13, 14, 17, 24, 36, 37, 38, 39, 41, 43, 50, 53, 56, 67, 71, 75, 81, 82, 85, 86, 89, 90, 94, 95, 97, 104, 106, 108, 110, 112, 113, 116, 118, 120, 123, 124, 125, 129, 136, 138, 139, 143, 145, 149, 157, 159, 160, 163, 170, 174, 175, 177, 178, 179, 181, 185, 190, 191, 192, 193, 196, 202, 203, 204, 207, 210, 211, 215, 216, 217, 219, 223, 230, 231, 232, 238, 239, 241, 243, 246, 254, 255, 257, 259, 260, 263, 264, 266, 268, 270, 279, 294, 304, 305, 307, 316, 321, 325, 333, 336, 337, 338, 341, 347, 349, 350, 353, 355, 357, 359, 361, 362, 364, 367, 369, 371, 374, 379, 380, 381, 382, 386, 388, 391, 392, 393, 394, 396, 402, 409, 415, 416, 419, 422, 429, 434, 435, 436, 437, 439, 442, 443, 444, 445, 446, 448, 449, 452, 454, 456, 463, 465, 468, 469, 470, 472, 473, 476, 492, 499, 501, 503, 504, 506, 520, 524, 525, 526, 531, 533, 536, 541, 542, 544, 547, 548, 549, 550, 552, 558, 569, 570.

In addition, Aromatherapy trainings are offered at the following locations:

CA: **Pacific Institute of Aromatherapy**, P.O. Box 903, San Rafael, CA 94915, (415) 479-9121

FL: **Atlantic Institute of Aromatherapy**, 16018 Saddlestring Dr., Tampa, FL 33618, (813) 265-2222

    Oil Lady Aromatherapy, 764 12th Avenue South, Naples, FL 34102, (941) 263-3451

    The National Coalition of Certified Aromatherapist and Aromatologist Practitioners (NCCAAP), P.O. Box 835025, Miami, FL 33283, (305) 595-4776

NJ: **Institute of Aromatherapy**, 3108 Route 10 West, Denville, NJ 07834, (201) 989-1999
www.aromatherapy4u.com

OR: **Australian College of Herbal Studies**, P.O. Box 57, Lake Oswego, OR 97034
1-800-48-STUDY (1-800-487-8839), www.herbed.com

WA: **Institute of Dynamic Aromatherapy**, 2000 Second Ave., Ste. 206, Seattle, WA 98121
(206) 374-8773 or 1-800-260-7401, www.fragrantearth.com

Aston-Patterning®

Aston-Patterning aims to increase the body's grace, resiliency and ease of movement by releasing layers of tension throughout the body. It uses movement education, bodywork, environmental design and fitness training. For information about trainings and certification, contact:

Aston-Patterning
P.O. Box 3568
Incline Village, NV 89450
(702) 831-8228

Aston-patterning is also taught at schools 143, 145 and 544.

Berrywork

This bodywork was created by the late Lauren Berry, PT. He was a contemporary of Trager, Feldenkrais and Rolf who devised a system of "correctives" that involve stretches and that work the fascia, cartilage and joints. His work is passed on through the teaching of his advanced students.

The following schools offer training in Berrywork: 193, 391, 426, 429, 544.

Bindegewebsmassage

Bindegewebsmassage is a type of connective tissue massage originated in Germany. It is an adjunctive therapy in the treatment of organic and musculo-skeletal disorders.

Bindegewebsmassage is taught at Schools 177, 193, 202, 276, 382, 396, 468, 532, 550, 551.
Also teaching Bindegewebsmassage is:

Patricia M. Donohue
Wholistic Pathways
152 N. Wellwood Ave., ste. 5
Lindenhurst, NY 11757
(516) 226-3898

Bioenergetics

Bioenergetics was created by Alexander Lowen, M.D., an outgrowth of his work with Wilhelm Reich, M.D. Bioenergetics is a way of understanding personality in terms of the body and its energetic processes. Bioenergetics therapy works with the mind and the body to release chronic stresses and chronic muscular tensions.

Dr. Lowen has written 14 books. An excellent introduction to bioenergetics is *Bioenergetics*, available at most bookstores and libraries.

For a brochure listing centers, workshops and books about bioenergetics, contact:

International Institute for Bioenergetic Analysis
144 E. 36th St.,
New York, NY 10016
(212) 532-7742

Bioenergetics is also taught at schools 52, 123, 145, 177, 307, 330, 355, 375, 393, 436, 449, 452, 540, 544.

Biokinetics/Hanna Somatics

Biokinetics uses a composite of techniques for rehabilitation through neuromuscular retraining. It is designed to release chronic muscular contraction and restore voluntary control of the muscular system. For complete information about Biokinetics and training, contact:

Biokinetics/Hanna Somatics
115 N. 5th St., suite 330
Grand Junction, CO 81501
(970) 245-4370

Biokinetics/Hanna Somatics is taught at schools 221, 550.

Body Logic^{SM}

Body Logic is a system of bodywork and body understanding developed by Yamuna Zake. It uses the principle of "space making" whereby space is created around joints and locked areas to allow the body to unfold and finds its own balance, enhancing freedom of movement, posture, strength and energy. For information on Body Logic, trainings and practitioners, contact:

Body Logic
295 West 11th Street, apt. 1F
New York, NY 10014
(212) 633-2143

Body Logic is taught at schools 75, 544.

Body-Mind (also see "Somatics")

"Body-mind" is a term used to acknowledge the intimate connection between the state of the mind and the state of the body. This is an awareness that is present in most forms of massage and bodywork, and many massage schools teach massage from a "body-mind" perspective. However, some forms make it the focus of the work. The programs listed below are designed as advanced programs for massage therapists, and focus on the body-mind connection.

Body Synergy Institute, Inc.
305 Bangor Rd.
Bala Cynwyd, PA 19004
(610) 667-3070

Curriculum includes deep tissue bodywork, body reading, using a floor-length mirror as an educational tool, working with postural history and attitudes, and using your body with awareness and case.

School for Body-Mind Centering
189 Pond View Dr.
Amherst, MA 01002
(413) 256-8615

The school, founded by Bonnie Bainbridge Cohen, offers introductory and certification training programs in many locations. The course includes study of the body systems and how they support and initiate movement, as well as movement re-education to correct problems at their root level.

Somatic Therapy Institute
546 Harkle Road, suite B
Santa Fe, New Mexico 87501
(505) 983-9695

Short intensives for CEU credit for psychologists, nurses and massage therapists.

The following schools include body-mind in their curriculum: 8, 10, 13, 26, 30, 39, 40, 41, 62, 69, 85, 95, 106, 108, 110, 112, 120, 124, 125, 126, 129, 132, 143, 145, 159, 165, 177, 180, 181, 202, 206, 207, 211, 216, 219, 220, 221, 223, 224, 232, 246, 278, 304, 307, 314, 316, 330, 336, 338, 355, 359, 369, 376, 377, 378, 380, 386, 393, 394, 417, 422, 436, 442, 468, 470, 473, 475, 482, 503, 506, 524, 533, 540, 542, 544, 546, 548, 550, 569.

Bowen Technique

This technique was developed in Australia by Thomas Bowen. It combines energy work with gentle soft tissue manipulation. www.bowtech.com is the home page of the founders of the Bowen Therapy Academy of Australia.

Bowen technique is taught at schools 36, 85, 113, 145, 165, 540.

Breema

Breema takes its name from the Kurdish mountain village of Breemava where it originated and was passed down from generation to generation. It is a comprehensive system of bodywork, done on the floor, with a variety of techniques ranging from simple holding points on the body to techniques requiring flexibility and dexterity. This work is taught at:

The Breema Center
6076 Claremont Ave.
Oakland, CA 94618
(510) 428-0937

Breema is also taught at Schools 43, 50, 53, 71, 94, 421.

Canadian Deep Muscle Massage

This work was created by Will Green, founder of the International Massage Association (IMA Group) and owner of Georgetown Bodyworks in Washington, DC. It is derived from a system of cross-fiber massage that began in northern Canada in the 1940's. Will added insights gained from the works of Therese Pfrimmer, Joseph Pliates, Ida Rolf, Dr. Samuel West, and Debra Smith.

Canadian deep muscle massage is taught at schools 154, 301, 390. Canadian deep tissue massage is taught at school 232.

Chair Massage (or on-site or seated massage)

This refers to a brief bodywork session, usually a shiatsu-based routine, done in a special chair in which the client sits facing toward the cushions, exposing the scalp, shoulders, neck, back and hips. Sessions may last between five and thirty minutes.

Originally pioneered as "on-site massage", a modality for the workplace, it has expanded into many other environments. Chair massage is now offered in storefronts, health food stores, airports, airplanes, health fairs, grand openings, sporting events, and other locations. It has therefore come to be called "chair massage" or "seated massage" instead of "on-site."

Because of the relatively low cost of a brief session, it is more affordable than the usual full-body massage. Because it is done fully clothed, it attracts some clients who would be too uncomfortable for table massage. Because it is done in locations where the client is already present, it is more convenient than table massage. For all these reasons, the practice of chair massage has grown so fast that many of the massage table companies report they are selling more on-site chairs than massage tables. The large number of massage schools including chair massage in their curriculum (see below) is another indication of the popularity and wide-spread acceptance of this branch of the profession.

The following schools offer training in chair massage, seated massage, or on-site massage: 3, 4, 8, 9, 11, 12, 13, 14, 17, 20, 23, 24, 29, 30, 31, 33, 36, 37, 38, 41, 43, 47, 49, 50, 51, 52, 53, 56, 57, 60, 61, 63, 64, 67, 69, 75, 76, 77, 79, 81, 82, 85, 86, 89, 91, 94, 95, 104, 106, 108, 110, 112, 113, 116, 117, 120, 124, 125, 126, 129, 131, 132, 136, 137, 139, 140, 144, 145, 149, 155, 157, 159, 160, 163, 165, 169, 170, 172, 174, 175, 177, 178, 179, 180, 181, 185, 190, 191, 192, 193, 196, 201, 202, 203, 204, 207, 209, 210, 211, 216, 219, 223, 226, 268, 270, 271, 272, 273, 276, 277, 278, 279, 285, 292, 296, 304, 305, 307, 314, 315, 318, 320, 321, 325, 327, 333, 334, 336, 337, 338, 341, 344, 347, 350, 351, 356, 357, 359, 360, 361, 362, 364, 365, 366, 367, 369, 370, 374, 377, 378, 379, 380, 381, 382, 384, 386, 388, 391, 393, 394, 396, 405, 409, 412, 415, 416, 417, 418, 419, 421, 422, 423, 424, 426, 427, 429, 430, 432, 434, 435, 436, 437, 439, 442, 444, 445, 448, 449, 452, 454, 456, 458, 459, 464, 465, 466, 467, 468, 469, 470, 471, 472, 473, 475, 476, 481, 482, 483, 487, 497, 499, 011, 501, 503, 504, 506, 515, 516, 520, 522, 524, 525, 526, 519, 531, 533, 536, 538, 541, 554, 546, 547, 548, 549, 550, 551, 557, 558, 560, 562, 563, 564, 567, 568, 569, 570, 571, 572.

Two companies conduct workshops on chair massage technique and marketing. These are:

TouchPro Chair Massage Seminars 1-800-999-5026
Instructors certified and supervised by David Palmer

Seated Massage Experience® 1-800-868-2448 / 1-800-TOUCH-4-U
Workshops are taught by Raymond Blaylock

Chi gong
See Qi gong

Colon Hydrotherapy (also called colonics or high colonics or colonic irrigation)

A cleansing procedure for the colon, using purified water at controlled temperature and controlled pressure, providing a gentle, deep cleansing of the colon. Practitioners often use massage, reflexology or visceral manipulation skills during a session. Of the 50 states, only Florida licenses colon hydrotherapy. Certification is available through:

International Association of Colon HydroTherapy
P.O. Box 461285
San Antonio, TX 78246
(210) 366-2888
www.healthy.net/iact.

Cranio-Sacral Therapy (also called cranial-sacral)

A technique for finding and correcting cerebral and spinal imbalances or blockages that may cause sensory, motor or intellectual dysfunction. Practitioners work with the subtle articulations of skull sutures, and the flow of cerebro-spinal fluid.

Cranio-sacral techniques are taught at the following schools: 3, 4, 10, 12, 13, 16, 23, 26, 29, 39, 41, 44, 47, 49, 50, 52, 53, 56, 57, 61, 67, 69, 71, 73, 75, 91, 95, 104, 106, 110, 112, 113, 117, 124, 126, 129, 132, 136, 139, 145, 155, 159, 165, 168, 170, 175, 177, 178, 179, 181, 190, 192, 193, 196, 201, 206, 209, 210, 211, 215, 216, 218, 219, 223, 226, 239, 241, 245, 246, 255, 257, 260, 263, 264, 270, 271, 272, 273, 279, 285, 292, 294, 298, 303, 304, 305, 307, 313, 316, 320, 321, 325, 336, 337,

346, 349, 350, 353, 356, 362, 366, 369, 370, 371, 374, 377, 379, 382, 386, 394, 407, 409, 415, 417, 418, 422, 424, 434, 435, 436, 441, 442, 449, 452, 466, 469, 473, 499, 501, 503, 506, 516, 524, 525, 526, 529, 533, 536, 538, 540, 544, 546, 548, 550, 551, 569, 570, 572.

In addition, Cranio-sacral techniques are taught by the following institutions:

Colorado Cranial Institute
1080 Hawthorne Ave.
Boulder, CO 80304
(303) 449-0322

National Institute of Craniosacral Studies, Inc.
7827 N. Armenia Av.
Tampa, FL 33604-3806
1-888-824-7025 or (813) 933-6335

Shea Educational Group
13878 Oleander Avenue
Juno Beach, FL 33408
1-800-717-SHEA(7432)
or (516) 627-3727

The Upledger Institute
11211 Prosperity Farms Road
Palm Beach Gardens, FL 33410
(561) 622-4334

Equine Sports Massage

Massage or other bodywork can adapted to horses for the purpose of enhancing performance and preventing injuries. This field has recently been developed and shows signs of gaining rapidly in popularity, as breeders are interested in any techniques that can give them a competitive edge.

According to Jack Meagher, author of *Beating Muscle Injuries for Horses* (available Horse Muscle Injuries, 667 Weathersfield St., Rowley, MA 01969), the practitioner applies techniques of human massage, especially sports massage, to horses. A pioneer in the fields of sports massage and equine sports massage, Jack Meagher turned to working with horses as a way of proving the value of sports massage techniques for athletes. By using the techniques on horses and achieving demonstrable results, he was able to rebut the contention that results with humans were due to psychological factors.

An instructional video about equine sports massage is available for $49.95 postpaid from Equissage, P.O. Box 447, Round Hill, VA 22141, 1-800-843-0224 or (540) 338-1917. At the same phone number, you can get information about the International Association of Equine Sports Massage Therapists, and about their quarterly newsletter "Stable Talk." Their educational program is listed below.

Equine sports massage is taught at the following locations:

Equinology, 13933 Village Ave. / P.O. Box 928, Windsor, CA 95492
(707) 431-8276, www.equinology.com

Equissage School, 15715 Southern Cross Lane / P.O. Box 447, Round Hill, VA 20141
1-800-843-0224 or (540) 338-1917

EquiTouch Systems, Rocky Mountain Lazy J Bar S Ranch / P.O. Box 7701,
Loveland, CO 80537, 1-800-483-0577 or (970) 635-0479

Optissage, 7041 Zane Trail Road, Circleville, OH 43113, 1-800-251-0007.

TT.E.A.M.SM Training International, P.O. Box 3793, Santa Fe., NM 87501,
(505) 455-2945 (Tellington-Touch Equine Awareness Method)

In addition, the following schools offer training in equine massage: 3, 4, 13, 129, 132, 145, 163, 170, 175, 178, 179, 192, 203, 226, 242, 260, 271, 279, 285, 336, 346, 349, 350, 402, 415, 436.

Esalen® Massage

Esalen is a variant of Swedish massage pioneered at Esalen Institute in Big Sur, California. Esalen is the place where many therapies were tested or launched in the 60's and 70's, including gestalt therapy and rolfing. The unique brand of massage practiced there typically involves total nudity and long flowing stokes. Esalen is known for its original, honest, nurturing and probing atmosphere. Esalen massage tends to be nurturing, trance-like and meditative, allowing the greatest possible unfoldment to take place in the client. For information contact:

Esalen Institute
Big Sur, CA 93920
(408) 667-3000

Esalen massage is taught at the following schools: 3, 4, 13, 14, 23, 28, 30, 44, 45, 47, 48, 51, 52, 53, 59, 60, 61, 62, 64, 69, 71, 73, 79, 81, 82, 85, 86, 94, 104, 124, 125, 138, 140, 175, 192, 202, 214, 219, 220, 221, 241, 249, 314, 315, 318, 326, 330, 336, 347, 348, 350, 369, 392, 428, 432, 466, 467, 468, 469, 471, 473, 483, 516, 527, 540, 541, 544.

Facial Rejuvenation

This bodywork was developed by Linda Burnham, N.D. It involves sculpting the face and affecting the twelve major nerve centers on the head. On another level, it involves shedding beliefs and thoughts that aren't ours and the emotions that no longer serve us. Professional certification is in three phases. For complete information contact:

Burnham Systems Facial RejuvenationSM
369 Montezuma, Suite 346
Santa Fe, NM 87501
(505) 989-1807

Feldenkrais®

Moshe Feldendrais was an Israeli physicist who began developing this system in mid-life. Feldenkrais work emphasizes having a coherent body image and thinking a movement through. It also uses micro-movements for neuromuscular re-education. The system is most effective for pain relief, and also promotes grace and ease of movement. For further information contact:

The Feldenkrais Guild of North America
524 Ellsworth St, SW / P.O. Box 489
Albany, OR 97321
1-800-775-2118

Some training in Feldenkrais is offered at the following schools: 71, 125, 129, 145, 149, 180, 181, 193, 219, 221, 232, 295, 316, 336, 374, 409, 422, 439, 442, 452, 458, 471, 524, 525, 527, 544, 546, 550, 568.

Geriatric Massage

Working with the elderly and the ill, often in a long-term care setting. A therapist doing geriatric massage should understand the physical and psychological characteristics of aging, and should also be familiar with the diseases that commonly afflict the elderly. Some resources in the field of geriatric massage are:

Daybreak Geriatric Massage Project, P.O. Box 1815, Sebastopol, CA 95473
(707) 829-2798, fax 829-2799 (videos and books available)

Irene Smith, Service Through Touch, c/o Inlight Productions, P.O. Box 1493
Kihei, HI 96753, 1-800-537-6767 (video and audio tapes available)

AllenTouch Productions, 706 S. Fremont, San Mateo, CA 94402
(650) 340-7885 (Videos and books available)

Foundation for Long Term Care, 150 State Street, Albany, NY 12207
(Carol Hegemen, Director).

Geriatric massage is taught at schools 11, 33, 36, 38, 43, 53, 67, 97, 124, 139, 145, 163, 170, 215, 217, 229, 231, 241, 263, 279, 313, 314, 326, 349, 350, 360, 361, 362, 365, 373, 393, 407, 417, 419, 439, 445, 449, 452, 456, 466, 475, 524, 543.

Hakomi bodywork

Hakomi bodywork regards body, mind and spirit as one, and blends bodywork and psychotherapy into a simultaneous process. The work serves to lead a person to an awareness of limitations in his physical and psychological patterns, bringing the possibility of new openness and freedom.

Hakomi Integrative Somatics is taught at schools 62, 94, 125, 132, 181, 221, 224, 316, 377, 386, 427, 544.

Healing Touch www.healingtouch.net.

Healing touch is an energy-based, hands-on technique done to balance and align the human energy field. The technique is approved by the American Holistic Nurses Association. Information about the technique, trainings, and organization membership can be obtained from:

Healing Touch International, Inc.
198 Union Boulevard, Suite 202
Lakewood, Colorado 80228
(303) 989-7982

Healing Touch is taught at the following schools: 10, 11, 14, 26, 41, 49, 57, 77, 85, 94, 95, 126, 129, 132, 136, 145, 157, 159, 178, 181, 196, 202, 209, 215, 221, 226, 231, 232, 246, 255, 271, 272, 273, 303, 305, 308, 314, 316, 318, 320, 321, 338, 341, 355, 369, 394, 415, 436, 442, 456, 470, 476, 538, 540, 544, 546, 548, 550, 567, 569.

Hellerwork® www.hellerwork.com

Hellerwork is an outgrowth of Rolfing (see below), created by Joseph Heller. It integrates movement and verbal communication with connective tissue work. Information about Hellerwork can be obtained from:

Hellerwork, Inc.
406 Berry Street
Mt. Shasta, CA 96067
(530) 926-2500

The following schools offer partial or complete training in Hellerwork: 458, 544, 550, 555.

Hoshino Therapy

A unique system of acupressure for the treatment of musculo-skeletal pain and sports injuries; physical fitness exercises are taught to complement the therapy. The training is offered in weekend workshops and intensives.

Training in Hoshino Therapy is offered at Schools 174, 529, 544.

Hydrotherapy

See Spa Treatments

Infant Massage

Infant massage instructors teach parents the art of infant massage. Trainings are offered to certify people as infant massage instructors. For information, contact:

International Association of Infant Massage
1-800-248-5432 or (415) 752-4920

International Loving Touch Foundation, Inc.
P.O. Box 16374
Portland, OR 97292
(503) 253-8482

Infant massage is taught at the following schools: 3, 4, 8, 10, 11, 12, 13, 16, 29, 30, 33, 36, 37, 38, 39, 56, 61, 67, 69, 85, 91, 95, 112, 120, 126, 129, 131, 132, 134, 136, 145, 155, 159, 160, 163, 165, 170, 174, 175, 178, 179, 180, 181, 191, 192, 193, 201, 203, 204, 210, 216, 229, 231, 241, 242, 243, 245, 246, 255, 259, 260, 261, 266, 270, 271, 276, 277, 279, 292, 304, 305, 307, 314, 315, 318, 325, 329, 334, 336, 337, 338, 341, 349, 350, 356, 359, 362, 366, 370, 375, 376, 377, 379, 380, 381, 382, 384, 388, 393, 394, 396, 402, 407, 409, 416, 422, 424, 426, 429, 435, 436, 445, 448, 452, 456, 463, 470, 471, 473, 476, 481, 497, 504, 508, 515, 524, 525, 526, 527, 531, 533, 548, 550, 563, 564, 567, 570, 572.

Jin Shin Do®

Jin Shin Do is a synthesis of acupressure theory, psychology, taoist philosophy, and breathing methods, which helps release physical and emotional tensions and armoring. The Jin Shin Do Foundation has information about trainings and practitioners, as well as books, charts, videos and audiotapes.

Jin Shin Do Foundation for Bodymind Acupressure
1084G San Miguel Canyon Rd.
Watsonville, CA 95076
(408) 763-7702

Jin Shin Do is taught at the following schools: 10, 13, 30, 66, 79, 86, 91, 106, 123, 124, 125, 129, 145, 159, 165, 193, 222, 241, 255, 263, 270, 347, 351, 442, 529, 538, 542, 544, 548, 569, 571.

Jin Shin Jyutsu®

This is an ancient art promoting harmony of life energy and the body. It was revived and systematized in the early 1900's by Master Jiro Murai. It was brought to the US in the 1950's by Mary Burmeister. It is an energy technique done with a light touch, and is often used as a self-treatment. For further information contact:

Jin Shin Jyutsu, Inc.
8719 E. San Alberto
Scottsdale, AZ 85258
(602) 998-9331

Jin shin jyutsu is also taught at school 351.

Lymphatic drainage (manual lymphatic drainage^SM or MLD®)

The lymphatic system is a vital part of the immune system in the body. Lymphatic drainage massage assists the operation of the lymphatic system. The system was devised in the 1930's by a Danish massage therapist, Dr. Emil Vodder, and is popular and well established as a health modality in Germany and Austria. Two organizations certify practitioners and teachers of manual lymphatic drainage:

North American Vodder Association of Lymphatic Therapy™ (NAVALT®)
1-888-4-NAVALT (1-888-462-8258)

NAVALT has certified individuals in Florida, Ohio and Texas to offer trainings in manual lymphatic drainage and will supply contact information upon request.

LLS Academy of Lymphatic Studies
12651 West Sunrise Blvd., Suite 101
Sunrise, FL 33323
(954) 846-7855

LLS Academy offers six trainings per year, each 135 hours over 14 days, most often in New Jersey and Florida.

Also offering trainings in lymphatic drainage is:

Dana Wyrick, BA, RMT, LMT
Wyrick Institute and Clinic
P.O. Box 99745
San Diego, CA 92109
(619) 273-9764

The following schools offer training in lymphatic drainage massage: 11, 12, 13, 14, 23, 24, 27, 28, 30, 35, 36, 37, 39, 44, 45, 49, 50, 51, 52, 53, 56, 58, 67, 73, 75, 85, 86, 90, 91, 96, 104, 108, 112, 113, 116, 118, 124, 125, 126, 129, 132, 139, 145, 157, 163, 165, 170, 174, 177, 178, 181, 190, 196, 203, 207, 211, 216, 217, 218, 219, 222, 229, 238, 239, 241, 246, 249, 254, 255, 270, 271, 273, 277, 279, 292, 304, 305, 314, 318, 321, 333, 338, 341, 346, 349, 350, 362, 367, 370, 371, 372, 373, 375, 378, 379, 380, 393, 396, 409, 418, 424, 426, 429, 432, 433, 435, 436, 438, 442, 445, 452, 456, 458, 469, 470, 471, 473, 476, 481, 492, 506, 525, 529, 538, 541, 548, 549, 550, 551, 558, 562, 563, 568, 569, 572.

Medical Massage (clinical massage)

Working with injuries, pathologies and rehabilitation; working by physician's prescription. A program of instruction in medical massage is very desirable for a therapist interested in working in the health care system and obtaining insurance reimbursement for massage services. (See Chapter 20)

The following schools offer instruction in medical massage or clinical massage: 3, 4, 11, 13, 17, 23, 24, 33, 37, 39, 43, 44, 75, 76, 77, 81, 82, 86, 97, 106, 108, 110, 120, 125, 128, 132, 133, 139, 145, 149, 155, 160, 163, 165, 169, 172, 175, 179, 181, 184, 191, 192, 193, 196, 203, 204, 207, 210, 218, 219, 220, 223, 226, 245, 246, 259, 263, 269, 270, 271, 278, 279, 285, 298, 308, 313, 314, 321, 330, 336, 338, 341, 346, 347, 349, 351, 353, 355, 356, 357, 361, 362, 367, 368, 374, 377, 379, 380, 381, 384, 385, 393, 394, 396, 400, 402, 404, 413, 415, 417, 422, 432, 435, 436, 438, 444, 445, 467, 468, 469, 471, 475, 476, 481, 504, 532, 533, 543, 544, 548, 549, 550, 551, 558, 569.

Also offering certification in Medical Dysfunction is:

Kurashova Institute for Studies in Physical Medicine
P.O. Box 6246
Rock Island, IL 61201
(309) 786-4888

Myofascial Release

Myofascial release (MFR) is a technique for working with fascia as a means of achieving pain relief, restoring function and reducing stress. The system is taught in a series of seminars in various locations. It is designed to be used by massage therapists and physical therapists. For information about trainings contact:

John F. Barnes' MFR Seminars
Rts. 30 and 252, 10 S. Leopard Rd., Ste 1
Paoli, PA 19301-1569
1-800-FASCIAL
(610) 644-0136

The following schools offer training in myofascial techniques of one kind or another: 3, 4, 9, 10, 12, 13, 14, 16, 20, 23, 24, 29, 31, 33, 37, 50, 51, 58, 67, 81, 85, 86, 91, 106, 112, 115, 124, 126, 129, 131, 132, 133, 137, 138, 145, 149, 157, 159, 160, 163, 165, 169, 170, 175, 177, 178, 180, 181, 184, 186, 191, 192, 193, 201, 202, 203, 204, 206, 207, 210, 211, 215, 216, 218, 220, 222, 223, 226, 228, 229, 234, 242, 246, 249, 254, 255, 260, 264, 271, 273, 275, 276, 277, 278, 279, 283, 285, 292, 294, 296, 298, 303, 304, 305, 307, 314, 316, 318, 325, 330, 336, 338, 346, 347, 349, 355, 356, 357, 362, 367, 370, 372, 377, 379, 380, 382, 386, 388, 392, 396, 399, 401, 402, 405, 407, 412, 413, 417, 418, 420, 421, 424, 426, 429, 432, 434, 435, 436, 438, 442, 443, 445, 448, 449, 501, 503, 504, 516, 524, 525, 532, 533, 536, 537, 540, 544, 546, 548, 550, 551, 567, 569, 570, 571, 572.

Myopractic®

This is a system of posture balancing and deep relaxation developed and taught by Robert Petteway. The three basic techniques are 1. releasing tension and holding patterns; 2. clearing scar tissue, trigger points and other obstructions in soft tissue; and 3. separating to release myofascial adhesions and balance muscles. The practitioner does deep muscle therapy while keeping her own body and hands relaxed, and the system relieves chronic pain and postural imbalances. Trainings are offered through:

The Myopractic Institute
5644 Westheimer, Suite 217
Houston, TX 77056
(713) 869-5151

Myopractic is also taught at school 276.

Myotherapy℠

See Trigger Point Therapies

Neuromuscular Therapy

See Trigger Point Therapies

On-Site Massage

See Chair Massage

Ortho-Bionomy™

This system seeks to remind the body of its ability to find balance. The work involves positioning the client, working with points of tension in the body, and using movement. Results can include relieving pain, promoting emotional release, and improving structural alignment. For information, contact:

Society of Ortho-Bionomy International
P.O. Box 869
Madison, WI 53701-0869
1-800-743-4890

or

Northwest Center for Ortho-Bionomy
P.O. Box 70384
Seattle, WA 98107
(206) 783-5404

or

Lives Unlimited School of Healing Arts
401 Wisconsin Ave.
Madison, WI 53703
(608) 256-3733 www.ortho-bionomy.org

The following schools teach Ortho-Bionomy: 13, 23, 41, 47, 49, 64, 79, 94, 123, 139, 180, 181, 241, 336, 337, 374, 377, 382, 401, 409, 418, 449, 452, 464, 533, 548, 568, 569, 570.

Orthopedic Massage

This term is used by Whitney W. Lowe and Benny Vaughn to describe their work. Ten modalities are combined to create a comprehensive approach to the treatment of soft-tissue pain and injury conditions. The work shares some elements of sports massage and some elements of medical massage. The Institute offers a 100-hour certification program several times each year at various locations, and also publishes a newsletter "Orthopedic & Sports Massage Reviews." For further information, contact:

Orthopedic Massage Education & Research Institute
P.O. Box 1468
Bend, OR 97709
(541) 317-9855
www.omeri.com

Pfrimmer Deep Muscle Therapy®

Pfrimmer Deep Muscle Therapy is a system of corrective treatment to aid in the restoration of damaged muscles and soft tissue. It is intended to be used as one aspect of treatment for a wide range of muscular and soft-tissue conditions. Information is available from the Therese C. Pfrimmer International Association of Deep Muscle Therapists at 1-800-484-7773, ext. 7368.

The following schools offering Pfrimmer deep muscle therapy trainings: 10, 91, 110, 177, 207, 232, 242, 313, 448.

Polarity

Developed by Dr. Randolph Stone, polarity focuses on the energy currents that exist in all life. The polarity therapist uses her hands as conductors of energy. The intention is to balance the electromagnetic energy in the body, toward the ultimate goal of uniting the body, emotions, mind and soul.

Polarity is commonly taught in massage schools, but programs also exist to teach polarity that have no connection to massage schools. Although many massage schools offer an introduction to polarity as part of their training, few offer a substantial amount of training.

The American Polarity Therapy Association (APTA) is a non-profit organization that distributes educational material, registers practitioners, hosts educational conferences and publishes a regular newsletter. The APTA also certifies schools as meeting their educational standards, and will supply a list of approved schools upon request. For further information contact:

American Polarity Therapy Association
2888 Bluff St., ste. 149
Boulder, CO 80301
(303) 545-2080

The following schools offer training in polarity: 3, 4, 8, 10, 13, 16, 17, 26, 28, 31, 35, 38, 39, 48, 50, 52, 60, 64, 67, 69, 71, 78, 79, 81, 86, 91, 112, 118, 126, 132, 133, 136, 145, 155, 165, 170, 172, 174, 175, 180, 181, 183, 192, 193, 196, 207, 209, 211, 215, 217, 218, 219, 222, 223, 224, 229, 238, 245, 249, 254, 263, 266, 270, 275, 278, 279, 280, 294, 295, 304, 305, 307, 308, 313, 316, 321, 325, 327, 336, 338, 341, 346, 349, 350, 355, 359, 369, 370, 371, 374, 376, 379, 381, 386, 388, 392, 394, 396, 401, 409, 413, 418, 420, 424, 426, 427, 429, 434, 435, 437, 438, 439, 441, 442, 443,

444, 452, 565, 473, 476, 481, 499, 504, 520, 522, 524, 526, 536, 540, 544, 546, 550, 558, 562, 563, 564, 567, 569, 570.

Postural Integration
See Structural Integration

Pregnancy Massage (or prenatal massage)
This is an adaptation of Swedish massage for the needs of pregnant women. It is sometimes called prenatal or perinatal massage, or massage for the child-bearing year. Two individuals offer regular trainings in pregnancy massage:

Carole Osborne-Sheets
11650 Iberia Place, #137
San Diego, CA 92128
(619) 748-8827
http://members.aol.com/cos9/index.html

Kate Jordan Seminars
8950 Villa La Jolla Dr., Suite 2162
La Jolla, CA 92037
(760) 436-0418

Pregnancy massage is taught at the following schools: 3, 4, 8, 9, 10, 11, 12, 13, 14, 16, 29, 31, 33, 36, 37, 39, 43, 49, 51, 52, 53, 57, 61, 67, 75, 79, 82, 85, 91, 94, 95, 106, 112, 120, 124, 126, 129, 132, 134, 139, 140, 143, 145, 155, 159, 160, 165, 170, 175, 179, 180, 191, 192, 193, 201, 202, 203, 204, 206, 207, 215, 216, 218, 219, 223, 224, 229, 231, 234, 241, 243, 245, 246, 249, 254, 255, 259, 260, 261, 263, 266, 268, 271, 276, 277, 278, 279, 292, 304, 305, 307, 314, 315, 318, 325, 328, 329, 334, 336, 337, 338, 341, 347, 348, 349, 350, 351, 356, 357, 360, 361, 362, 365, 366, 367, 369, 370, 373, 374, 375, 376, 377, 378, 379, 381, 382, 384, 388, 393, 394, 402, 409, 416, 417, 419, 421, 422, 424, 427, 430, 432, 435, 436, 437, 444, 445, 448, 449, 452, 456, 458, 464, 466, 470, 471, 473, 475, 476, 481, 497, 501, 503, 504, 508, 515, 521, 524, 525, 526, 529, 531, 533, 536, 538, 541, 543, 548, 549, 550, 551, 560, 562, 563, 564, 567, 569, 570.

Qi Gong
Also called Chinese Medical Massage, this may be the most commonly practiced modality in the world. It is routinely used in Chinese hospitals as a healing modality. The name literally means "skill with life energy" and it evolved over two thousand years ago in Tibet and China.

Qi gong is taught at schools 67, 229, 527, 533.

Radiance Technique
The Radiance Technique was formerly called The Official Reiki Program. For further information, contact:

Radiance Stress Management Association International, Inc
P.O. Box 86425
St. Petersburg Fl 33738
(813) 347-3421

Radiance Technique is also taught at schools 499 and 544.

Rebirthing
Rebirthing is a technique of conscious breathing that can help in releasing physical, emotional or mental blockages. It is best learned by participating as a client in rebirthing sessions with a certified rebirther. Several books are available that describe the process. The leading author on rebirthing is Sondra Ray.

Rebirthing is taught at schools 52, 56, 59, 181, 206, 221, 224, 255, 357, 465, 526, 540.

Reflexology

Reflexology is a system of massaging the feet, or feet and hands, with the intention of affecting other parts of the body. The feet and hands are regarded much like maps of the body, with points on the feet and hands corresponding to organs and tissues in the body. It is thought that sensitivity or tenderness in the feet or hands indicates imbalances in the corresponding body part, and by working with the point on the foot or hand, beneficial results can be achieved in the corresponding body part.

While many reflexologists spend an entire therapy session working only on the hands and feet (and sometimes ears), some spend approximately half of their time on the feet, and half on Swedish massage. Reflexology is taught at more US massage schools than any other form of bodywork.

Independent certification in reflexology is offered by:

American Reflexology Certification Board (ARCB)
P.O. Box 620607
Littleton, CO 80162
(303) 933-6921

The ARCB certifies the competency of reflexology practitioners. It does not accredit schools or endorse curricula. To become ARCB certified, a reflexologist must be 18 years old or older, have a high school diploma or equivalent, live and practice in the United States, complete a "hands on" reflexology course beyond the introductory level, and pass the written, practical and documentation portions of the ARCB exam.

Reflexology training is usually a brief program. For information about trainings, contact:

Laura Norman and Associates
Reflexology Center
41 Park Ave.
New York, NY 10016
(212) 532-4404

International Academy for
Reflexology Studies
4759 Cornell Rd., Suite D.
Cincinatti, OH 45241
(513) 489-9328
(600 hour training plus advanced programs)

International Institute of Reflexology
P.O. Box 12642
St. Petersburg, FL 33733-2642
(813) 343-4811

Modern Institute of Reflexology
7043 West Colfax
Denver, CO 80215
1-800-533-1837 or (303) 237-1530
www.reflexologyinstitute.com

The following schools teach reflexology: 3, 4, 7, 8, 10, 12, 13, 14, 16, 17, 18, 20, 23, 24, 27, 28, 29, 36, 37, 38, 39, 41, 43, 44, 45, 46, 47, 48, 49, 50, 51, 52, 53, 56, 57, 60, 61, 63, 64, 67, 71, 72, 75, 76, 77, 82, 85, 8, 90, 91, 94, 95, 96, 97, 106, 108, 110, 112, 113, 114, 118, 119, 120, 123, 124, 126, 129, 130, 131, 132, 136, 138, 139, 140, 143, 145, 152, 155, 156, 157, 159, 160, 163, 165, 168, 170, 174, 175, 176, 177, 178, 179, 180, 181, 183, 190, 192, 193, 196, 201, 203, 204, 206, 207, 208, 209, 210, 211, 216, 217, 218, 219, 220, 221, 222, 223, 224, 228, 229, 231, 232, 234, 236, 238, 239, 241, 242, 243, 246, 254, 255, 259, 260, 261, 263, 266, 268, 270, 271, 272, 273, 274, 275, 276, 277, 278, 279, 285, 286, 292, 294, 295, 296, 304, 305, 307, 308, 311, 313, 316, 318, 320, 321, 325, 327, 328, 329, 334, 336, 337, 338, 346, 346, 348, 349, 350, 351, 353, 355, 356, 357, 360, 361, 362, 364, 366, 367, 368, 369, 370, 372, 373, 374, 375, 376, 377, 378, 379, 380, 381, 382, 386, 391, 393, 394, 399, 401, 402, 407, 409, 412, 415, 416, 417, 418, 419, 421, 422, 424, 426, 427, 428, 429, 432, 433, 434, 435, 436, 437, 438, 439, 441, 442, 443, 444, 445, 446, 448, 449, 452, 454, 456, 457, 458, 463, 464, 465, 466, 467, 468, 469, 471, 472, 473, 476, 481, 484, 492, 497, 499, 501, 504, 506, 508, 515, 516, 520, 521, 522, 524, 526, 527, 531, 533, 536, 537, 538, 541, 542, 543, 544, 546, 547, 548, 550, 551, 552, 563, 564, 567, 571, 572.

Reiki

Reiki is an energy process for restoring and balancing life energy and promoting healing and personal transformation. The approach is thousands of years old, and was systematized in the 1800's by Dr. Mikao Usui. The practitioner attunes to and transmits reiki energy. Further information can be obtained from:

Reiki Alliance
P.O. Box 41
Cataldo, ID 83810-1041
(208) 682-3535

Reiki is taught at the following schools: 3, 4, 10, 12, 13, 14, 17, 36, 51, 57, 67, 81, 85, 94, 95, 112, 120, 124, 126, 129, 132, 138, 139, 141, 145, 155, 157, 159, 170, 175, 177, 178, 192, 216, 217, 218, 219, 223, 226, 229, 231, 238, 246, 255, 257, 263, 270, 286, 292, 304, 307, 314, 316, 321, 333, 337, 338, 341, 345, 346, 351, 353, 356, 361, 362, 366, 380, 392, 393, 394, 401, 409, 427, 429, 433, 437, 439, 442, 446, 452, 456, 503, 524, 526, 536, 541, 544, 548, 549, 550, 558, 567, 569, 572.

Rolfing®

Ida Rolf was the first to create, practice and teach a system of bodywork aimed toward working with the connective tissue of the body to achieve structural changes in the client. She originally called her system Structural Integration, but it came to be called Rolfing and is taught by:

The Rolf Institute
205 Canyon Blvd.
Boulder, CO 80302
1-800-530-8875 or (303) 449-5903

Some exposure to Rolfing is offered at the following schools: 159, 163, 168, 178, 179, 211, 232, 308, 458, 536.

Rosen Method Bodywork®

Developed by Marion Rosen, this work emphasizes simplicity. The practitioner contacts contracted muscles and matches the muscle tension. The practitioner follows changes in the client's breathing as a means of guiding the client's inner process. The work can bring up buried feelings and memories, and can be a tool for pain relief and personal growth.

Below are the three centers that teach Rosen Method Bodywork. These centers can give you information about trainings and practitioners in their areas.

Rosen Method: The Berkeley Center
2550 Shattuck Ave., Box 49
Berkeley, CA 94704
(510) 845-6606

Rosen Center East
P.O. Box 5004
Westport, CT 06881-5004
(203) 319-1090

Rosen Method Center Southwest
P.O. Box 344
Santa Fe, NM 87504
(505) 982-7149

Some training in Rosen Method Bodywork is offered at schools 94, 113, 145.

Rubenfeld Synergy™

This method integrates elements of Alexander, Feldenkrais, gestalt and hypnotherapy into a body-mind therapy that helps clients contact and release energy blocks, tensions and imbalances. Rather than treating illnesses, the practitioner treats the psychophysical problems people carry with them. By dealing with the emotional body, the practitioner can often abate physical symptoms. For information, contact:

The Rubenfeld Center
115 Waverly Place
New York, N.Y. 10011
(212) 254-5100 (10:00 to 6:00 weekdays)

Rubenfeld Synergy is taught at school 149.

Seated Massage

See Chair Massage

Shiatsu or acupressure

Shiatsu is a Japanese bodywork which uses pressure to points on acupuncture meridians. Practice of shiatsu is usually accompanied by study of Chinese five-element theory and meridians, and it involves a way of looking at the body that is completely different from the "muscles, bones and blood" view of Western science, focusing instead on the flow of life energy through meridians.

The name "Acupressure" is sometimes used to mean shiatsu, and is sometimes used to describe a finger-pressure technique similar to shiatsu but not identical.

Massage schools offering shiatsu instruction: 3, 4, 7, 8, 9, 10, 11, 12, 13, 14, 16, 18, 20, 23, 24, 26, 30, 31, 35, 37, 38, 41, 43, 46, 47, 50, 52, 53, 57, 61, 63, 66, 67, 70, 72, 75, 76, 78, 79, 81, 85, 89, 90, 91, 94, 96, 106, 108, 110, 111, 112, 114, 118, 119, 120, 124, 125, 128, 129, 131, 132, 133, 136, 137, 138, 139, 140, 143, 144, 145, 150, 157, 160, 168, 169, 170, 172, 174, 175, 177, 179, 180, 183, 190, 191, 192, 193, 196, 201, 203, 207, 209, 210, 211, 212, 214, 215, 216, 217, 218, 219, 220, 221, 222, 223, 226, 228, 231, 232, 234, 239, 241, 246, 249 254, 255, 257, 260, 266, 268, 271, 272, 273, 274, 275, 276, 277, 278, 279, 295, 296, 298, 304, 307, 308, 315, 316, 318, 320, 321, 325, 327, 330, 333, 336, 338, 341, 346, 347, 348, 349, 350, 351, 353, 357, 359, 360, 361, 362, 364, 365, 369, 370, 371, 373, 374, 375, 376, 377, 378, 379, 380, 381, 382, 384, 386, 392, 394, 407, 409, 417, 420, 422, 424, 426, 427, 428, 429, 434, 435, 436, 437, 438, 442, 443, 444, 448, 452, 454, 458, 464, 465, 469, 473, 476, 497, 499, 501, 503, 504, 515, 520, 521, 522, 524, 525, 526, 527, 529, 530, 536, 540, 541, 542, 543, 544, 546, 548, 549, 550, 551, 552, 557, 563, 564, 568, 569, 570, 571, 572.

Massage schools offering acupressure instruction: 3, 4, 9, 10, 12, 13, 14, 17, 18, 20, 24, 26, 27, 29, 30, 31, 35, 36, 38, 41, 43, 46, 49, 50, 52, 57, 58, 60, 61, 63, 64, 67, 69, 71, 72, 75, 77, 78, 79, 81, 82, 86, 89, 91, 94, 96, 97, 103, 104, 105, 106, 108, 110, 112, 113, 114, 116, 118, 119, 120, 123, 124, 125, 126, 129, 130, 131, 136, 138, 140, 144, 145, 147, 157, 158, 160, 170, 175, 177, 179, 181, 190, 192, 202, 203, 207, 209, 215, 216, 218, 220, 221, 222, 223, 226, 231, 232, 234, 241, 246, 254, 255, 257, 259, 260, 261, 263, 265, 268, 270, 271, 272, 273, 304, 305, 307, 308, 313, 315, 316, 318, 320, 321, 333, 336, 337, 338, 341, 344, 345, 346, 347, 350, 355, 356, 357, 359, 362, 366, 367, 372, 375, 378, 380, 391, 392, 393, 394, 396, 402, 416, 417, 418, 421, 428, 434, 435, 436, 437, 439, 442, 444, 445, 454, 456, 457, 458, 463, 465, 469, 473, 476, 501, 516, 520, 524, 525, 526, 527, 529, 531, 533, 536, 543, 544, 548, 551, 558, 563, 569, 571, 572.

Some schools that offer independent shiatsu training

Acupressure Institute
1533 Shattuck Avenue
Berkeley, CA 94709
(510) 845-1059
1-800-442-2232

Aisen Shiatsu School
1314 South King Street, room 601
Honolulu, HI 96814
(808) 596-7354

Associates for Creative Wellness
Executive Mews, suite G-38
1930 E. Marlton Pike
Cherry Hill, NJ 08003
(609) 424-7501

International School of Shiatsu
10 South Clinton St., suite 300
Doylestown, PA 18901
(215) 340-9918

Minnesota Center for Shiatsu Study
1313 5th St., SE, suite 336
Minneapolis, MN 55414
(612) 379-3565

Ohashi Institute
12 West 27th Street, 9th Fl.
New York, NY 10001
(212) 684-4190
1-800-810-4190

Santa Barbara College of Oriental Medicine
1919 State Street, suite 204
Santa Barbara, CA 93101
(805) 898-1180

Shiatsu School of Canada, Inc.
547 College Street
Toronto, Ont., M6G 1A9, Canada
(416) 323-1818

Tsuko Therapy School
239 Seal Beach Blvd., Unit C
Seal Beach, CA 90740
(562) 493-0890

Somatics (also called Somatics Psychology or Somatic Therapy)

"Somatic" literally means "of or pertaining to the body." In the context of Somatics Psychology, it refers to the mind-body connection and makes use of techniques to bring awareness of the mind and the body to each other. It is therefore related to the form "Body-Mind" which is described above.

The Lomi School offers professional training that includes psychotherapeutic techniques and meditative practices. Breath, movement, sound, touch, sitting meditation, Gestalt, Reichian and developmental theories are all presented. The program spans one year, beginning with a 5-day intensive, continuing one weekend per month, and concluding with an intensive. For complete information, contact:

Lomi Clinic
600 B Street
Santa Rosa, CA 95401
(707) 579-0465

Body Synergy Institute teaches Body Psychology to psychotherapists and body therapists. Trainings are offered in 2-day, 40-hour, or 3-year formats. Postural analysis and client communication are combined to allow practitioners to use body awareness and touch as educational tools with their clients. The Institute also teaches Postural Integration. For complete information, contact:

Body Synergy Institute
305 Bangor Rd.
Bala Cynwyd, PA 19004
(610) 667-3070

The following schools offer training in Somatics or a similar approach: 8, 12, 26, 30, 38, 50, 57, 61, 62, 64, 67, 71, 73, 79, 90, 106, 110, 112, 125, 129, 145, 155, 159, 168, 206, 221, 222, 224, 230, 246, 263, 271, 272, 273, 275, 279, 313, 314, 320, 330, 333, 347, 349, 355, 366, 369, 386, 427, 435, 436, 442, 449, 452, 466, 503, 522, 540, 544, 550, 561, 567, 569.

Spa Treatments

Spa, or Health Spa, refers to an establishment that provides rejuvenating treatments in a residential setting (or non-residential at a day spa). Often at a resort and often luxurious in setting, spas aim for relaxation, therapeutic treatments, and beautification treatments. Modalities such as herbal wraps, seaweed wraps, mud baths, loofa scrubs and salt glows are designed to detoxify and refresh the system.

Related to spa treatments is Hydrotherapy, meaning "water therapy." It includes treatments like contrast baths (alternating hot and cold water), and wet sheet wraps. Hydrotherapy is a required course for massage licensure in Texas and Florida.

Spa treatments are taught at the following massage schools: 39, 43, 53, 104, 118, 129, 138, 146, 169, 170, 203, 207, 221, 249, 309, 311, 320, 336, 365, 416, 417, 426, 432, 454, 504, 526, 547.

Sports Massage

Sports massage is an adaptation of Swedish massage. Its purpose is to prepare athletes for sporting activity and help them recover from the exertion of sporting activity.

Sports massage trainings vary widely in length, and there is no standard training length, although the American Massage Therapy Association and the United States Sports Massage Federation both have standards for approving trainings.

The following massage schools offer sports massage training: 3, 4, 8, 9, 10, 11, 12, 13, 14, 16, 17, 18, 20, 23, 24, 26, 31, 33, 36, 37, 38, 39, 41, 43, 46, 49, 50, 52, 53, 58, 61, 63, 66, 67, 70, 71, 72, 75, 76, 78, 81, 82, 84, 85, 86, 91, 94, 95, 96, 97, 104, 107, 108, 110, 112, 113, 115, 116, 117, 118, 119, 120, 125, 126, 129, 131, 132, 133, 134, 136, 1367, 138, 129, 142, 145, 155, 156, 157, 160, 163, 165, 168, 169, 170, 171, 172, 174, 175, 177, 178, 179, 180, 181, 186, 190, 191, 192, 193, 196, 201, 202, 203,. 204, 207, 210, 214, 215, 216, 217, 218, 219, 220, 221, 222, 223, 226, 228, 229, 231, 234, 238, 241, 242, 243, 245, 246, 249, 254, 255, 259, 260, 263, 264, 266, 268, 270, 271, 272, 273, 274, 275, 276, 277, 278, 279, 283, 285, 286, 292, 294, 295, 296, 298, 304, 305, 307, 308, 309, 313, 315, 316, 318, 320, 321, 325, 326, 327, 328, 329, 334, 336, 338, 341, 344, 345, 346, 347, 348, 349, 350, 351, 353, 356, 357, 359, 360, 361, 362, 364, 366, 367, 368, 369, 370, 374, 376, 378, 379, 380, 381, 382, 383, 384, 386, 388, 391, 394, 396, 402, 405, 409, 412, 415, 416, 417, 419, 422, 424, 426, 427, 429, 430, 432, 433, 434, 435, 436, 437, 439, 441, 442, 443, 444, 448, 449, 452, 454, 463, 464, 465, 466, 468, 469, 470, 471, 472, 473, 476, 481, 482, 499, 500, 501, 503, 504, 506, 515, 520, 524, 525, 526, 527, 529, 533, 536, 538, 540, 541, 542, 543, 544, 546, 547, 548, 549, 550, 551, 558, 560, 562, 563, 564, 567, 570, 571, 572.

Training in Russian Clinical Sports Massage is offered at Kurashova Institute, P.O. Box 6246, Rock Island, IL 61201 (309) 786-4888

Structural Integration (or Postural Integration)

This is a generic term for therapies that are related to Rolfing, in that they aim to improve the structure or posture of the client. See also Hellerwork and Berrywork.

The following schools offer introductory or advanced structural integration trainings: 8, 39, 56, 67, 106, 124, 125, 139, 145, 155, 160, 163, 165, 170, 172, 177, 180, 181, 203, 204, 221, 224, 279, 303, 330, 349, 375, 380, 381, 386, 392, 393, 401, 417, 426, 441, 471, 546, 551, 569.

The following schools offer introductory or advanced postural integration trainings: 39, 85, 106, 120, 124, 132, 139, 145, 165, 177, 181, 193, 204, 207, 221, 246, 277, 279, 307, 314, 336, 337, 349, 369, 380, 409, 415, 417, 422, 426, 439, 442, 452, 469, 544, 546, 551, 569.

The schools listed below offer independent structural integration or postural integration training.

Body Synergy Institute
305 Bangor Rd.
Bala Cynwyd, PA 19004
(610) 667-3070

**Institute for Integrative
Body Therapies**
2822 Newport Circle
Grand Junction, CO 81503
(970) 242-9224

Soma Institute
730 Klink St.
Buckley, WA 98321
(360) 829-1025
(300 hours of training over a 12-week period)

Florida Institute of Psychophysical Integration
5837 Mariner Drive
Tampa, FL 33609
(813) 286-2273 www.QuantumBalance.com
(Intensive residential program includes about
150 hours over a three-week period)

International Center for Release & Integration
450 Hillside Avenue
Mill Valley, CA 94941
(415) 383-4017
(Program takes about two years to complete)

Thai Massage

The traditional massage of Thailand.

Schools teaching Thai massage: 7, 26, 39, 57, 82, 96, 112, 120, 125, 172, 208, 211, 216, 217, 218, 222, 255, 263, 304, 330, 351, 439, 499.

Therapeutic Touch (TT)

TT is a means of attuning to and directing the universal life energy. The goal is to release congestion and balance areas where the flow of life energy has become disordered. Removal of these blockages facilitates the person's intrinsic healing powers.

TT is most commonly taught to, and used by nurses. However, some massage therapists study TT and incorporate it into their work.

Several books are available on TT, including *Therapeutic Touch: A Practical Guide* by J. Macrae, Knopf, 1988; *The Therapeutic Touch* by D. Krieger, Prentice-Hall 1979; *Therapeutic Touch* by Borelli and Heidt, Springer Co., 1981.

The following schools offer instruction in Therapeutic Touch: 3, 4, 10, 11, 12, 13, 14, 26, 43, 69, 108, 113, 126, 132, 145, 149, 152, 165, 172, 175, 178, 179, 181, 192, 196, 210, 221, 226, 231, 232, 239, 249, 254, 255, 295, 304, 305, 313, 321, 325, 338, 341, 355, 356, 362, 367, 371, 372, 388, 394, 409, 413, 435, 436, 439, 442, 446, 452, 456, 476, 520, 524, 538, 540, 541, 544, 546, 548, 550, 558, 566, 568, 569.

Touch For Health (see also Applied Kinesiology)

This is a system for using applied kinesiology to aid the bodyworker. Applied kinesiology makes use of the fact that certain conditions result in weakening of specific muscles. Through muscle testing, the bodyworker gains information about the specifics of the client's condition. Further information and a catalogue of books and other products are available from the Touch for Health Association:

Touch for Health Kinesiology Association
11262 Washington Blvd.
Culver City, CA 90230
1-800-466-8342

The following schools offer training in Touch for Health: 14, 30, 41, 48, 50, 56, 57, 91, 108, 110, 123, 124, 126, 130, 145, 149, 152, 157, 170, 177, 210, 211, 215, 216, 217, 219, 221, 231, 241,

246, 255, 261, 263, 279, 304, 307, 308, 314, 327, 338, 349, 364, 377, 378, 379, 394, 402, 409, 434, 435, 442, 444, 446, 452, 470, 473, 524, 525, 527, 533, 536, 544, 548, 552, 567, 568, 569.

Trager®

Dr. Milton Trager, M.D., had a gift for bodywork from a young age, and developed his own system of bodywork which emphasizes gentle rocking of the client, and rolling body parts to encourage release and loosening and softening.

Some massage schools offer brief introductory trainings in Trager bodywork, giving the massage therapist a glimpse into the system. Massage therapists with introductory training often integrate a bit of the Trager awareness into their massage work. However, Trager practitioners practice only Trager, at least during a Trager session. Information about becoming a Trager practitioner can be obtained from:

The Trager Institute
21 Locust Ave.
Mill Valley, CA 94941
(415) 388-2688

The following schools offer an introduction to Trager bodywork: 3, 4, 41, 64, 113, 145, 155, 159, 163, 172, 174, 175, 178, 192, 211, 226, 292, 307, 316, 327, 353, 355, 356, 362, 369, 381, 386, 392, 439, 442, 501, 536, 541, 548, 551, 568.

Trigger Point Therapies (Myotherapy[SM] or neuromuscular therapy)

This refers to any of several systems of working with trigger points. Trigger points are tender congested spots in muscle tissue, which may radiate pain to other areas. Significant relief results when the trigger point is treated.

The techniques used in trigger point therapies are similar to those used in Shiatsu or acupressure, but trigger point therapies are based on western anatomy and physiology. Several institutions have refined the art of trigger point therapy into a self-contained modality, and teach their therapy in a non-massage context. These schools are:

Bonnie Prudden™ School of Physical Fitness and Myotherapy
7800 E. Speedway
Tucson, AZ 85710
(520) 529-3979
Nine-month, 1,300-hour program

International Academy of NeuroMuscular Therapies
C/O NMT Center
900 14th Ave N.
St. Petersburg, FL 33705
(813) 821-7167
Four-weekend series for NMT certification, given at various locations (massage diploma or other professional training preferred before admission).

St. John Neuromuscular Therapy Seminars
10710 Seminole Blvd., Suite #1
Largo, FL 33778
1-888-NMT-HEAL
http://webfx4u.com/stjohnnmt
Seminars in various locations; home-study videos also available.

Many schools listed in the State-by-State directory offer training in trigger-point therapies. The lists that follow divide the schools into those that teach "trigger point," and those that teach "neuromuscular" (NMT), and those that teach "myotherapy."

Trigger point: 3, 4, 9, 10, 12, 13, 14, 26, 27, 29, 31, 33, 36, 37, 39, 43, 50, 61, 67, 71, 76, 85, 86, 90, 91, 95, 97, 108, 112, 113, 115, 117, 125, 129, 132, 133, 137, 138, 139, 143, 145, 149, 157, 159, 160, 163, 165, 169, 172, 175, 177, 178, 179, 180, 181, 184, 185, 186, 191, 192, 203, 206, 207, 210, 217, 218, 219, 222, 223, 224, 226, 228, 229, 232, 234, 238, 241, 243, 246, 254, 260, 263, 270, 276, 277, 278, 279, 292, 295, 296, 298, 304, 307, 308, 314, 315, 316, 318, 325, 327, 329, 330, 333, 334, 336, 338, 341, 344, 346, 347, 349, 350, 361, 362, 367, 369, 370, 372, 373, 374, 375, 376, 378, 379, 380, 381, 388, 392, 394, 401, 402, 415, 417, 420, 421, 422, 424, 432, 434, 435, 436, 442, 443, 445, 458, 467, 470, 471, 472, 473, 481, 482, 499, 503, 504, 515, 516, 520, 524, 526, 527, 532, 540, 541, 543, 544, 546, 548, 549, 550, 551, 569, 571.

Neuromuscular or NMT: 3, 4, 8, 9, 11, 20, 23, 26, 50, 82, 91, 112, 113, 115, 117, 124, 125, 126, 129, 131, 132, 133, 136, 137, 139, 143, 145, 149, 155, 157, 159, 160, 165, 168, 170, 172, 174, 175, 177, 178, 179, 180, 181, 183, 191, 192, 193, 196, 201, 203, 204, 206, 207, 209, 210, 211, 217, 220, 221, 223, 224, 234, 248, 246, 249, 268, 271, 272, 273, 274, 276, 277, 278, 285, 296, 298, 3030, 307, 314, 316, 318, 320, 321, 330, 334, 336, 337, 338, 347, 350, 353, 356, 357, 359, 365, 366, 369, 370, 371, 376, 377, 378, 380, 381, 382, 383, 388, 392, 393, 401, 402, 405, 407, 409, 412, 415, 417, 424, 432, 434, 435, 436, 438, 439, 441, 442, 444, 445, 448, 449, 454, 456, 467, 468, 469, 471, 473, 475, 482, 499, 516, 526, 532, 533, 538, 540, 544, 549, 550, 551, 557, 564, 567, 569, 570, 572.

Myotherapy: 13, 20, 33, 37, 61, 108, 110, 131, 132, 140, 145, 149, 157, 159, 165, 202, 220, 223, 256, 259, 276, 279, 298, 308, 314, 335, 336, 338, 347, 349, 361, 401, 435, 445, 533, 544, 546, 550, 551, 569, 570.

Tui Na

Tui Na is an Oriental bodywork related to Qi Gong.

Schools that teach Tui Na: 13, 39, 57, 69, 77, 90, 114, 118, 120, 124, 125, 127, 145, 180, 181, 228, 231, 241, 263, 330, 346, 371, 378, 382, 426, 529, 544, 549, 569.

Vibrational Healing Massage Therapy®

This modality was developed by Patricia Cramer, founder of the World School of Massage in San Francisco (school #56). It is based on the Fluid Body Model, and brings liquid consciousness to movement and breathing. Focusing on fluidity frees up tensions and stresses which have been held in the body. Thinking, speaking, listening and bodywork are all part of the system.

Vibrational healing is taught at schools 56, 123, 325, 333.

Watsu™ (aquatic shiatsu) www.waba.edu

Watsu (from "water" and "shiatsu") began when Harold Dull started floating people, applying the moves and stretches of the zen shiatsu he had studied in Japan. Physical and emotional blocks are removed by the work, which can be done even by small individuals since the client's body in water is buoyant. It is done in chest-high, 94-degree water.

Certification can be obtained by taking three week-long workshops at:

School of Shiatsu and Massage
P.O. Box 889
Middletown, CA 95461
(707) 987-3801

Watsu is also taught at schools 3, 4, 16, 46, 132, 143, 145, 175, 181, 192, 221, 226, 230, 377, 422, 436, 468, 544.

Yoga therapy

In this method, yoga asanas are used to facilitate healing.

Yoga therapy is taught at schools 3, 4, 12, 13, 26, 30, 43, 52, 71, 85, 108, 112, 123, 124, 125, 129, 132, 145, 175, 177, 178, 179, 192, 202, 211, 221, 224, 226, 231, 242, 245, 246, 255, 279, 285, 304, 314, 336, 341, 346, 349, 356, 359, 374, 378, 381, 349, 356, 359, 374, 378, 381, 386, 392, 393, 407, 426, 436, 438, 442, 452, 465, 467, 506, 520, 540, 548, 567, 570.

Zero-Balancing www.zerobalancing.com

Developed by Fritz Smith, MD, osteopath, Rolfer and acupuncturist, zero balancing works with the relationship between a person's physical structure and their energy. The practitioner works with fulcrums, points where structure and energy can be accessed together, to bring about change.

For fuller information about zero-balancing, trainings or practitioners, contact:

The Zero Balancing Association
P.O. Box 1727
Capitola, CA 95010
(408) 476-0665

Introductory training in Zero Balancing is offered at schools 132, 217, 283, 452, 501, 538, 546.

VII

State-by-State
Directory

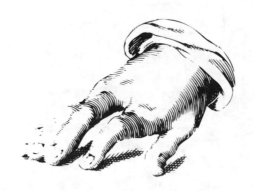

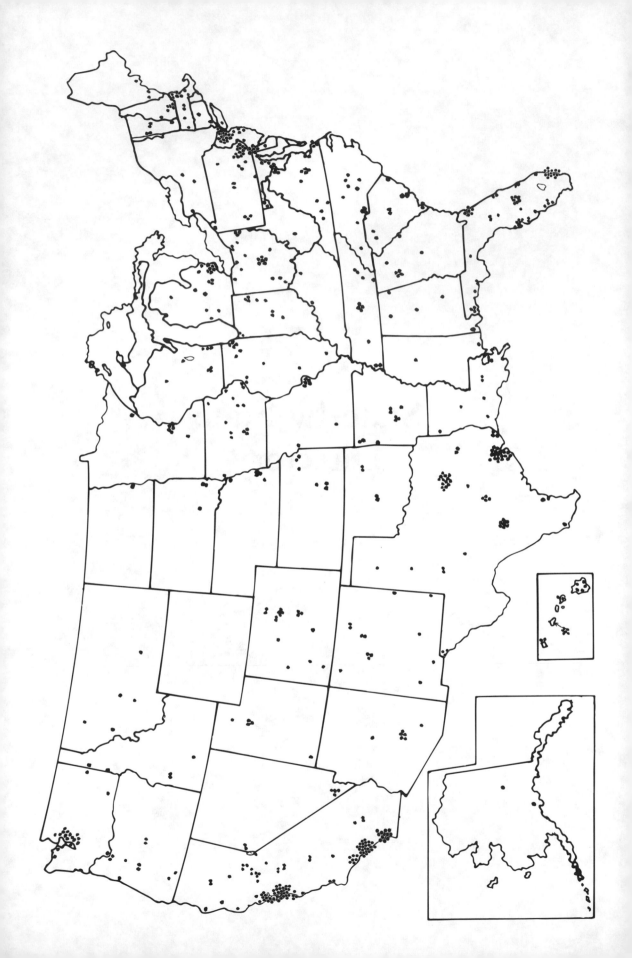

How to Use the State-by-State Directory

For those familiar with earlier editions, please note the following important change:
In the listing for each school's "Modalities and subjects," all subjects taught at the school are listed in one alphabetical list. This single list includes the school's main program, continuing education, and advanced courses, unless specifically noted otherwise. Please inquire of the school if you want to find out whether a specific course is part of the main curriculum or not.

Conventions used in this Directory:

1. "Hours of training" means in-class hours unless otherwise noted. "In-class hour" means a period of 50 to 60 minutes during which a teacher is present, and it includes teacher-supervised practice sessions.

2. "Cost" includes any mandatory fees, including registration fee or application fee. If books or other supplies are included in the cost, the items included are noted in the listing.

3. Some schools offer financing plans that include fees or interest. These have not been included in the Directory. Only no-fee, no-interest financing plans are listed.

4. The "accreditations or approvals" section lists COMTA (AMTA's accrediting arm), IMSTAC (ABMP's accrediting arm), ACCET and ACCSCT (federal accrediting boards). COMTA accreditation is required by some state licensing authorities, and ACCET or ACCSCT accreditation opens the way for federal loans and grant eligibility.

5. "Modalities and Subjects" includes all subjects taught at the school, including continuing education and advanced programs, in one alphabetical listing. All schools in the Directory teach Swedish massage and anatomy & physiology (unless otherwise noted), so these items are not listed in any school's description.

6. Unless otherwise noted, all schools in licensed states prepare students for their own state's licensing. If schools also prepare students for licensing in one or more other states, that is noted in the school's listing.

7. Each school was invited to submit a self-description of up to 25 words, which is printed under the heading "School statement."

Degree-granting schools:

Seven schools listed in the directory grant Associate, Bachelors, or Masters degrees in massage: 70, 76, 96, 125, 178, 382, 422. In addition, school 446 is approved for transfer credit.

Is every entry in this Directory 100% accurate?

The information published in this Directory was supplied by the massage schools. The listed information is the school's description of its own program, and has not been independently verified by the publisher. Every effort has been made to print exactly the information that was supplied by the school, but mistakes do happen. Please verify information with the school before relying upon it.

This information was accurate as of 1998. Curriculum, price, and other information can change over time, so please confirm any crucial information with the school before relying on it.

Alphabetical List of Schools

ALABAMA

State licensing requires 650 hours until 1/1/02, and 1,000 hours thereafter.

National Certification Exam not accepted.

Board: (334) 269-9990

SCHOOLS:

#1 Alabama School of Massage Therapy
201 Beacon Parkway West, suite 400
Birmingham, AL 35209
(205) 941-1718

Contact school for program information.

#2 Massage Therapy Institute
1403 Beltline Road SW, suite 1
Decatur, AL 35603
(205) 306-0444

Contact school for program information.

#3 Mobile School of Massage Therapy
3995 Cottage Hill Road, suite B
Mobile, AL 36609
(334) 665-9900 or 1-888-699-6768
www.msmt.com

HOURS OF TRAINING: 650 (500 in-class hours).

DURATION OF COURSE: 5 months full-time, 11 months part time.

COST: $4,275 includes all books, oil & bottles. Payment plan without interest is available.

FINANCIAL AID: Scholarships or discounts, Veteran's Administration, State Vocational Rehab., Indian Affairs.

YEAR FOUNDED: 1994.

GRADUATES PER YEAR (APPROX.): 60.

MODALITIES AND SUBJECTS: acupressure, AIDS awareness, applied kinesiology, aromatherapy, business practices & development, chair massage, connective tissue, CPR, cranio-sacral therapy, equine sports massage, esalen, fitness, infant massage, joint mobilization, kinesiology, massage theory & practice, medical massage, meridian therapy, myofascial release, neuromuscular therapy, nutrition, PNF stretching, polarity, pregnancy massage, reflexology, reiki, shiatsu, sports massage, statutes & rules, therapeutic touch, trager, trigger point therapy, watsu, yoga therapy.

SCHOOL STATEMENT: MSMT believes therapeutic massage is a viable alternative healing method for neuromuscular problems as well as general relaxation and stress relief.

#4 Montgomery School of Massage Therapy
620-C Oliver Rd.
Montgomery, AL 36117
(334) 396-1600

HOURS OF TRAINING: 650 (500 in-class hours).

DURATION OF COURSE: 5 months full-time, 11 months part time.

COST: $4,275 includes all books, oil & bottles. Payment plan without interest is available.

FINANCIAL AID: Scholarships or discounts, Veteran's Administration, State Vocational Rehab., Indian Affairs.

YEAR FOUNDED: 1994.

GRADUATES PER YEAR (APPROX.): 60.

MODALITIES AND SUBJECTS: acupressure, AIDS awareness, applied kinesiology, aromatherapy, business practices & development, chair massage, connective tissue, CPR, cranio-sacral therapy, equine sports massage, esalen, fitness, infant massage, joint mobilization, kinesiology, massage theory & practice, medical massage, meridian therapy, myofascial release, neuromuscular therapy, nutrition, PNF stretching, polarity, pregnancy massage, reflexology, reiki, shiatsu, sports massage, statutes & rules, therapeutic touch, trager, trigger point therapy, watsu, yoga therapy.

SCHOOL STATEMENT: MSMT believes therapeutic massage is a viable alternative healing method for neuromuscular problems as well as general relaxation and stress relief.

#5 Valley School of Therapeutic Massage
P.O. Box 88
Valley Head, AL 35989
(205) 638-7696 or 635-0840

Contact school for program information.

ALASKA

No State Licensing.

State Business License required, contact:

Department of Commerce and Economic Development
Business Licensing Section
P.O. Box D-LIC
Juneau, AK 99811-0800
(907) 465-2534

SCHOOLS:

#6 GateKey School of Mind-Body Integration Studies
4041 B Street, suite 302
Anchorage, AK 99503
(907) 561-7327

Contact school for program information.

#7 School of Integrating Shiatsu
101 College Rd., suite 354
Fairbanks, AK 99701
(907) 479-3820

HOURS OF TRAINING: 400, 500 (1,000 hour program planned).

DURATION OF COURSE: 500 hours approx. one year.

YEAR FOUNDED: 1992.

GRADUATES PER YEAR (APPROX.): 12 to 15.

MODALITIES AND SUBJECTS: barefoot shiatsu, integrating shiatsu (created by the school's founder, Tarika Lea), reflexology, thai massage.

ARIZONA

No State licensing.

Many cities regulate the practice of massage, and requirements for city licensing range from 100 to 1,000 hours.

For the city of Phoenix, contact:

Special Business Licenses
251 West Washington, 3rd floor
Phoenix, AZ 85003
(602) 262-6786

SCHOOLS:

#8 Arizona School of Integrative Studies
753 N. Main St.
Cottonwood, AZ 86326
(520) 639-3455

HOURS OF TRAINING: 650 (530 in-class hours).

DURATION OF COURSE: 6 months (days).

COST: $5,250 including books. Payment plan without interest is available.

YEAR FOUNDED: 1995.

GRADUATES PER YEAR (APPROX.): 32.

MODALITIES AND SUBJECTS: aromatherapy, body-mind, chair massage, connective tissue therapy, hydrotherapy, infant massage, neuromuscular therapy, polarity, pregnancy massage, reflexology, shiatsu, somatic therapy, sports massage certification, structural integration, teacher training.

SCHOOL STATEMENT: ASIS offers a wholistically presented program in an awareness oriented format. Peace through knowledge.

#9 Desert Institute of the Healing Arts
639 North Sixth Ave.
Tucson, AZ 85705
(520) 882-0899 or (800) 733-8098

HOURS OF TRAINING: 1,000.

DURATION OF COURSE: one year, days.

COST: $8,725.

FINANCIAL AID: Pell grants, Federal Direct Loans, PLUS Loans, approved for veterans' benefits. Payment plan without interest is available.

YEAR FOUNDED: 1982.

ACCREDITATIONS/APPROVALS: COMTA/Accredited, ACCSCT.

GRADUATES PER YEAR (APPROX.): 100.

MODALITIES AND SUBJECTS: acupressure, addictions recovery, Anatomiken, body mechanics and self-care, business and professionalism, chair massage, clinic, communication skills, gerontology, hydrotherapy, journaling for ourselves, massaging people with AIDS, massaging physically challenged clients, medical center externship, movement integration, myofascial strokes, neuromuscular therapy, prenatal massage, rocking, senior massage, shaking and rolling technique, shiatsu, sports massage, stretching and joint mobilization, t'ai chi, teaching aids, treatments for specific conditions, trigger point, women in transition, yoga. Advanced program: 650-hour zen shiatsu program.

SCHOOL STATEMENT: Dedicated to providing quality personal instruction in the art and science of massage therapy and shiatsu, thereby providing the public with highly skilled professionals.

#10 Institute for Natural Therapeutics, Inc.
217 West University
Mesa, AZ 85201
(602) 844-2255
(call 844-1959 Wednesdays)

HOURS OF TRAINING: 200, 500, 1,000 (100, 380, 750 in-class hours).

DURATION OF COURSE: 3 months, 9 months, 14 months (day & evening programs available).

COST: 200 hours $1,415 including books, 500 hours $3,215 including books. Payment plan without interest is available for 3-month program.

FINANCIAL AID: Discount for pre-payment, loans through TFC Credit Corp.

YEAR FOUNDED: 1988.

GRADUATES PER YEAR (APPROX.): 95.

MODALITIES AND SUBJECTS: accounting, acupressure, advanced massage, aromatherapy, body-mind, business, cranio-sacral therapy, deep tissue, empowering the practitioner, healing touch, holistic health, hydrotherapy, infant massage, iridology,

jin shin do, myofascial release, nutrition I & II, pfrimmer deep muscle, polarity, pregnancy massage, preventative & developmental care, reflexology, reiki, shiatsu, sports massage, tao, therapeutic touch, trigger point therapy.

SCHOOL STATEMENT: "The drugless healer is one of the best things that has come into the live of the present." – Charles Mayo

#11 Phoenix Therapeutic Massage College
2225 N. 16th Street
Phoenix, AZ 85006
(602) 254-7002
www.ptmc-az.com

HOURS OF TRAINING: 735 or 1,110 classes offered days, afternoons, and evenings.

COST: 735 hours $6,506; 1,110 hours $9,316 (includes massage table, books, uniform & supplies).

FINANCIAL AID: Pell Grants, Federal SEOG and Federal Family Education Loans.

YEAR FOUNDED: 1981.

ACCREDITATIONS/APPROVALS: COMTA/approved, ACCET, approved for veterans training.

GRADUATES PER YEAR (APPROX.): 175.

MODALITIES AND SUBJECTS: applied kinesiology, career development, chair massage, deep tissue massage, externship, healing touch, health care, hospice/geriatric massage, kinesiology, lymphatic/immune system, massage theories, medical massage, neuromuscular therapy, nutrition, pathology, pregnancy/infant massage, psychology, shiatsu, sports massage, therapeutic touch, traditional chinese medicine.

SCHOOL STATEMENT: Our college is complying with major natural health care services toward a possible prevention of some diseases, through human soft tissue management with massage therapy.

#12 RainStar College
RainStar Campus
4110-4130 N. Goldwater Blvd.
Scottsdale, AZ 85251
(602) 423-0375 or 1-888-RAINSTAR
www.rainstargroup.com

HOURS OF TRAINING: 200, 500, 750 or 1,000.

DURATION OF COURSE: 2 to 14 months, classes offered days, afternoons, evenings & weekends.

COST: $1,895 to $7,995 plus approximately $250 for books and supplies.

FINANCIAL AID: Scholarships, Veteran's Administration, JPTA, Vocational Rehabilitation.

ACCREDITATIONS/APPROVALS: IMSTAC.

MODALITIES AND SUBJECTS: acupressure, aromatherapy, business, chair massage, chi gong, cranio-sacral therapy, health, infant massage, lymphatic drainage, myofascial release, pregnancy massage, reflexology, reiki, shiatsu, somatic therapy, sports massage, therapeutic touch, trigger point therapy, yoga therapy; over 150 continuing education courses offered.

SCHOOL STATEMENT: Our mission is to elevate the stature of massage and alternative health care to the same level of acceptance as other mainstream health-care providers.

#13 Southwest Institute of Healing Arts
1402 N. Miller Rd., #D
Scottsdale, AZ 85257
(602) 994-9244
www.dream@swiha.org

HOURS OF TRAINING: 4 to 1,000 hours.

DURATION OF COURSE: 1 day to 1 year; day & evening & weekend programs available.

COST: $7.50 to $10.00 per clock hour. Payment plan without interest is available.

FINANCIAL AID: Scholarships or discounts available.

YEAR FOUNDED: 1992.

GRADUATES PER YEAR (APPROX.): 300.

MODALITIES AND SUBJECTS: acupressure, AMMA, aromatherapy, body-mind, chair massage, chi gong, clinic nutritionist certification, cranio-sacral therapy, equine sports massage, esalen, holistic health care practitioner certification, infant massage, jin shin do, lymphatic drainage, medical massage, myofascial release, myotherapy, nutrition & chinese herbology, ortho-bionomy, polarity, pregnancy massage, reflexology, reiki, shiatsu, sports massage, therapeutic touch, trigger point therapy, tui na, yoga therapy.

SCHOOL STATEMENT: We are a state-licensed, degree-granting private college providing a wide range of continuing education classes and diploma courses.

#14 West Valley Massage College
518 N. 35th Avenue
Phoenix, AZ 85009
(602) 269-1741 or 269-3310

HOURS OF TRAINING: 200, 300, 500, 1,000.

DURATION OF COURSE: 200 hours 5 weeks or 10 weeks; 300 hours 8 weeks or 15 weeks; 500 hours, 13 weeks or 25 weeks; 1,000 hours 25 weeks or 50 weeks.

COST: 200 hours $1,600, 300 hours $2,350, 500 hours 3,850, 1,000 hours $7,600.

YEAR FOUNDED: 1997.

SUBJECTS AND MODALITIES: acupressure, aromatherapy, business practices, chair massage, chi gong, classification & application of massage movements, cryotherapy, effects & benefits & equipment & products, esalen, face & scalp massage, healing touch, hydrotherapy, lymphatic drainage, myofascial release, orientation & historical overview, pregnancy massage, professional ethics, reflexology, reiki, safety & sanitation, shiatsu, specialized massage, sports massage, therapeutic exercise, therapeutic touch, touch for health, trigger point therapy.

ARKANSAS

State Licensing: 500 hours.

National Certification Exam not accepted.

APPROVED OUT-OF-STATE SCHOOL:

Massage Institute of Memphis, TN.

Reciprocity for accredited out-of-state schools with minimum 500 hour programs.

Board: (501) 623-0444

SCHOOLS:

#15 A Healing Touch Inc.
Clinic & School of Alternative Healing
2201 Rogers Ave., Ste. F
Fort Smith, AR 72901
(501) 783-7566

HOURS OF TRAINING: 525.

DURATION OF COURSE: 6 months, day and evening programs available.

COST: $3,000 Payment plan without interest is available.

#16 American Academy of Healing Arts
1501 N. University, ste. 570
Little Rock, AR 72207
(Classroom: 1405 N. Pierce, ste. 210)
(501) 666-9100 or 1-888-666-9101

HOURS OF TRAINING: 500.

DURATION OF COURSE: 6 months days or weekends, 24 months evenings.

COST: $3,525 including books.

YEAR FOUNDED: 1996.

GRADUATES PER YEAR (APPROX.): 24.

MODALITIES AND SUBJECTS: business & marketing skills, CPR, cranio-sacral therapy, hydrotherapy, hygiene, infant massage, myofascial therapy, polarity, pregnancy massage, reflexology, shiatsu, sports massage, watsu.

#17 Body Wellness Therapeutic Massage Academy
11323 Arcade Dr., suite D
Little Rock, AR 72212
(501) 219-2639 or 1-800-280-6138

HOURS OF TRAINING: 500.

DURATION OF COURSE: 6 months, day and evening programs available.

COST: $3,325 including books. Payment plan without interest is available.

FINANCIAL AID: Veteran's Administration, Rehabilitation.

YEAR FOUNDED: 1995.

GRADUATES PER YEAR (APPROX): 50.

MODALITIES AND SUBJECTS: acupressure, aromatherapy, business management & ethics, chair massage, deep tissue massage, hydrotherapy, heliotherapy & electrotherapy, medical massage, polarity, reflexology, reiki, sports massage, structural kinesiology.

SCHOOL STATEMENT: Endeavoring to teach wholeness of mind, wellness of body and completeness of spirit, while encouraging dedication to the healing process of the whole person.

#18 Hot Springs School of Therapy Technology
1415 North Moore Road
Hot Springs, AR 71913
(Classroom in Little Rock)
1-800-844-0667

HOURS OF TRAINING: 500.

DURATION OF COURSE: 4 months minimum, usually 5 months.

COST: $3,000 including textbooks. Payment plan without interest is available.

FINANCIAL AID: contact school.

YEAR FOUNDED: 1957.

GRADUATES PER YEAR (APPROX.): 20 to 50.

MODALITIES AND SUBJECTS: acupressure, british sports massage, business & marketing, electrotherapy, heliotherapy, hydrotherapy, reflexology, shiatsu.

#19 Ida's Massage Therapy School
418 N. Hickory St.
Pine Bluff, AR 71601
(501) 535-1675

HOURS OF TRAINING: 500 (in-class hours not specified).

COST: $900.

#20 Jean's School of Therapy Technology, Inc.
655 Park Ave.,
Hot Springs, AR 71901
(501) 623-9686

HOURS OF TRAINING: 500.

DURATION OF COURSE: four to six months, days.

COST: $3,000 (includes required books) Payment plan without interest is available.

ACCREDITATIONS/APPROVALS: veterans training program.

YEAR FOUNDED: 1985.

GRADUATES PER YEAR (APPROX.): 50.

MODALITIES AND SUBJECTS: acupressure, applied kinesiology, business, chair massage, electrotherapy, hydrotherapy, myofascial release, myotherapy, neuromuscular therapy, pathology, range of motion, reflexology, shiatsu, sports massage, state law.

#21 Medicine Mountain Massage
4810 Central-Sunbay Resort
Hot Springs, AR 71913
(501) 525-8209

Contact school for program information.

#22 Northwest Arkansas School of Massage Therapy
28 S. College, suite 8
Fayetteville, AR 72701
(501) 582-4341

Contact School for program information.

#23 White River School of Massage
48 Colt Square, suite B
Fayetteville, AR 72703
(501) 521-2550
www.avey.com/wrs

HOURS OF TRAINING: 500.

DURATION OF COURSE: summer intensive 4 months, days 7 months, weekends 10 months.

COST: $3,460 (includes books) ($160 discount for tuition paid two weeks before classes start). Payment plan without interest is available.

FINANCIAL AID: payment plans, approved for veterans training, vocational rehabilitation and other state assistance.

YEAR FOUNDED: 1991.

GRADUATES PER YEAR (APPROX.): 60 - 80.

MODALITIES AND SUBJECTS: assessment skills, business marketing/ethics, chair massage, chi gong, clinical practice, cranio-sacral therapy, esalen massage, hygiene/CPR, integrative therapy, lymphatic drainage, medical massage, myofascial therapy, neuromuscular therapy, ortho-bionomy, reflexology, self-care, shiatsu, sports massage, therapeutic modalities.

SCHOOL STATEMENT: Course places equal emphasis on scientific knowledge, competent hands-on skills and compassionate care. Hospital externship program available. Highly qualified faculty. Beautiful facility. Supportive learning environment.

CALIFORNIA

No State licensing.

Licensing of massage practitioners in California is done only by city and county governments. A State of California law (Chapter 6, sections 51030 through 51034) gives authority to cities and counties to regulate massage. The law states what aspects of the practice may and may not be regulated. Section 51034 states that local laws may not restrict massage to same-sex massage only.

Some southern California jurisdictions exempt Holistic Health Practitioners from their massage laws. This is usually defined as someone with demonstrable training and experience in massage.

The following table of municipal and county licensing requirements was compiled in 1991. While most of this information is still accurate, it is the nature of such information that it slowly goes out of date. Nonetheless, this table provides a useful picture of the diverse state of massage licensing in California.

Aside from the educational requirements listed below, most cities have some practical requirements for a person who wants to practice massage. For example, some towns prohibit "outcall" massage, or house calls, and some regulate it separately and require a special outcall massage license.

The amount charged for business or professional licenses varies tremendously from place to place, from a few dollars to over two thousand dollars. Some towns require a business license but no professional credentials. Some regulate massage as "adult entertainment." Some prohibit the practice of massage altogether.

For updated information about local laws, inquire at the city hall or county government building in the county seat. If you cannot locate a city government, contact the League of California Cities, 1400 K Street, Sacramento, CA 95814.

1,000 HOURS (6): Orange, San Clemente, Santa Paula, Thousand Oaks, Tustin, Vista.

600 HOURS (3): Fontana, Rialto, San Bernardino.

500 HOURS (4): Brea, Cupertino, Palm Desert, Seal Beach.

300 HOURS (1): Newport Beach.

225 HOURS (1): Marina.

200 HOURS (42): Alhambra, Auburn, Bakersfield, Big Bear Lake, Camarillo, Carlsbad, Carson, Chula Vista, Covina, Cudahy, Cypress, El Segundo, Fairfield, Glendale, Grover City, Hayward, Hercules, Highland, Imperial, Imperial Beach, Kern County, Laguna Beach, Loma Linda, Los Alamitos, Huntington Park, Marysville, Montebello, Ontario, Orange County, Placentia, Ridgecrest, San Bernardino County, San Buenaventura, Santa Barbara, Signal Hill, Solano Beach, Torrance, Twentynine Palms, Union City, Ventura County, West Sacramento, Yuba County.

180 HOURS (7): Atwater, Ceres, Dublin, Livingston, Merced, Modesto, Turlock.

100 HOURS (20): Corona, Desert Hot Springs, Dublin, El Dorado County, Escondido, Fresno, Gardena, Hollister, La Mesa, Livermore, Merced County, Monterey, Monterey County, Novato, Palm Springs, Redlands, San Francisco, San Leandro, San Luis Obispo, Santa Monica.

70 HOURS (20): Alameda, Burlingame, Colma, Contra Costa County, Daly City, Half Moon Bay, Lakewood, Manteca, Milpitas, Pacifica, Palo Alto, Portola Valley, Richmond, San Mateo County, San Pablo, San Ramon, Santa Clara, Santa Clara County, Saratoga, Selma.

ANY APPROVED OR RECOGNIZED SCHOOL (37): Adelanto, Arroyo Grande, Azuza, Beaumont, Belmont, Beverly Hills, Cloverdale, Encinitas, Eureka, Foster City, Fullerton, Glendora, Healdsburg, Imperial County, Lemon Grove, Millbrae, Napa, Oceanside, Oxnard, Pacific Grove, Pleasanton, Poway, Rancho Mirage, Sacramento County, San Bruno, San Diego County, San Marcos, San Mateo, Santa Rosa, Santee, Simi Valley, South Lake Tahoe, Stockton, West Covina, West Hollywood, Westmoreland, Whittier.

NO EDUCATIONAL REQUIREMENT BUT OTHER REQUIREMENTS (12): Anaheim, Bell Gardens, Burbank, Commerce, Culver City, Hemet, Long Beach, Los Angeles, Manhattan Beach, Riverside, Riverside County, Santa Fe Springs.

SCHOOLS:

CALIFORNIA, FAR NORTHERN

#24 Chico Therapy: Wellness Center Institute of Healing Arts
1215 Mangrove Ave. #B
Chico, CA 95926
(530) 891-4301

HOURS OF TRAINING: 100 to 500 (31/2 to 8 hours in-class).

DURATION OF COURSE: days 3 months, weekends 1½ months, 2 week intensive.

COST: 100 hours $1,000 including notebook. Payment plan without interest is available, discount for full payment in advance.

YEAR FOUNDED: 1992.

GRADUATES PER YEAR (APPROX.): 100.

MODALITIES AND SUBJECTS: acupressure, body mechanics, business and marketing, general anatomy.

ADVANCED OR CONTINUING EDUCATION: aromatherapy, deep tissue, hospital internship, lymphatic massage, medical massage, myofascial release, neuro-muscular therapy, chair massage, reflexology, shiatsu, sports massage.

SCHOOL STATEMENT: Teaching and educating students about bodywork. Taking Eastern and Western techniques and incorporating them into our everyday lifestyle.

#25 Conscious Choice School of Massage and Integral Healing Arts
670 Azalea Ave.
Redding, CA 96002
(916) 224-0957

Contact school for program information.

#26 Heartwood Institute
220 Harmony Lane
Garberville, CA 95542
(707) 923-5000 reception

HOURS OF TRAINING: 120, 240, 570, 750 or 1,000.

DURATION OF COURSE: 2 weeks, 11 weeks, 6 months, 9 months, one year.

COST: $1,140 to $8,755.

YEAR FOUNDED: 1978.

ACCREDITATIONS/APPROVALS: COMTA/approved, APTA, AOBTA.

PREPARATION FOR OUT-OF-STATE LICENSING EXAM: OR, WA.

GRADUATES PER YEAR (APPROX.): 100

MODALITIES AND SUBJECTS: acupressure, advanced massage, body-mind, deep tissue, cranio-sacral therapy, emotional clearing, energy healing, healing touch, neo-reichian, neuromuscular therapy, orthopedic massage, polarity, shiatsu, somatic therapy, sports massage, thai, therapeutic touch, trigger point therapy, yoga therapy. Programs offered: Heartwood Massage Technician, Massage Practitioner, Massage Therapist, Advanced Massage Therapist, Somatic Therapist, Holistic Health Practitioner, Oriental Healing & Awareness Arts.

SCHOOL STATEMENT: Celebrating 20 years of love in action, Heartwood honors the dreams of those who want to bring their hearts fully into their lives and work.

#27 Loving Hands Institute of Healing Arts
639 11th St.
Fortuna, CA 95540
(707) 725-9627

HOURS OF TRAINING: holistic massage therapy (HMT) 120 (96 in-class hours); advanced holistic massage therapy (AHMT) 100; teacher training certification program (TTCP) 120; universal concepts of health and holism (UCH&H) 140; holistic health educator (HHE) 140.

DURATION OF COURSE: 2 weeks to 8 weeks evenings and weekends.

COST: HMT $1,000; AHMT $1,300; TTCP $600; UCH&H $600; HHE $400 (all include books, workbooks, handouts and lotion. Payment plan without interest is available; approved for VA funding.

YEAR FOUNDED: 1989.

ACCREDITATIONS/APPROVALS: approved for nursing CEU's.

GRADUATES PER YEAR (APPROX.): 20 to 40.

MODALITIES AND SUBJECTS: acupressure massage, deep tissue, introduction to homeopathy, lymphatic massage, reflexology, trigger point therapy.

SCHOOL STATEMENT: We support self-care, natural therapeutics, personal growth and healing, and facilitate personal growth and development by the practice of spiritual expression in all daily activities.

#28 Mendocino School of Holistic Massage and Advanced Healing Arts
2680 Road B
Redwood Valley, CA 95470
(707) 485-8197

HOURS OF TRAINING: massage therapist (HMT) 120 (96 in-class hours); advanced massage therapist (AHMT) 220 (186 in-class hours); holistic health practitioner (HHP) 500 (in-class hours not specified).

DURATION OF COURSE: HMT: 3 months some evenings & weekends, AHMT: 3 months some weekends, most classes meet from 1:00 p.m. Friday to 6:00 p.m. Sunday.

COST: HMT $1,380; AHMT $1,275, HHP $1,300 plus prerequisites.

YEAR FOUNDED: 1993.

ACCREDITATIONS/APPROVALS: approved for nursing CEU's.

GRADUATES PER YEAR (APPROX.): 60 to 85.

MODALITIES AND SUBJECTS: body mapping, business, conscious breathwork, core energy work, counseling, emotional point release, energy field anatomy & theory, esalen, ethics, hypnosis for bodyworkers, integrative holistic massage, intuitive development, lymphatic drainage, mind-body principles, organ revitalization, polarity, polarity yoga, private instruction, reflexology, relaxation & balancing techniques, self-care. Advanced programs: rebirther training, holistic health practitioner.

SCHOOL STATEMENT: small classes, holistic orientation with emphasis on personal growth, rural setting, no charge for accommodations.

#29 New Life Institute of Massage Therapy
1159 Hilltop Dr.
Redding, CA 96002
(530) 222-1467

HOURS OF TRAINING: Basic 180 (160 in-class); Advanced 120 (100 in-class).

DURATION OF COURSE: Basic 3½ months, Advanced 4 months, day and evening classes available.

COST: Basic $1,436; Advanced $973 (both courses include texts and materials). Payment plan without interest is available.

YEAR FOUNDED: 1990.

GRADUATES PER YEAR (APPROX): 40.

MODALITIES AND SUBJECTS: acupressure, applied kinesiology, chair massage, cranio-sacral therapy, ethics and business practices, infant massage, medical massage, myofascial release, pregnancy massage, reflexology, theory and history of massage, trigger point therapy hygiene.

SCHOOL STATEMENT: We stress the therapeutic nature of massage and encourage cooperation between the medical profession and the massage therapist.

#30 Pacific School of Massage & Healing Arts
44800 Fish Rock Road
Gualala, CA 95445
(707) 884-3138

HOURS OF TRAINING: 110.

DURATION OF COURSE: two six-day sessions separated by one month of independent study and practice.

COST: $1,700.

FINANCIAL AID: County Vocational Rehab. programs.

YEAR FOUNDED: 1978.

ACCREDITATIONS/APPROVALS: approved for nursing CEU's.

GRADUATES PER YEAR (APPROX.): 36.

MODALITIES AND SUBJECTS: acupressure, applied kinesiology, body-mind, chair massage, esalen massage, infant massage, jin shin do, lymphatic drainage, shiatsu, shen, somatic therapy, touch for health, Transformational Bodywork, yoga therapy. Coursework is eligible for academic credit at Summit University of Louisiana.

SCHOOL STATEMENT: In residential retreat, we blend an eclectic and 'down to earth' East-West curriculum of hands-on modalities, psycho-emotional, and spiritual aspects of healing and transformation.

CALIFORNIA: SACRAMENTO – LAKE TAHOE AREA

#31 The Body Institute – A School of Massage Therapy
8331 Sierra College #210
Granite Bay, CA 95746
(916) 791-1951

HOURS OF TRAINING: 500 (in-class hours not specified).

DURATION OF COURSE: 18 months; day, evening and weekend programs available.

FINANCIAL AID: Scholarships, Department of Rehabilitation.

YEAR FOUNDED: 1996.

GRADUATES PER YEAR (APPROX.): 70.

MODALITIES AND SUBJECTS: acupressure, breathwork, business, chair massage, deep tissue, joint mobilization, myofascial release, polarity, pregnancy massage, shiatsu, sports massage, trigger point therapy.

SCHOOL STATEMENT: To empower the individual to be both a student and a teacher of touch.

#32 Calaveras College of Therapeutic Massage
P.O. Box 274
(classroom: 96 Court Street)
San Andreas, CA 95249
(209) 754-4876

HOURS OF TRAINING: 100 (in-class hours not specified).

DURATION OF COURSE: 2 weeks, days & weekends.

COST: $750 including coloring workbook Payment Plan without interest is available.

YEAR FOUNDED: 1996.

GRADUATES PER YEAR (APPROX.): 50.

SCHOOL STATEMENT: Learn the basic fundamental of massage in a peaceful environment conducive to learning.

#33 Clinical Touch School of Massage Therapy
1365 Cobblestone Drive
Lincoln, CA 95648
(Classroom: 6809 Five Star Blvd.,
Rocklin, CA 95677)
(916) 536-0700

HOURS OF TRAINING: 130 to 260.

DURATION OF COURSE: 2 to 6 months, evenings & weekends.

COST: 130 hours $894.00, 260 hours $1,950.00; both including registration, books and supplies. Payment plan without interest is available.

YEAR FOUNDED: 1997.

GRADUATES PER YEAR (APPROX.): 50.

MODALITIES AND SUBJECTS: chair massage, deep tissue, geriatric massage, infant massage, medical massage, myofascial release, myotherapy, pediatric massage, pregnancy massage, sports massage, trigger point therapy.

SCHOOL STATEMENT: We offer a practical curriculum. Strong emphasis is put on proper technique, body mechanics, and "hands-on" supervised practice.

#34 Federico College of Hairstyling
2100 Arden Way, suite 265
Sacramento, CA 95825
(916) 929-4242

Contact school for program information.

#35 Foothills Massage School
P.O. Box 826
North San Juan, CA 95959
(classes at North Columbia Schoolhouse and Cultural Center)
(530) 292-3123

HOURS OF TRAINING: 100.

DURATION OF COURSE: 10 weeks, evenings.

COST: $520 includes books and materials.

YEAR FOUNDED: 1996.

GRADUATES PER YEAR (APPROX.): 50-60.

MODALITIES AND SUBJECTS: acupressure, business, legal aspects, lymphatic drainage, meridians, nutrition, polarity, professional ethics & communication, range of motion, reflexology, shiatsu. The massage certification program provides 30 continuing ed. Credits for nurses.

SCHOOL STATEMENT: FMS offers quality training for working and limited-income people to explore hidden healing abilities and use these skills to generate revenues in their communities.

#36 Healing Arts Institute
112 Douglas Blvd.
Roseville, CA 95678
(916) 782-1275
www.abundanthealth.com

HOURS OF TRAINING: 126.

DURATION OF COURSE: day class 3 weeks, morning class 6 weeks, evening class 12 weeks.

COST: $967.16 including books.

YEAR FOUNDED: 1990.

GRADUATES PER YEAR (APPROX.): 200+.

MODALITIES AND SUBJECTS: acupressure, aromatherapy, Bowen Technique, chair massage, deep tissue, infant massage, pregnancy massage, reflexology, reiki, sports massage, trigger point, joint mobilization, stretches, lymphatic massage, massage for children and elderly clients, business and ethics, stress management, deep relaxation techniques. Advanced programs: acupressure certification training, deep tissue, sports massage, geriatric massage, aromatherapy, marketing, reflexology.

#37 Institute of Therapeutic Massage
5777 Madison Ave. #180
Sacramento, CA 95841
(916) 334-7393

HOURS OF TRAINING: Basic 135, Advanced 115.

DURATION OF COURSE: Basic, 11 weeks evenings or 5 weeks days; Advanced 5 weeks days.

COST: Basic $1,300; Advanced $1,300, both including textbooks and study manual. Payment plan without interest is available.

YEAR FOUNDED: 1996.

GRADUATES PER YEAR (APPROX.): 100.

MODALITIES AND SUBJECTS: applied kinesiology, aromatherapy, body mechanics, business legalities, business theory & marketing, chair massage, chronic conditions, client communication, cross fiber, deep tissue, designer massage, hands on injury, infant massage, integrative massage, kinesiology, lymphatic drainage, massage theory and applications, medical massage, myofascial release, myotherapy, nutrition, physical therapy modalities, pregnancy massage, reflexology, shiatsu, SOAP note documentation, specific health conditions, sports massage, teaching clinic, trigger point therapy.

SCHOOL STATEMENT: Quality of graduates, not quantity. Our intense, diversified, and comprehensive course insures graduates have the skills necessary to be effective and successful therapists and educators.

#38 Integrative Therapy School
3000 T. St., suite 104
Sacramento, CA 95816
(916) 739-8848

HOURS OF TRAINING: 130 or 500.

DURATION OF COURSE: 130-hour course 3 months or 1-month intensive, 500-hour course 9 months full-time or 15 months part time. Day and evening/weekend programs available.

COST: 130 hours $1,236; 500 hours $4,461 (including supplies).

YEAR FOUNDED: 1982.

ACCREDITATIONS/APPROVALS: COMTA/approved, City and State Departments of Vocational Rehabilitation, approved for nursing CEU's.

GRADUATES PER YEAR (APPROX.): 130.

MODALITIES AND SUBJECTS: acupressure, body mechanics, breath awareness, business & marketing, clinical practices, communication skills, contraindication for massage, deep tissue, muscle balancing, nutrition, polarity, reflexology, shiatsu, somatic movement, sports massage, tai chi. Advanced programs: advanced acupressure. Continuing ed: infant massage, chair massage, aromatherapy, geriatric, Upledger cranial.

SCHOOL STATEMENT: Aspects of body, mind and spirit are integrated fully into the I.T.S. curriculum. Community outreach program gives students experience in a variety of settings.

#39 Lake Tahoe Massage School & Seasons Spa
1034 Emerald Bay Rd., #401
So. Lake Tahoe, CA 96150
(Classroom: 1970 Highway 50)
(530) 544-1227

HOURS OF TRAINING: 30 to 575 hours.

DURATION OF COURSE: one weekend to one year, day & evening & weekend programs available.

COST: $225 to $3,000, including manuals and books. Payment plan without interest is available.

FINANCIAL AID: Private Credit Company offers loans.

YEAR FOUNDED: 1996.

GRADUATES PER YEAR (APPROX.): 70.

MODALITIES AND SUBJECTS: applied kinesiology, aromatherapy, body-mind, chinese orthopedic massage, cranio-sacral therapy, deep tissue, infant massage, lymphatic drainage, medical massage, medical "think tank" certification, polarity, postural integration, pregnancy massage, reflexology, spa certification, sports massage, structural integration, thai massage certification, trigger point therapy, tui na.

SCHOOL STATEMENT: Lake Tahoe Massage School promotes excellence through education, combining soft tissue techniques with classes of sensitivity, intuitiveness and awareness.

#40 Makoto Kai Healing Arts
443 First St.
Woodland, CA 95695
(530) 662-5662

HOURS OF TRAINING: 150.

DURATION OF COURSE: 6 months, weekends.

COST: $780.

YEAR FOUNDED: 1996.

GRADUATES PER YEAR (APPROX.): 15.

MODALITIES AND SUBJECTS: Okazaki Restorative Massage.

SCHOOL STATEMENT: ORM was taught by Master therapist and Jujitsu founder Henry Okazaki. His heirs balance martial arts with healing arts. The technique is deep, invigorating massage.

#41 Phillips School of Massage
P.O. Box 1999
Nevada City, CA 95959
(Classroom: 101 Broad St., suite B)
(530) 265-4645

HOURS OF TRAINING: 230 and 600 (in-class hours not specified).

DURATION OF COURSE: 230 hours 7 weeks days or 8½ months evenings, 600 hours 5½ months—2 years.

COST: $1,650 to $3,300 including books.

YEAR FOUNDED: 1983.

ACCREDITATIONS/APPROVALS: approved for CA nursing CEU's.

GRADUATES PER YEAR (APPROX.): 100.

MODALITIES AND SUBJECTS: active isolated stretching, acupressure, aromatherapy, body-mind, chair massage, chi gong, circulatory, cranio-sacral therapy, deep tissue, healing touch, ortho-bionomy, reflexology, shiatsu, sports massage, touch for health, trager.

SCHOOL STATEMENT: PSM training offers a bridge between technical and intuitive perspectives, combining understanding of various forms of bodywork with the importance of attitude, presence and respect.

CALIFORNIA, NAPA AND SONOMA COUNTIES

#42 The Alchemy Institute of Healing Arts
567A Summerfield Rd. Santa Rosa, CA 95405
Classroom: 20889 Geyserville Ave., Geyserville
(707) 537-0495

Contact school for program information.

#43 California Institute of Massage & Spa Services
P.O. Box 673 / 730 Broadway
Sonoma, CA 95476
(707) 939-9431

HOURS OF TRAINING:
- Massage Technician 165 (120 in-class) $1,150 (all prices include books and materials).
- Advanced Massage I 100 (75 in-class) $895.
- Advanced Massage II 135 (100 in-class) approx. $1,200.
- Advanced Massage III (medical massage) 250 (200 in-class) $1,995.
- Spa Services Certification 100 (80 in-class) $950. Payment plan without interest is available, scholarships and discounts may be available.

FINANCIAL AID: approved by state vocational rehabilitation.

DURATION OF COURSE: 14 weeks to 2 years. Day, evening and weekend programs offered.

YEAR FOUNDED: 1992.

GRADUATES PER YEAR (APPROX.): 60.

MODALITIES AND SUBJECTS: acupressure, aromatherapy, breema, business practices, chair massage, cranio-sacral therapy, energy work, ethics, geriatric massage, injury prevention, medical massage, pregnancy massage, reflexology, shiatsu, spa services, sports massage, therapeutic touch, trigger point therapy, yoga therapy.

SCHOOL STATEMENT: Our programs blend the principles of bodywork with techniques for self-awareness. We emphasize keen observation, good body mechanics and the healing power of touch.

#44 Calistoga Massage Therapy School
5959 Commerce Blvd., suite 13
Rohnert Park, CA 94928
(707) 586-1953

HOURS OF TRAINING: 100.

DURATION OF COURSE: 7 weeks evenings or 10 weeks days.

COST: $800 (includes books and materials). Payment plan without interest is available.

YEAR FOUNDED: 1981.

GRADUATES PER YEAR (APPROX.): 50.

MODALITIES AND SUBJECTS: esalen massage, lymphatic drainage, medical massage, reflexology.

SCHOOL STATEMENT: Class size maximum 14 students. The program emphasizes body mechanics, intuitive awareness of client's energy blocks, and a spiritual awareness of the therapist's healing potential.

#45 Jupiter Hollow School for Massage
P.O. Box 8043
Santa Rosa, CA 95407
(707) 584-7903

HOURS OF TRAINING: 101.

COST: $1,000.

YEAR FOUNDED: 1979.

GRADUATES PER YEAR (APPROX.): 30.

MODALITIES AND SUBJECTS: accident and sports rehabilitation, body mechanics, Edgar Cayce therapies, esalen, lymphatic & circulatory massage, reflexology.

SCHOOL STATEMENT: Massage can be a moving meditation for the practitioner. We teach body centered awareness to bring integration of body mind spirit to giver and receiver.

#46 School of Shiatsu and Massage at Harbin Hot Springs
P.O. Box 570
Middletown, CA 95461
(707) 987-3801
www.waba.edu

HOURS OF TRAINING: Training is offered in 50 and 100 hour segments. Certificates are given for 100-hour Practitioner Course and 500-hour Therapist Course. The school also offers 1,000-hour Practitioner Course and 1,000-hour Advanced Therapist Program.

DURATION OF COURSE: 50 hour segments 6 days; 100 hour segments 11 days.

COST: Each 50-hour segment costs $600, inclusive of lodging and use of the facilities.

YEAR FOUNDED: 1977.

GRADUATES PER YEAR (APPROX.): 400 to 750.

MODALITIES AND SUBJECTS: acupressure, deep tissue, healing intimate trauma, NLP, pain relief, rebalancing, shiatsu, sports massage, tantsu, watsu (aquatic shiatsu), wassertantzen™.

SCHOOL STATEMENT: located at a hot springs retreat and resort, is a center for the teaching of watsu® (aquatic shiatsu).

#47 Sebastopol Massage Center
108 North Main St. #5
Sebastopol, CA 95472
(707) 823-3550

HOURS OF TRAINING: 150 (100 in-class).

DURATION OF COURSE: 6 weeks, day or evening or weekend courses available.

COST: $800. Payment plan without interest is available.

FINANCIAL AID: Rehab.

YEAR FOUNDED: 1983.

GRADUATES PER YEAR (APPROX): 100.

MODALITIES AND SUBJECTS: business practices, chair massage, cranio-sacral therapy, documented practice, esalen, ethics, marketing, ortho-bionomy, reflexology, shiatsu.

SCHOOL STATEMENT: The program is a well-rounded one, with emphasis on swedish/esalen, that stresses the development of the therapist's own natural awareness and intuition.

#48 Wellness Holistic School of Massage
345 South "E" St
Santa Rosa, CA 95404
(707) 546-8115

HOURS OF TRAINING: 120.

COST: $940.

YEAR FOUNDED: 1983.

GRADUATES PER YEAR (APPROX.): 12.

MODALITIES AND SUBJECTS: brain gym for bodyworkers, business & ethics, esalen, polarity, reflexology, touch for health, wellness counseling. Additional trainings: Natural Health Counselor (70 hours), Holistic Health Educator (100 hours).

CALIFORNIA: MARIN COUNTY

#49 Aesclepion Massage Institute, Inc.
     1314 Lincoln Ave., suite B
     San Rafael, CA 94901
     (415) 453-6196

HOURS OF TRAINING: 130 (48 in-class hours).

DURATION OF COURSE: 3 months, evenings.

COST: $900. Payment plan without interest is available.

YEAR FOUNDED: 1993.

GRADUATES PER YEAR (APPROX): 20.

MODALITIES AND SUBJECTS: business practices & marketing strategies, chair massage, cranio-sacral therapy, healing touch, introduction to acupressure, introduction to hydrotherapy, introduction to reflexology, joint mobilization, kinesiology, lymphatic drainage, meditation & the healing arts, ortho-bionomy, pregnancy massage, reflexology, sports massage, therapeutic techniques in swedish massage, using your own healing energy; healing yourself while healing others.

SCHOOL STATEMENT: AMI recognizes the physical and energetic aspects of massage. Students learn therapeutic massage techniques and what they personally have to bring to the healing arts.

#50 Alive & Well!
     Institute of Conscious BodyWork
     100 Shaw Drive
     San Anselmo, CA 94960
     (415) 258-0402

HOURS OF TRAINING: 140 hours, 300 hours, 570 hours, 1,000 hours.

DURATION OF COURSE: 140 hours 3-week intensive, 12 weeks or longer, 300 hours 6 to 8 months, 570-hours 18 to 24 months, 1,000 hours 36 months. Courses offered days, evenings and weekends.

COST: 140 hours $1,250, 300 hours $2,900, 570 hours $5,500, 1,000 hours $10,800 (books included). Payment plan without interest is available, some scholarships available, VA approved and eligible for local education fund from county.

YEAR FOUNDED: 1987.

GRADUATES PER YEAR (APPROX.): 100.

MODALITIES AND SUBJECTS: acupressure, advanced techniques for the neck, applied kinesiology, aromatherapy, bodywork for abuse survivors, brain function facilitation, breema bodywork, carpal tunnel and wrist problems, chair massage, chi gong, continuum, Conscious BodyWork, conscious breathwork, counseling for bodyworkers, cranio-sacral therapy, deep tissue, energetic tune-ups, establishing a business, ethics and communication, eucapnic breathing for asthmatics, face and head massage, insurance billing, kinesiology, lymphatic drainage, massage ergonomics, movement education, myofascial release, neuro-muscular reprogramming, neuromuscular therapy, nutrition, polarity, primary movement, reflexology, rocking and shaking, self-care, shiatsu, skydancing tantra, somatic technique, sports massage, stretching and massage, touch for health, trigger point therapy.

SCHOOL STATEMENT: The focus is on the power of conscious attention and intention as an agent of change within.

#51 Diamond Light School of Massage & Healing
     P.O. Box 5443
     Mill Valley, CA 94942
     (415) 454-6651

HOURS OF TRAINING: 150.

IN-CLASS HOURS: 100.

DURATION OF COURSE: 6 weeks intensive or ten weeks (classes meet evenings and weekends).

COST: $1,195 (up to $70 discount for early payment).

FINANCIAL AID: Scholarships available.

YEAR FOUNDED: 1987.

GRADUATES PER YEAR (APPROX.): 80.

MODALITIES AND SUBJECTS: business practices, chair massage, deep tissue, energy and chakra work, esalen, foot reflexology, hygiene and ethics, hypnotherapy, laying on of hands, lymphatic drainage, meditation, movement, myofascial release, pregnancy massage, reflexology, reiki, sound healing, transforming emotions, working with the elements.

ADVANCED PROGRAMS: deep bodywork specialization, spiritual healing certification, hypnotherapy certification.

SCHOOL STATEMENT: We emphasize the practice of bodywork as a spiritual art and a path to facilitate spiritual awakening in the client as well as the therapist.

#52 Wind Walk Institute of Natural Healing
     and Beauty
     1001 Bridgeway, #505
     Sausalito Anchorage, *The Enterprise*
     (510) 525-0446

HOURS OF TRAINING: 100 basic, 500 total.

DURATION OF COURSE: 100 hours, two-week intensive.

COST: $895.

YEAR FOUNDED: 1992.

GRADUATES PER YEAR (APPROX): 10.

MODALITIES AND SUBJECTS: acupressure, bioenergetics, chair massage, cranio-sacral therapy, esalen, gravitational leverage, intuitive response, kali & quan yin dancing, lymphatic drainage, pattern detachment, pele's mouth wide open, polarity, pregnancy massage, rebirthing, reflexology, retropressure, shiatsu, sports massage, sunhawk, the devotion of hera's hearth, yoga therapy.

SCHOOL STATEMENT: Intuition frames our teaching as we gain body awareness aboard our ship, *The Enterprise*.

CALIFORNIA, SAN FRANCISCO

#53 San Francisco School of Massage
     1327 A Chestnut St.
     San Francisco, CA 94123
     (415) 474-4600

HOURS OF TRAINING: 102 basic, 201 advanced.

DURATION OF COURSE: 102 hours six weeks to 17 weeks; 201-hour advanced course 4 months, day and evening and weekend programs are available.

COST: 102-hour $950; 201-hour advanced $2,010. Payment plan without interest is available.

YEAR FOUNDED: 1969.

ACCREDITATIONS/APPROVALS: approved for nursing CEU's.

GRADUATES PER YEAR (APPROX.): 200.

MODALITIES AND SUBJECTS: aromatherapy, barefoot shiatsu, breathwork, breema, business, chair massage, chi gong, cranio-sacral massage, deep tissue massage, energy work, esalen, geriatric massage, light touch, lymphatic massage, marketing, massage for clients with physical limitations, nutrition, pregnancy massage, reflexology, shiatsu on a table, spa massage, sports massage.

ADVANCED PROGRAMS: 103-hour zen shiatsu, 103-hour insight

bodywork, 201-hour advanced swedish. 30 hours continuing education free to students who take the basic course.

SCHOOL STATEMENT: We believe the key to training outstanding bodyworkers is instructors with a wealth of knowledge and a special ability to make learning fun and interesting.

#54 School for Self-Healing
1718 Taraval St.
San Francisco, CA 94116
(415) 665-9574

HOURS OF TRAINING: Segment A, 80 hours; Segment B, 80 hours; Level two, 100 hours; Apprenticeship 500 hours.

DURATION OF COURSE: Segment A, 8 days; Segment B, 8 days; Level two, 2 weeks; Apprenticeship at student's pace.

COST: $6,743.10 for entire training. Payment plan without interest is available.

FINANCIAL AID: discount for payment in full and for domestic partners.

YEAR FOUNDED: 1984.

GRADUATES PER YEAR (APPROX): 150 world-wide.

MODALITIES AND SUBJECTS: The Meir Schneider Self-Healing Method: breathing, cultivating intuition & inventiveness, empowering the client, kinesthetic awareness, massage, movement, vision improvement, visualization/imagery.

SCHOOL STATEMENT: Meir Schneider, born blind, used his unique method to gain functional eyesight and has helped thousands overcome pain, injury, limited movement and poor vision problems.

#55 Trinity Business College
939 Market St.
San Francisco, CA 94103
(415) 541-7777

Contact school for program information.

#56 The World School of Massage and Advanced Healing Arts
401-32nd Avenue
San Francisco, CA 94121
(415) 221-2533

PROGRAMS OFFERED:
- Holistic Massage Therapist (HMT)
- Advanced Massage Therapist (AMT)
- Holistic Health Counselor (HHC)
- Master Bodyworker/Holistic Health Educator (MB/HHE)

HOURS OF TRAINING: HMT 172 (130 in-class); AMT 222 (153 in-class); HHC 350 (315 in-class); MB/HHE 804 (682 in-class).

DURATION OF COURSE: HMT 4 months; AMT 5 months; HHC 9 months; MB/HHE 12 to 14 months, day & evening & weekend programs available.

COST: HMT $1,250; AMT $1,875; HHC $3,750; MB/HHE $6,650.

YEAR FOUNDED: 1982.

ACCREDITATIONS/APPROVALS: approved for nursing continuing education contact hours.

GRADUATES PER YEAR (APPROX.): 150–200.

MODALITIES AND SUBJECTS: alternative theories of healing, aromatherapy, consciousness: breath, birth & being, chair massage, death & dying/how to be really alive!, cranio-sacral therapy, educational kinesiology, emotional let-go-lab, energy body's awakening, expression leadership program, flower essence consulting, foot bone rehabilitation, holistic business skills, holistic fitness & nutrition, holistic movement, infant massage, liquid consciousness! liquid bodies!, lymphatic drainage, power

of language and communication, rebirthing, reflexology, structural integration, touch for health, vibrational healing massage therapy levels I–IV.

SCHOOL STATEMENT: The school offers Vibrational Healing Massage Therapy, developed by the school's founder, Patricia Cramer. The school's focus is on self-responsibility and communication.

CALIFORNIA, BERKELEY & OAKLAND AREA

#57 Acupressure Institute
1533 Shattuck Ave.
Berkeley, CA 94709
(510) 845-1059 or (800) 442-2232
www.acupressure.com and www.healthy.net/acupressure

HOURS OF TRAINING: 150 to 1,000.

DURATION OF COURSE: four-week intensive or, six months to one year part-time.

COST: $1,100 to $6,400. Payment plan without interest is available.

FINANCIAL AID: work trade.

YEAR FOUNDED: 1976.

ACCREDITATIONS/APPROVALS: AOBTA, approved for nursing CEU's.

MODALITIES AND SUBJECTS: acupressure apprenticeship trainings, acupressure for menopause, acupressure teacher training, acu-yoga teacher training, advanced acupressure oil massage, arthritis relief, ashiatsu, ashiatsu skills clinic, balancing the 5 elements with food, body psychology, chair massage, chakra healing, chi gong, chinese healing imagery, chinese massage (tui na), counseling skills, cranio-sacral therapy, creating a successful practice, dealing with abuse, emotion balancing using meridians, emotional release, healing touch, herbal patent formula, hypnosis & somatic healing, iridology, kinesiology, major medical disorders, moxa & cupping & magnets, practical teaching skills, practical treatment points, pregnancy & birthing, reflexology, reiki, shiatsu, somatic therapy, spirit of the points, thai massage program, touch for health, touching spirit, traditional chinese theory, western herbology, women's health issues, zen shiatsu for common complaints.

SCHOOL STATEMENT: Learn hands-on healing skills through comprehensive trainings in Asian bodywork, Shiatsu, and massage. Instructional videos and workbooks available through our Hands-On Health Care Catalog.

#58 American Institute of Massage Therapy
1661 Tice Valley Blvd., suite 102
Walnut Creek, CA 94595
(925) 945-8976

HOURS OF TRAINING: 400 (additional offerings planned).

COST: under $4,000.

YEAR FOUNDED: 1979.

GRADUATES PER YEAR (APPROX.): 110.

MODALITIES AND SUBJECTS: abdominal stress release, acupressure, biofeedback, business practices & ethics, cervical-scapular release, distal myofascial release, history & ethics of massage, introduction to medical & wholistic therapies, lumbar-sacral release, lymphatics, nutrition, preventative maintenance, self-expansion breathing, stress analysis, temporo-mandibular joint, therapeutic exercises for you & your clients, therapist communication skills.

SCHOOL STATEMENT: Myro Therapy Deep Tissue Massage is a successful neuromuscular release for sports massage and injuries. Our dedication is to graduate the best massage therapist.

#59 Body Electric School
6527A Telegraph Ave.
Oakland, CA 94609
(510) 653-1594

HOURS OF TRAINING: 100.

DURATION OF COURSE: two weeks.

COST: $1,095. Payment plan without interest is available.

FINANCIAL AID: scholarships.

YEAR FOUNDED: 1984.

GRADUATES PER YEAR (APPROX.): 50.

MODALITIES AND SUBJECTS: bodywork for people with life-threatening illnesses, conscious breathwork, deep tissue massage, esalen, rebirthing.

SCHOOL STATEMENT: Body Electric welcomes students of all sexual orientations and spiritual paths. The work is holistic and emphasizes the integration of mind/body and spirit.

#60 Care Through Touch Institute
2401 LeConte Ave.
Berkeley, CA 94709
(510) 548-0418

HOURS OF TRAINING: 160 to 500 (130 to 420 in-class hours).

DURATION OF COURSE: 160 hours 4 weeks, 500 hours 18 months, program offered days or evenings/weekends.

COST: 160 hours $1,500 (includes books). Payment plan without interest is available, scholarships or discounts are available.

YEAR FOUNDED: 1989.

ACCREDITATIONS/APPROVALS: Graduate Theological Union of Berkeley, CA; CA approved for nursing CEU's.

GRADUATES PER YEAR (APPROX.): 45.

MODALITIES AND SUBJECTS: acupressure, advanced therapeutic modalities, applied anatomy, breathing and introspection, business and ethics, chair massage, deep tissue, esalen, hydrotherapy, movement, pastoral ministry, polarity, reflexology, special skills for working with children, the elderly, sick, disabled and abused, supervised pastoral internship, theological reflection.

SCHOOL STATEMENT: We teach massage within the context of contemporary Christian spirituality. Students are prepared for work with the elderly, poor, dying, disabled, addicted, and AIDS patients.

#61 McKinnon Institute of Professional Massage and Bodywork
2940 Webster St.
Oakland, CA 94609-3407
(510) 465-3488

HOURS OF TRAINING: 100 to 920.

DURATION OF COURSE: 2 weeks to 2 years, day or evening or weekend or intensive programs available.

COST: $10 per hour of class (average). Payment plan without interest is available.

YEAR FOUNDED: 1973.

GRADUATES PER YEAR (APPROX.): 400 to 500 for all programs combined.

MODALITIES AND SUBJECTS: acupressure (shiatsu), business—ethics—hygiene, chair massage, cranio-sacral therapy, deep tissue—sports massage, esalen, infant massage, myotherapy, pregnancy massage, reflexology, shiatsu, somatic therapy, specialized settings, subtle touch, trigger point therapy. Certificate programs offered: swedish/esalen, sports/deep tissue I & II, asian systems I & II, subtle systems, advanced modalities.

SCHOOL STATEMENT: The McKinnon approach acknowledges body, mind and spiritual life. Certificate programs provide a learning atmosphere grounded in technical competence while inspiring intuition, creativity and individuality.

#62 Moving On Center School for Participatory Arts and Research
1428 Alice St., #201
Oakland, CA 94612
(510) 834-0284

HOURS OF TRAINING: 100 massage; 1,000 (750 in-class) full training.

DURATION OF COURSE: 100 hours 2 weeks.

COST: 100 hours $750; full training $11,000. Payment plan without interest is available.

FINANCIAL AID: Some scholarships or discounts available.

YEAR FOUNDED: 1994.

GRADUATES PER YEAR (APPROX.): 10.

MODALITIES AND SUBJECTS: action thither, alexander, authentic movement, bartneiff fundamentals, body-mind centering, contact improvisation, daban movement analysis (introduction), embodying the archetypes of health, hakomi, somatic movement therapy training, vocal motion.

SCHOOL STATEMENT: Massage emphasizes Tai Chi body usage, Swedish and Esalen massage. The full training integrates performing arts and somatic research, bridging health, education and the arts.

#63 National Holistic Institute
5900 Hollis St. J
Emeryville, CA 94608
1-800-315-3552
www.nhimassage.com

HOURS OF TRAINING: 720 (664 in-class hours).

DURATION OF COURSE: day program 9 months, evening/weekend program approx. 12–15 months.

COST: $8,838.85 (includes books, massage table and supplies).

FINANCIAL AID: federally guaranteed grants and loans available (contact admissions office).

YEAR FOUNDED: 1979.

ACCREDITATIONS/APPROVALS: COMTA/approved, ACCET.

GRADUATES PER YEAR (APPROX.): 500.

MODALITIES AND SUBJECTS: acupressure/shiatsu, body mechanics, business skills, chair massage, communication skills, customization of massage sessions, deep tissue, energy massage, first aid, CPR, foot reflexology, hydrotherapy, joint mobilization, kinesiology, marketing, massage for people with injuries, massage for pregnant women, postural analysis, record-keeping, resume writing and interviewing, rocking and shaking massage, sports massage, stress management, time management.

SCHOOL STATEMENT: Students participate in a real-world clinic and a non-profit agency for indigent clients. Students receive extensive training in building a successful massage therapy practice.

#64 re Source
Box 5398
Berkeley, CA 94705
(classroom: 825 Bancroft Way)
(510) 433-7917

HOURS OF TRAINING: 200, 500 or 1,000 (in-class hours not specified).

DURATION OF COURSE: Students proceed at their own pace.

COST: 200 hours $900 plus cost of electives. Advanced trainings are comprised of individual courses. Payment plan without interest is available.

YEAR FOUNDED: 1982.

GRADUATES PER YEAR (APPROX.): 15.

MODALITIES AND SUBJECTS: acupressure, advanced practice class, advanced practitioner seminars, bodymind survey course, bodyreading, chair massage, deep tissue, esalen, massage & anatomy, massage & kinesiology, ortho-bionomy, polarity, professional issues & skills & development, reflexology, somatic therapy, trager.

SCHOOL STATEMENT: re Source offers comprehensive education in bodywork to individuals who want a program which values their intuition and acknowledges their physical intelligence.

> **#65 Silicon Valley College**
>   41350 Christy St.
>   Fremont, CA 94538
>   (510) 623-9966

Contact the school for program information.

CALIFORNIA, SAN JOSE – SANTA CRUZ – SALINAS AREA

> **#66 Body Therapy Center**
>   368 California Ave.
>   Palo Alto, CA 94306
>   (650) 328-9400

HOURS OF TRAINING: 125 to 1,000.

COST: $1,050 to $1,275 per 125-hour professional course.

YEAR FOUNDED: 1983.

GRADUATES PER YEAR (APPROX.): 500.

MODALITIES AND SUBJECTS: 125-hour courses: fundamentals of massage, advanced massage symposium, advanced massage & bodywork, fundamentals of shiatsu, intermediate shiatsu, sports massage, clinical deep tissue, jin shin do. Shorter continuing education courses and community workshops are also offered.

SCHOOL STATEMENT: Well-known and respected, BTC provides dynamic, superior training in massage. We cherish and develop our students fully. We offer professional, community and continuing education courses.

> **#67 The Center for Body Harmonics**
>   1210 Memorex Dr.
>   Santa Clara, CA 95050
>   1-800-700-1993 or (408) 727-1939
>   www.alternativehealing.com

HOURS OF TRAINING: 100, 500, 750, 1,000.

DURATION OF COURSE: 100 hours: 3 weeks days, six weeks evenings or 5 weekends.

COST: $1,395, $5,495, $7,495, $9,495 All include textbooks and massage table.

YEAR FOUNDED: 1994.

GRADUATES PER YEAR (APPROX.): 150.

MODALITIES AND SUBJECTS: acupressure for emotional release, applied kinesiology, aromatherapy, basic acupressure, basic qi gong, basic shiatsu floor massage, beginning & advanced hypnotherapy, body wrap, breathwork, cranio-sacral therapy, creating the life you desire, deep tissue, face & scalp techniques, geriatric massage, holistic approach to personal empowerment, hydrotherapy, hypnosis 101, introduction to asian medicine theory, introduction to herbology, introduction to infant massage,

introduction to myofascial techniques, introduction to polarity, introduction to pregnancy massage, introduction to somatic practices, lomilomi, lymphatic drainage, massage instructor training, massage techniques refresher, massage therapy billing, new beginnings, reflexology, rehabilitation techniques, reiki, residency program, safety procedures, shiatsu chair massage, somato emotional release, sports massage, stress reduction & relaxation, structural integration, trigger point therapy.

SCHOOL STATEMENT: At the Center for BodyHarmonics we pride ourselves in offering a supportive, family-like atmosphere where the needs and comfort of the student come first.

> **#68 Central Coast Massage Institute**
>   1263 S. Padre Dr.
>   Salinas, CA 93901
>   (408) 422-8240

Contact school for program information.

> **#69 Cypress Health Institute**
>   P.O. Box 2941
>   Santa Cruz, CA 95063
>   (Classroom: 200 7th Ave., Santa Cruz, CA 95062)
>   (408) 476-2115

HOURS OF TRAINING: 170.

DURATION OF COURSE: 3 months, evenings & weekends.

COST: $1,150 includes all texts and manuals. Payment plan without interest is available.

YEAR FOUNDED: 1982.

GRADUATES PER YEAR (APPROX.): 70.

MODALITIES AND SUBJECTS: acupressure, AMMA, body-mind, chair massage, counseling skills for bodyworkers. cranio-sacral therapy, esalen, five element balances, infant massage, nutrition, polarity, professional studies, therapeutic touch, tui na. A 500-hour training is also available which includes cranio-sacral therapy, deep tissue, intermediate and advanced polarity, pregnancy massage and several oriental massage modalities.

SCHOOL STATEMENT: Training in a broad spectrum of therapeutic modalities; environment of physical, mental, emotional and spiritual awareness; commitment to professional integrity and personal growth.

> **#70 DeAnza College**
>   21250 Sevens Creek Blvd.
>   Cupertino, CA 95014
>   (408) 864-5678

DEGREE OFFERED: Associate of Arts degree—Massage Therapy.

MODALITIES AND SUBJECTS: advanced massage skills, care & prevention of athletic injuries, clinical practicum in massage therapy, emergency response, exercise science, internship in massage therapy, introduction to adaptive & remedial PE assisting, intermediate massage, introduction to athletic injuries, introduction to massage, nutrition & athletic performance, personal fitness trainer, sports massage, stress management, stretching, table shiatsu, tai chi.

> **#71 Esalen Institute**
>   Coast Rt. 1
>   Big Sur, CA 93920
>   (408) 667-3000
>   www.esalen.org

HOURS OF TRAINING: 12 to 26 continuing ed.; 130 to 250-hour certification; 500-hour advanced.

DURATION OF COURSE: continuing ed. 12 hours – weekend, 26 hours five days; certification one month; advanced six months. All programs are residential.

COST: 12 hours $425, 26 hours $795, certification $3,600, advanced program varies.

FINANCIAL AID: scholarships or discounts are available.

YEAR FOUNDED: 1963.

GRADUATES PER YEAR (APPROX): 100.

MODALITIES AND SUBJECTS: acupressure, aromatherapy, breema, chi gong, cranio-sacral therapy, esalen massage, feldenkrais, polarity, reflexology, somatic therapy, sports massage, trigger point therapy, upledger, yoga therapy, zero-balancing.

SCHOOL STATEMENT: "Esalen" is a registered mark. A 28-day certification in Esalen Massage is offered. The school emphasizes sensitive contact and a whole person approach.

#72 Just for Your Health College of Massage
2075 Lincoln Ave., suite E
San Jose, CA 95125
(408) 723-2570

HOURS OF TRAINING: 100 or 500 (in-class hours not specified).

DURATION OF COURSE: 12 days to 5½ months, day and evening programs available.

COST: 100 hours $850; 500 hours $4,300 (both include books and supplies).

FINANCIAL AID: JPTA.

MODALITIES AND SUBJECTS: acupressure, business practices, chinese medicine, deep tissue, focusing, magnetic fields, nutrition, pediatric massage, professional ethics, reflexology, shiatsu, sound and color therapy, sports massage, student apprenticeship, tai chi, tuina.

SCHOOL STATEMENT: We teach self healing and manifestation of the body's memory, and the mechanics of massage. We assist our students in healing and changing their lives.

#73 Lupin Massage Institute
The Center for Conscious Touch
P.O. Box 1274
Los Gatos, CA 95031
(408) 353-4231
www.lupin.com/lmi.html

HOURS OF TRAINING: 125 (105 in-class hours).

DURATION OF COURSE: two weeks or five weekends.

COST: $995 intensive; $1,100 weekends, includes anatomy text, binder with detailed notes, oils, linens, snacks and beverages.

FINANCIAL AID: discounts for couples and certified practitioners.

YEAR FOUNDED: 1993.

GRADUATES PER YEAR (APPROX): 40–50.

MODALITIES AND SUBJECTS: cranio-sacral therapy, cybersomatics: the anatomy of consciousness, esalen massage, lomilomi, lymphatic drainage, professional ethics & business development, somato-emotional & viscero-emotional therapies.

SCHOOL STATEMENT: The body is not a machine—it's a miracle of conscious form. Our classes explore how skilled touch can inspire physical, emotional and spiritual healing.

#74 Milpitas Electrolysis College
500 E. Calaveras Blvd. #202-204
Milpitas, CA 95035
(408) 946-9522

YEAR FOUNDED: 1982.

#75 Monterey Institute of Touch
27820 Dorris Dr.
Carmel, CA 93923
(408) 624-1006

HOURS OF TRAINING: massage practitioner 200; massage therapist 500.

DURATION OF COURSE: 200-hour course varies from 5-week intensive to 18 weeks part-time; 500-hour course takes one to two years, day and evening programs available.

COST: 200-hour program $1,100 (includes books); 500-hour program contact school.

YEAR FOUNDED: 1983.

GRADUATES PER YEAR (APPROX.): 100.

MODALITIES AND SUBJECTS: advanced anatomy & physiology, advanced massage, aromatherapy, body handling, body logic, business practice & ethics, chair massage, clinical massage, CPR & emergency medical practice, cranio-sacral therapy, hand & wrist & forearm care, hawaiian massage, healing and meditation, intuitive massage, lymphatic and visceral massage, massage for couples, massage in the chiropractic setting, movement awareness, pathology, polarity, pregnancy massage, range of motion, reflexology, self-care, shiatsu, skilled touch for the seriously ill, soft tissue release, sports massage, supervised internship. Advanced programs: Three different 100-hour programs are available to graduates of 200-hour course; intermediate massage, advanced massage, and specialized massage (specialized massage may be craniosacral therapy or sports massage). Taking all three advanced 100-hour programs qualifies student for 500-hour certificate.

SCHOOL STATEMENT: The school stresses movement to help students do massage without creating stress in their own bodies.

#76 Monterey Peninsula College
Massage Therapy Program
Physical Fitness Department, 980 Fremont St.
Monterey CA 93940
(831) 646-4220 or 649-8873

HOURS OF TRAINING: 160 to 824 (Associate in Science degree in Massage Therapy).

DURATION OF COURSE: 8 weeks to 2 years.

COST: 160 hours $100 ($750 for non-residents); 800 hours or 30 units $450 or $3,500 for non-residents; 800 hours or 60 units (including electives) $800 or $6,800 for non-residents.

FINANCIAL AID: Federal student aid program loans and grants.

YEAR FOUNDED: 1994.

ACCREDITATIONS/APPROVALS: Western Association of Colleges and Schools.

GRADUATES PER YEAR (APPROX.): 75.

MODALITIES AND SUBJECTS: advanced first aid & emergency care, chair massage, clinical massage, fitness anatomy & kinesiology, general education electives, health psychology, massage therapy skills lab, reflexology, shiatsu sports massage, therapeutic massage I & II, trigger point therapy.

SCHOOL STATEMENT: Quality. Value. Environment. Monterey Peninsula College offers professional training, exceptional affordability, and is located in one of the most beautiful areas on the planet.

#77 Pacific College of Alternative Therapies
19997 Stevens Creek Blvd.
Cupertino, CA 95014
(408) 777-0102

HOURS OF TRAINING: five 100-hour programs: Fundamental Acupressure, Fundamental Massage, Fundamental Tui Na, Intermediate Massage, Intermediate Tui Na.

DURATION OF COURSE: 100 hours 15 days or five weekends.

COST: $960 each 100 hour program including hand-outs.

YEAR FOUNDED: 1993.

GRADUATES PER YEAR (APPROX.): 80.

MODALITIES AND SUBJECTS: acupressure, chair massage, chi gong, healing touch, lomilomi, medical massage, reflexology, tui na.

SCHOOL STATEMENT: We offer five different state certificate programs (fundamental and intermediate massage, acupressure and tui na), specialized in combination of the techniques of Chinese and Western.

#78 Twin Lakes College of the Healing Arts
1210 Brommer St.
Santa Cruz, CA 95062
(408) 476-2152

HOURS OF TRAINING: 200, 500 or 750.

DAY/EVENING/WEEKEND: day and evening programs available.

COST: 200 hours $1,325 (can vary with electives chosen); advanced classes are priced individually.

YEAR FOUNDED: 1982.

GRADUATES PER YEAR (APPROX.): 100.

MODALITIES AND SUBJECTS: acupressure I and II, counseling & communications skills, integrative swedish, internship & practice, massage-a-thon event, polarity I and II, shiatsu I and II, subtle body energywork. 500-hour concentration choices: integrative swedish + sports massage, integrative swedish + deep tissue, oriental + ayurvedic massage, or oriental + acupressure, shiatsu, or polarity. Graduates of other state-licensed massage programs may be eligible for advanced standing in the 500-hour program. The school also offers an annual Winter certificate program for women only. Advanced program: hypnotherapy.

SCHOOL STATEMENT: The 750-hour program offers a unique independent design option for the Natural Health Counselor and Massage Therapist Certificate Program.

#79 Western College of Therapeutic Massage
P.O. Box 1992
San Jose, CA 95109-1992
(408) 379-9750

HOURS OF TRAINING: 100 to 1,000 hours.

DURATION OF COURSE: 10 days to 2 years, classes offered days, evenings and weekends.

COST: $795 up, depending on length of program.

YEAR FOUNDED: 1983.

GRADUATES PER YEAR (APPROX.): 100.

MODALITIES AND SUBJECTS: advanced massage, applied kinesiology, chair massage, chi gong, clinical aspects of somatic practice, esalen massage, foundations of acupressure, foundations of massage, foundations of remobilization, jin shin do, orthobionomy, polarity, pregnancy massage, remobilization breathwork, shiatsu.

SCHOOL STATEMENT: Scheduling can be flexible to adapt to the needs of the individual student.

CALIFORNIA, STOCKTON TO BAKERSFIELD

#80 Abrams College
101 College Ave., suite 4
Modesto, CA 95354
(209) 527-7777

Contact school for program information.

#81 Body Tuneup School of Massage Therapy
1955 Lucile, Ste. D
Stockton, CA 95209
(209) 473-4993 or (800) 622-9766

HOURS OF TRAINING: Basic 100, advanced 100, additional programs to 500-hour total.

DURATION OF COURSE: Basic course—6 weekends or 10 weeks days or 14 weeks evenings; advanced course 6 weekends or 10 weeks days.

COST: Basic 100-hour course $850 including workbooks; advanced 100-hour course $750.

ACCREDITATIONS/APPROVALS: approved for nursing CEU's.

MODALITIES AND SUBJECTS: acupressure, acu-roma massage, aromatherapy, barefoot shiatsu, body mechanics, business, care giving massage for the elderly, caring touch massage, chair massage, cranio therapy, deep tissue massage, esalen, insurance billing, iridology, joint mobilization, lumbar sciatic pain relief, massage marketing, myofascial work, polarity, pre-natal massage, reiki, shiatsu, t'ai chi, wrist & forearm & shoulder massage. Advanced programs: advanced therapeutic massage, diagnosis in massage, massage in the chiropractic office, paramedical massage (100 hours), sports massage (100 hours).

#82 Central California College of Massage Therapy
1407 Standiford Ave., A-3
Modesto, CA 95350
(209) 549-2111

HOURS OF TRAINING: 500.

DURATION OF COURSE: one year, evenings & weekends.

COST: $4,000 including books. Payment plan without interest is available.

FINANCIAL AID: Scholarships or discounts, Private Industry Council

YEAR FOUNDED: 1996.

GRADUATES PER YEAR (APPROX.): 60.

MODALITIES AND SUBJECTS: acupressure, aromatherapy, chair massage, esalen, neuromuscular therapy, pregnancy massage, reflexology (100 hours), sports massage & soft tissue rehabilitation (100 hours), thai medical massage (100 hours).

SCHOOL STATEMENT: Teaching the art, science and practice of massage therapy professionally and ethically, to produce a well-trained and caring massage therapist.

#83 Massage Training Institute
1527 19th St., suite 428
Bakersfield, CA 93301
(805) 632-2823

YEAR FOUNDED: 1993.

#84 Quality College of Health Care Careers
1570 N. Wishon Ave.
Fresno, CA 93728
1-800-542-2225 or (209) 497-5050

HOURS OF TRAINING: 150 (in-class hours not specified).

COST: $1,700.

YEAR FOUNDED: 1994.

GRADUATES PER YEAR (APPROX): 100.

MODALITIES AND SUBJECTS: clinical therapeutic massage, deep friction, joint mobilization, rocking, sports massage.

SCHOOL STATEMENT: 75 of the 150 program hours are supervised practice on patients who are receiving chiropractic treatment.

#85 Therapeutic Learning Center
3636 N. First, suite 154
Fresno, CA 93726
(209) 225-7772

HOURS OF TRAINING: 200 or 100.

DURATION OF COURSE: 14 weeks or 12 weeks, days and evening & weekends classes offered.

COST: 200 hours $1,600; 100 hours $800 (includes required texts).

YEAR FOUNDED: 1986.

GRADUATES PER YEAR (APPROX.): 60–75.

In addition to the 200-hour Massage Practitioner course, 100-hour certifications are offered in Advanced Massage, Shiatsu and Reflexology.

MODALITIES AND SUBJECTS: aromatherapy, body-mind, bowen technique, business administration, chair massage, esalen massage, ethics, healing touch, infant massage, law, lymphatic drainage, myofascial release, neuromuscular therapy, postural Integration, pregnancy massage, reflexology, reiki, shiatsu, sports massage, trigger point therapy, yoga therapy.

SCHOOL STATEMENT: Training individuals to improve their capacity for hands-on healing and to open to greater self-realization by promoting body therapies through love and high professional standards.

#86 Touching for Health Center
School of Professional Bodywork
628 Lincoln Center
Stockton, CA 95207
(209) 474-9559

HOURS OF TRAINING: 105 or 500.

DURATION OF COURSE: 105 hours 7 to 11 weeks, 500 hours up to 3 years, evenings & weekends.

COST: 105 hours $876 including anatomy coloring book, 500 hours fee will vary but will not exceed $5,000. Payment plan without interest is available.

YEAR FOUNDED: 1990.

GRADUATES PER YEAR (APPROX): 60–80.

MODALITIES AND SUBJECTS: acupressure, applied kinesiology, aromatherapy, assessment and treatment planning, business ethics and documentation, business practice, chair massage, clinical treatments, CPR, deep tissue, esalen massage, history and psychology of massage, human behavior, hydrotherapy, indications/contraindications, introduction to other modalities, jin shin do, kinesiology, lymphatic drainage, massage theory and hygiene, massage theory practice, medical massage, myofascial release, polarity, reflexology, sports massage, trigger point therapy.

SCHOOL STATEMENT: Our goals, standard of practice are committed to excellence. We are dedicated to the highest standards of teaching, personal growth, through education, clarity and intuition.

CALIFORNIA, SAN LUIS OBISPO AREA

#87 Central California School of Body Therapy
1330 Southwood Dr. #7
San Luis Obispo, CA 93401
(805) 783-2200

YEAR FOUNDED: 1991.

ACCREDITATIONS/APPROVALS: COMTA/Accredited.

#88 Pacific Coast School of Massage
P.O. Box 7124, Halcyon, CA 93421
(Classroom: 3220 S. Higuera St., suite 302,
San Luis Obispo)
(805) 481-3828

Contact school for program information.

CALIFORNIA, SANTA BARBARA AND VENTURA

#89 Caring Hands School of Massage
1691 Spinnaker, suite 105
Ventura, CA 93001
(805) 568-0691

HOURS OF TRAINING: 200 (100 in-class hours).

DURATION OF COURSE: 14 weeks, plus time for outside practice. Evening and weekend programs.

COST: $700 including all required study materials Payment plan without interest is available.

FINANCIAL AID: Some partial scholarships available.

YEAR FOUNDED: 1993.

GRADUATES PER YEAR (APPROX.): 56.

MODALITIES AND SUBJECTS: acupressure, aromatherapy, body mechanics, business, chair massage, chakra system, energy anatomy & healing, shiatsu Also offered: six-week Acupressure & Chinese Healing Techniques program.

SCHOOL STATEMENT: Warm, supporting learning environment. Students are encouraged to be fully present to the needs of their own bodies and the person they are working on.

#90 Lu Ross Academy
470 East Thompson Blvd.
Ventura, CA 93001
(805) 643-5690
www.lurossacademy.com

HOURS OF TRAINING: 200 (165 in-class hours) 400 additional hours are available in three advanced programs: oriental studies (tui na), neuro-structural, and energetic therapies.

COST: 200 hours $1,495.

YEAR FOUNDED: 1954.

GRADUATES PER YEAR (APPROX.): 200.

MODALITIES AND SUBJECTS: aromatherapy, herbology, lymphatic drainage, neuro-structural, reflexology, shiatsu, somatic therapy, trigger point therapy.

SCHOOL STATEMENT: Provide our students with an excellent education—assist in career placement—develop entrepreneurial skills or the student—transforming lives through the art of touch.

#91 Santa Barbara Body Therapy Institute
835 N. Milpas St.
Santa Barbara, CA 93103
(805) 966-5802

HOURS OF TRAINING: 200 (125 in-class hours), 650 or 1,000.

DURATION OF COURSE: 13 weeks, 1-2 years, 2 years; day & evening & weekend programs available.

COST: $1,100, $4,600, $6,600 including nature retreat, books, oil.

YEAR FOUNDED: 1985.

GRADUATES PER YEAR (APPROX.): 50.

MODALITIES AND SUBJECTS: acupressure, beyond active listening, building a practice, chair massage, chi gong, clinic, cranio-sacral therapy, deep tissue, ethics, holistic health practitioner, holistic massage, infant massage, jin shin do, leadership, living in love, lymphatic drainage, mentorship, myofascial release, neuromuscular therapy, nutrition, pfrimmer deep muscle, polarity, pregnancy massage, private sessions, reflexology, regenerative massage, shiatsu, sports massage, subtle body structures, touch for health, touching AIDS, trigger point therapy, unity in motion, women's cycles.

SCHOOL STATEMENT: We are a community based center dedicated to the principles and practices of wholistic health. Our approach blends compassion, anatomical understanding and energy-based massage.

#92 Santa Barbara College of Oriental Medicine
1919 State St., suite 204
Santa Barbara, CA 93101
(805) 898-1180

YEAR FOUNDED: 1987.

#93 Santa Barbara School of Massage
1018 Garden St., suite 104
Santa Barbara. CA 93101
(805) 962-4748

Contact school for program information.

#94 School of Intuitive Massage and Healing
503 Foxen Drive
Santa Barbara, CA 93105
(classroom: 1911-D de la Vina)
(805) 687-2917

HOURS OF TRAINING: 200 to 1,000 (120 to 600 in-class hours) Five 200-hour courses offered.

DURATION OF COURSE: 3½ months to 16 months or longer, evenings and weekends.

COST: $1,100 to $5,500, including handouts and oil.

FINANCIAL AID: Fee waivers and payment plans are available.

YEAR FOUNDED: 1984.

GRADUATES PER YEAR (APPROX): 150.

MODALITIES AND SUBJECTS: The five courses offered are "Massage Therapist I", "Massage Therapist II", "Professional Skills", "Intuitive Massage and Healing—Energy Skills" and "Intuitive Massage and Healing—Emotional Skills"; which include acupressure, aromatherapy, breema, chair massage, chi gong, cranio-sacral therapy, energy work, esalen massage, hakomi bodywork, healing touch, infant massage, intuitive massage, massage of children, massage of elderly, ortho-bionomy, pregnancy massage, reflexology, reiki, rosen method, shiatsu, sports massage.

SCHOOL STATEMENT: Massage as profession, service and ministry. In addition to modalities, through intuition and healing energy, we open to the Love that heals all.

CALIFORNIA, LOS ANGELES AREA

#95 Advanced School of Massage Therapy
1414 E. Thousand Oaks Blvd., suite 213
Thousand Oaks, CA 91362
(805) 495-1353

HOURS OF TRAINING: 200 to 750 (150 hours to 750 hours in-class).

DURATION OF COURSE: 3 months to 16 months, day & evening & weekend programs available.

COST: 200 hours $1,350 including books & materials, 500 hours $3,700, 750 hours $6,200. Payment plan without interest is available.

FINANCIAL AID: Scholarships or discounts available.

YEAR FOUNDED: 1997.

GRADUATES PER YEAR (APPROX.): 100.

MODALITIES AND SUBJECTS: advanced massage moves, aromatherapy, body-mind, chair massage (basic & advanced), craniosacral therapy, deep tissue, defense lecture, energy work for bodyworkers, ethical practices & responses, facial massage, healing touch, herbology, hydrotherapy, hygiene & sanitation, infant massage, nursing & health care, nutrition, practical experience, pregnancy massage, psychology for bodyworkers, reflexology, reiki, sports massage, trigger point therapy.

SCHOOL STATEMENT: We provide you with the best education in Massage Therapy and the knowledge it takes to become a healer and make a living from it.

#96 American Institute of Massage Therapy
2156 Newport Ave.
Costa Mesa, CA 92627-1710
(714) 642-0735

HOURS OF TRAINING: 1,029 (624 plus 405 hours clinical Sports-Massage internship).

DURATION OF COURSE: 11 to 12 months, day and evening programs available.

COST: $5,100.

FINANCIAL AID: scholarships or discounts available.

YEAR FOUNDED: 1983.

ACCREDITATIONS/APPROVALS: COMTA/Accredited, approved for nursing CEU's.

PREPARATION FOR OUT-OF-STATE LICENSING EXAM: Washington.

GRADUATES PER YEAR (APPROX.): 40.

MODALITIES AND SUBJECTS: acupressure, business practices and marketing, Chinese and Russian techniques, clinical practice, counterstrain, CPR/first aid, functional muscle testing, hydrotherapy, hygiene, immediate injury care, lymphatic drainage, medical ethics, nutrition, pathology, PNF stretches, pre-event massage, post-event massage, psychology and philosophy, reflexology, remedial exercises, restoration/rehabilitation, shiatsu, sports kinesiology, sports pathology and psychology, Thai stretches, training and conditioning.

SCHOOL STATEMENT: Graduates receive dual certificates as massage therapist and sports massage specialist. Specialized associate degree in massage therapy granted, hospital-based massage therapy program offered.

#97 California College of Physical Arts
18582 Beach Boulevard, suite 14
Huntington Beach, CA 92648
(714) 964-7744

32332 Camino Capistrano, suite 206
San Juan Capistrano, CA 92675
(714) 240-7744

HOURS OF TRAINING: 300 to 1,000.

DURATION OF COURSE: 3 months to 12 months.

DAY/EVENING/WEEKEND: day, evening and weekend classes available.

COST: registration fee $75, each 100-hour segment $875.

YEAR FOUNDED: 1980.

GRADUATES PER YEAR (APPROX.): 100.

MODALITIES AND SUBJECTS: acupressure, aromatherapy, botanical modalities choreography, clinical massage, color modalities, externship, geriatric massage, history, hydrotherapy, injury care, introduction to holistic theory, joint movement, massage for the physically challenged, music modality, nutrition, oriental health systems, postural re-education, practitioner's well-being, professionalism, reflexology, sports massage, symptomatic assessment, theory and ethics of massage, trigger points, visualization modality. Programs offered: massage technician, massage therapist, advanced massage therapist, sports massage therapist I, sports massage therapist II, clinical massage therapist I (medical massage), clinical massage therapist II (each 100 hours), massage practitioner (600 hours), massage instructor (600 hours), myotherapist (700 hours), holistic health practitioner I (1,000 hours), holistic health practitioner II (1,200 hours).

SCHOOL STATEMENT: Placement department is actively involved with the medical community. Externships are available with athletic teams.

#98 California Healing Arts College
12217 Santa Monica Blvd., suite 206
West Los Angeles, CA 90025
(310) 826-7622 or 1-800-246-8878

YEAR FOUNDED: 1988.

#99 California Health Institute, Inc.
1529 E. Palmdale Blvd., #150
Palmdale, CA 93550
(805) 947-4069

Contact school for program information.

#100 California School of Medical Sciences
291 S. Lacienega Blvd., suite 200
Beverly Hills, CA 90211
(310) 657-9495

Contact school for program information.

#101 Cerritros College Center for Lifelong Learning
11110 East Alondra Blvd.
Norwalk, CA 90650
(562) 860-2451 ext. 2521

Contact school for program information.

#102 Educorp Career College
236 E. Third St.
Long Beach, CA 90802
(562) 437-0501

Program is 9 months, evenings. Contact school for program information.

#103 The Institute of Progressive Physical Therapy
School of Massage & Physical Therapy Aiding
4333 Admiralty Way, Marina Del Rey, CA 90292
(Classroom: 11911 Washington Blvd. Culver City)
(310) 823-6533

HOURS OF TRAINING: 120 (advanced 150 hour acupressure course also offered).

DURATION OF COURSE: day & evening and weekend programs available.

COST: $1,100 (Advanced acupressure course $1,550). Payment plan without interest is available.

YEAR FOUNDED:1994.

GRADUATES PER YEAR (APPROX.): 120.

SCHOOL STATEMENT: Also offered is a program in Certified Physical Therapy Aide, which may be combined with the massage training.

#104 Institute of Psycho-Structural Balancing
3767 Overland Avenue, suite 103
Los Angeles, CA 90034
(310) 815-3675
www.ipsb.com

HOURS OF TRAINING: 150 or 500.

COST: 150 hours $1,415 including registration fee, books and supplies.

YEAR FOUNDED: 1980.

GRADUATES PER YEAR (APPROX.): 275.

MODALITIES AND SUBJECTS: 150 hour program: body psychology, energy balancing, esalen, introduction to chiropractic & chair & spa massage, joint mobilization, tai chi. 500-hour program adds acupressure, advanced circulatory massage, business for bodyworkers, CPR/first aid, deep tissue, healthy boundaries for bodyworkers, human energy systems, hydrotherapy, hygiene, pathology and electives (active & passive stretching techniques, archetypes & the body, aromatherapy certification, body mechanics, healing the relationship with gravity, cranio-sacral balancing, lymphatic clearing certification, sports massage certification).

SCHOOL STATEMENT: Holistic orientation recognizes the importance of self-exploration and cultivates a balance between body, mind and spirit that is expressed in the quality of care.

#105 J.H.J. Education College
638 S. Van Ness, 1st floor
Los Angeles, CA 90010
(213) 384-0414

HOURS OF TRAINING: 100 to 1,350.

DURATION OF COURSE: 4 to 52 weeks, day and evening classes available.

YEAR FOUNDED: 1992.

MODALITIES AND SUBJECTS: acupressure technician, acupressure therapist, acupressure advanced therapist, massage technician, massage therapist, massage advanced therapist.

#106 Massage School of Santa Monica
1453 Third St. Promenade, suite 340
Santa Monica, CA 90401
(310) 393-7461 or (310) 453-2386

MSSM Extension
6422½ Coldwater Canyon
North Hollywood, CA 91605
(818) 763-4912

HOURS OF TRAINING: 150 to 800.

DURATION OF COURSE: 12 weeks to 12 months, classes available days, evenings and weekends.

DAY/EVENING/WEEKEND: day and evening programs available.

COST: 150 hours $1,144 (includes book); additional courses priced individually. Payment plan without interest is available, discount for prepayment of tuition.

FINANCIAL AID: Rehabilitation Department, Workman's Compensation.

YEAR FOUNDED: 1979.

GRADUATES PER YEAR (APPROX.): 350.

MODALITIES AND SUBJECTS: acupressure, applied kinesiology, aromatherapy, body-mind, chair massage, cranio-sacral therapy, ethical, legal & business aspects of massage practice, hygiene, jin shin do, medical massage, myofascial release, nutrition, postural integration, pregnancy massage, reflexology, self-care, shiatsu, somatics, sports massage, structural integration.

SCHOOL STATEMENT: Before you can respectfully enter the intimate arena of physical contact with another human being… you must first explore, accept and understand your own world.

#107 **Meridian Institute of Massage**
     6363 Santa Monica Blvd., suite 235
     Los Angeles, CA 90038
     (213) 467-3671

Contact school for program information.

#108 **Mesa Institute**
     150 N. Feldner
     Orange, CA 92868
     (714) 660-6222

HOURS OF TRAINING: 500, 1,000 (day & evening & weekend programs available).

YEAR FOUNDED: 1995.

GRADUATES PER YEAR (APPROX.): 50.

MODALITIES AND SUBJECTS: acupressure, applied kinesiology, aromatherapy, body-mind, chair massage, lymphatic drainage, medical massage, myotherapy, reflexology, shiatsu, sports massage, therapeutic touch, touch for health, trigger point therapy, yoga therapy. Programs offered: Holistic Health Practitioner (500 hours), Sports Massage Therapist (500 hours), Holistic Health Practitioner (1,000 hours), Sports Massage Therapist (1,000 hours).

#109 **Montebello Career College**
     2465 W. Whittier Blvd., suite 201
     Montebello, CA 90640
     (213) 728-9636

Contact school for program information.

#110 **Nova Institute**
     520 N. Euclid Ave.
     Ontario, CA 91762
     (909) 974-5027
     www.NOVAINSTITUTE.COM/

HOURS OF TRAINING: 648.

DURATION OF COURSE: 9 months, day or evening programs available.

COST: $6,913 includes books, uniforms and supplies. Payment plan without interest is available.

FINANCIAL AID: Scholarships, Pell Grants, Stafford Loans, VA Benefits.

YEAR FOUNDED: 1986.

ACCREDITATIONS/APPROVALS: ACCSCT.

GRADUATES PER YEAR (APPROX.): 165.

MODALITIES AND SUBJECTS: acupressure, applied kinesiology, aromatherapy, body-mind, chair massage, cranio-sacral therapy, fitness, medical massage, myotherapy, nutrition, pfrimmer deep muscle, reflexology, shiatsu, somatic therapy, sports massage, touch for health, traumatology, TREP/EXT.

#111 **Shiatsu Massage School of California**
     2309 Main St.
     Santa Monica, CA 90405
     (310) 396-4877

YEAR FOUNDED: 1983.

#112 **Southern California School of Massage**
     12702 Magnolia Ave., ste. 21
     Riverside, CA 92504
     (909) 340-3336

HOURS OF TRAINING: 100 (massage technician); 250 (massage specialist); 500 (massage therapist); 1,000 (holistic health practitioner); 1,150 (massage instructor); total 1,400 hours available.

DURATION OF COURSE: 100-hour course may be taken in 10-day intensive format or 5 weekends. Other programs are completed at the student's pace. Courses offered days, evenings, weekends.

COST: 100 hours $795; 250 hours $1,950; 500 hours $3,695; 1,000 hours $6,495; 1,400 hours $7,495.

FINANCIAL AID: Rehabilitation, Alliance.

YEAR FOUNDED: 1984.

ACCREDITATIONS/APPROVALS: approved for nursing CEU's.

MODALITIES AND SUBJECTS: acupressure, acupressure facelift, all about headaches, aromatherapy, body-mind, body wraps, business and marketing, cellulite massage, chair massage, color therapy, CPR, cranio-sacral therapy, deep tissue, ear acu-reflex, energy systems, ethics, face reading, healing with charcoal, health and hygiene, history, hospital massage, hydrotherapy, infant massage, integral body balancing, manual lymphatic drainage, mind/body dynamics, myofascial release, neuromuscular therapy, nutrition, polarity, powder massage, pregnancy massage, reflexology, reiki, shiatsu, social psychology, somatics, sports massage, structural kinesiology, thai massage, trigger point therapy, tui-na, yoga therapy.

SCHOOL STATEMENT: SCSM's curriculum, a synthesis of Eastern and Western concepts of bodywork, emphasizes the "holistic model" regarding dependent interactions of body functions, beliefs and emotions.

#113 **The Touch Therapy Institute**
     15720 Ventura #101
     Encino, CA 91436
     (818) 788-0824
     www.wholistictouch.com

HOURS OF TRAINING: 200, 500, 1,000, day, evening and weekend programs available.

COST: 200 hours $1,675 plus one book; 500 hours $2,400 to $4,225 (depending on courses selected), 1,000 hours $2,900 to $6,418 (depending on courses selected). Payment plan without interest is available.

YEAR FOUNDED: 1989.

ACCREDITATIONS/APPROVALS: approved for nursing CEU's, GI Bill, department of vocational rehabilitation.

GRADUATES PER YEAR (APPROX): 320.

MODALITIES AND SUBJECTS: acupressure, advanced communication skills, alexander, aromatherapy, basic communication skills, beginning movement, body awareness & seeing, body reading, bowen technique, breath and toning, chair massage, chakra massage, color therapy, connective tissue massage, CPR, cranio-sacral work, ethics, fascial anatomy, fibromyalgia & muscle pain, fieldwork projects, functional anatomy, history & business management, hygiene and nutrition, kinesiology, lomilomi, lymphatics for the immune system, neuromuscular therapy, nutrition, palpation, pathology, practice massage, psycho-energetic movement, reflexology, rosen method, rotator cuff solutions, sports massage, therapeutic touch I, II & III, trager, trigger points.

SCHOOL STATEMENT: 200, 500, 1,000 hour certifications, sports massage, advanced swedish massage, acupressure and reflexology; classes start monthly; job board; volunteer opportunities; small classes; language assistance available.

#114 USA Pain Care College
19093 Colima Road
Rowland Hts., CA 91748
(626) 854-2898

HOURS OF TRAINING: 100 to 1,000 hours.

DURATION OF COURSE: five weeks to 60 weeks, day & weekend programs available.

COST: $800 to $9,050.

YEAR FOUNDED: 1995.

GRADUATES PER YEAR (APPROX.): 100.

MODALITIES AND SUBJECTS: acupressure, reflexology, shiatsu, tui na. Programs: acupressure technician, professional acupressure technician, acupressure massage therapist, acupressure massage practitioner, acupressure massage instructor.

SCHOOL STATEMENT: We provide the opportunity to develop knowledge and skills, self-discipline and confidence, a professional attitude, and ability to meet employer expectations in the field.

#115 Western Institute of Neuromuscular Therapy
22981 Mill Creek Dr., suite A
Laguna Hills, CA 92653
(714) 830-6151
www.wintherapy.com

HOURS OF TRAINING: 500 or 1,000.

DURATION OF COURSE: 500 hours 12 months, 1,000 hours 16 months, evening and weekend programs available.

COST: 500 hours $5,904; 1,000 hours $6,860 including books and cadaver lab. Payment plan without interest is available.

FINANCIAL AID: FTPA, TRA, EDD.

YEAR FOUNDED: 1994.

GRADUATES PER YEAR (APPROX.): 70.

MODALITIES AND SUBJECTS: accounting & marketing, active isolated stretching, business practice, client history & evaluation, clinical & event sports massage, kinesiology, muscle testing, myofascial release, neuromuscular therapy, orthopedic testing, pathology, pre & post event & intercompetition massage, post isometric relaxation, prevention & rehabilitation techniques, proprioceptive neuromuscular facilitation, sports medicine, strain/counterstrain, trigger point therapy.

SCHOOL STATEMENT: We emphasize palpation skills, evaluation of musculoskeletal aspects of the body, and a variety of modalities, training therapists at the forefront of the health profession.

#116 West Pacific Institute of Body Therapy
434 N. Lakeview Ave.
Anaheim, CA 92807
(714) 998-8079

HOURS OF TRAINING: 100 to 500.

DURATION OF COURSE: one month to 6 months, day & evening & weekend programs available.

COST: $450 and up. Payment plan without interest is available.

YEAR FOUNDED: 1996.

GRADUATES PER YEAR (APPROX.): 20.

MODALITIES AND SUBJECTS: acupressure, aromatherapy, chair massage, circulatory massage (basic & advanced), deep tissue, lymphatic drainage, sports massage.

SCHOOL STATEMENT: Smaller class sizes and flexible hours—with personalized training at the student's pace—emphasis towards business training included.

CALIFORNIA, SAN BERNARDINO AREA

#117 Banning Massage School
66-705 E. 6th Street
Desert Hot Springs, CA 92240
(760) 329-5066

HOURS OF TRAINING: 100 or 500.

DURATION OF COURSE: 100 hours four weeks, 500 hours five months (day program).

COST: 100 hours $851.98, 250 hours $1,278, 500 hours $2,130. Payment plan without interest is available.

YEAR FOUNDED: 1986.

GRADUATES PER YEAR (APPROX.): 32.

MODALITIES AND SUBJECTS: applied kinesiology, business, chair massage, cranio-sacral therapy, deep tissue, ethics, home health aide, hydrotherapy, kinesiology, neuromuscular therapy, nutrition, physical therapy aide, sports massage, therapeutic massage, trigger point therapy.

SCHOOL STATEMENT: Banning Massage School is committed to assist students to develop the fullest possible potential by providing experienced, dedicated Christian teachers, professional equipment and peaceful environment.

#118 Desert Resorts School
13090 Palm Drive
Desert Hot Springs, CA 92240
(760) 329-1175 or 1-800-329-1175
www.somatherapy.com

HOURS OF TRAINING:
- massage technician (M.tech) 300
- massage therapist (M.Th) 600
- acupressure therapist (AT) 120
- comprehensive decongestive therapy (MLD) 160
- holistic health practitioner (HHP) 1000
Day and weekend programs available.

COST: M.Tech $1,815; M.Th $3,885; AT $1,,250; MLD $1,995; HHP $5,790.

YEAR FOUNDED: 1991.

GRADUATES PER YEAR (APPROX.): 120.

MODALITIES AND SUBJECTS: advanced anatomy, aromatherapy, business and ethics, communication skills, deep tissue, history and theory of massage, holistic theory, hydrotherapy, kinesiology, manual lymphatic drainage, massage clinic, nutrition, polarity, reflexology, shiatsu, sports events, sports massage, tui na.

SCHOOL STATEMENT: The program is spa oriented and provides travel opportunities, including study in China and Ironman in Hawaii.

#119 Just for Your Health College of Massage
    15888 Main St. #211
    Hesperia, CA 92345
    (760) 956-6655 or 956-3266

HOURS OF TRAINING: 200 or 300 (in-class hours not specified).

DURATION OF COURSE: 200 hours 12 weeks, 300 hours 5½ months, day and evening programs available.

COST: 200 hours $1,500; 300 hours $4,200.

FINANCIAL AID: JPTA, Rehab, San Jose and Hesperias College.

YEAR FOUNDED: 1986.

GRADUATES PER YEAR (APPROX): 130.

MODALITIES AND SUBJECTS: acupressure, business practices, chinese medicine, deep tissue, focusing, magnetic fields, medical billing course, nutrition, pediatric massage, professional ethics, reflexology, shiatsu, sound and color therapy, sports massage, student apprenticeship, tai chi, tuina.

SCHOOL STATEMENT: We teach self healing and manifestation of the body's memory, and the mechanics of massage. We assist our students in healing and changing their lives.

CALIFORNIA, SAN DIEGO AREA

#120 The Academy of Health Professions
    8376 Hercules St.
    La Mesa, CA 91942
    (619) 461-5100

    6784 El Cajon Blvd.
    San Diego, CA 92115
    (619) 464-3570

HOURS OF TRAINING: 1,000.

DURATION OF COURSE: 40 weeks, day or evening/weekend programs available.

COST: $9,952 including books, massage table, linens and oil. Payment plan without interest is available.

FINANCIAL AID: Scholarships or discounts, Federal Title IV programs—grants and loans.

YEAR FOUNDED: 1993.

ACCREDITATIONS/APPROVALS: ACCET.

GRADUATES PER YEAR (APPROX.): 55.

MODALITIES AND SUBJECTS: acupressure, applied kinesiology, aromatherapy, body mechanics, body-mind, body wrapping, business management, chair massage, chi gong, clinical practice internship & externship, CPR & first aid, deep tissue, energetic techniques, hawaiian back & frontal techniques, hawaiian body mapping, herbology, holistic awareness, hypnotherapy, infant massage, NCE review, neuromuscular practicum, nutrition, passive joint movement, postural integration, pregnancy massage, professional development, reflexology, reiki, shiatsu, sports massage, structural alignment I & II, thai medical massage, trager, tui na.

SCHOOL STATEMENT: HHP program designed to produce employable, competent therapists. Emphasis on Western methods with some Oriental modalities included.

#121 Advanced Career Training
    5125 Convoy St., suite 304
    San Diego, CA 92111
    (619) 279-2236

Contact school for program information.

#122 Body Mind College
    4050 Sorrento Valley Blvd. #L
    San Diego, CA 92121
    (619) 453-3295 or (800) BDY-MIND

YEAR FOUNDED: 1988.

#123 California Naturopathic College
    1011 Camino Del Mar, Ste. 204
    Del Mar, CA 92014
    (619) 259-8716 or 1-800-354-8166

HOURS OF TRAINING: 100, 1,000 or 1,500.

DURATION OF COURSE: 100 hours 12 weeks, 1,000 or 1,500 hours 2 years.

COST: $925 to $22,500 including books and handouts.

FINANCIAL AID: Scholarships or discounts available.

YEAR FOUNDED: 1996.

GRADUATES PER YEAR (APPROX.): 25.

MODALITIES AND SUBJECTS: acupressure, aromatherapy & botanical medicine, ayurveda, bioenergetics, body therapies & exercise physiology, clinical practicum, health psychology, herbology, homeopathy, human body systems, human pathology, jin shin do, mind-body integration, nutrition & diet & lifestyle, ortho-bionomy, principles of pharmacology, reflexology, touch for health, vibrational healing, yoga therapy.

SCHOOL STATEMENT: Our goal is to provide students with practical skills and individual healing. To assist others in healing the practitioner must address his/her own issues first.

#124 Healing Hands School of Holistic Health
    11064 Pala Loma Drive
    Valley Center, CA 92082
    Classrooms: Escondido, Laguna Hills
    1-800-355-6463 (in CA) or (760) 746-9364

HOURS OF TRAINING: 100, 500, 1,000.

DURATION OF COURSE: 3 weeks to 2 years, day & evening & weekend programs available.

COST: 100 hours $480, 500 hours $2,500, 1,000 hours $4,950

FINANCIAL AID: discounts for prepayment.

ACCREDITATIONS/APPROVALS: CA Board of Registered Nursing.

YEAR FOUNDED: 1993.

GRADUATES PER YEAR (APPROX): 30.

MODALITIES AND SUBJECTS: acupressure, aromatherapy, body-mind, chair massage, chi gong, cranio-sacral therapy, deep tissue, esalen, geriatric massage, hypnotism, jin shin do, lymphatic drainage, myofascial release, neuromuscular therapy, postural integration, pregnancy massage, reflexology, reiki, shiatsu, structural integration, touch for health, tui na, yoga therapy.

SCHOOL STATEMENT: Well-rounded curriculum affordable price, and an environment where students feel secure in their learning and growth processes. All courses may be taken individually.

#125 International Professional School of Bodywork (IPSB)
    1366 Hornblend St.
    San Diego, CA 92109
    (619) 272-4142 or 1-800-748-6497

HOURS OF TRAINING: 150 (essentials), 330 (essentials & contemporary), 1,260 (associate-masters degrees).

DURATION OF COURSE: 3 weeks to 30 months, day & evening & weekend programs available.

COST: application fee $100; 150 hours $900, 180 hours $1,125, Associate of Science $8.704.

YEAR FOUNDED: 1977.

ACCREDITATIONS/APPROVALS: COMTA/approved, CPPVE, Department of Vocational Rehabilitation, approved for veterans' training, approved for nursing CEU's.

GRADUATES PER YEAR (APPROX.): 200.

MODALITIES AND SUBJECTS: acupressure, alexander, applied kinesiology, aromatherapy, body-mind, business & legal issues, chair massage, chi gong, circulatory, deep tissue—muscle sculpting, esalen, ethics, feldenkrais, hakomi, hygiene, jin shin acutouch, lymphatic drainage, neuromuscular therapy, oriental theories, passive joint movement, shiatsu, somatic therapy, sports massage, structural integration, thailand medical massage, trigger point therapy, tui na, yoga therapy. Degree programs: Associate, Bachelors, Masters. Certificate programs in Essentials of Massage, Contemporary Methods, Relational Somatics, Sensory Repatterning, Somato-Emotional Integration, Structural Integration, Sports Massage, Neuromuscular Therapy, Therapeutic Applications, Tui Na, Jin Shin Acutouch, Thailand Medical Massage, Seitai Shiatsu, Teacher Aide Training, Teacher Training.

SCHOOL STATEMENT: IPSB's curriculum is designed to integrate and harmonize the student's body/mind and cultivate attitudes, techniques and skills which support their clients' growth and change.

#126 Mueller College of Holistic Studies
4607 Park Blvd.
San Diego, CA 92116
(619) 291-9811 or (800) 245-1976
www.muellercollege.com

HOURS OF TRAINING: 100, 512, 626, 1000 (minimum 702 in-class), 1000 (minimum 792 in-class).

DURATION OF COURSE: 10 days to 2 years; day, evening and weekend programs are available.

COST: 100 hours $960; 512 hours $5,180; 626 hours $6,280; 1000 hours $6,500 (prices include books and supplies).

Limited work-study is available for advanced programs.

YEAR FOUNDED: 1976.

ACCREDITATIONS/APPROVALS: COMTA/approved, AOBTA.

PREPARATION FOR OUT-OF-STATE LICENSING EXAM: preparation can be arranged for most states' exams; contact school for particulars.

GRADUATES PER YEAR (APPROX.): 320 to 365 all programs combined.

MODALITIES AND SUBJECTS: acupressure, advanced techniques active, advanced techniques passive, applied kinesiology, ayurveda, body-mind, business, cell biology, chair massage, chi gong, cranio-sacral therapy, cryotherapy, healing touch, hydrotherapy, kinesiology, infant massage, lymphatic drainage, myofascial release, neuromuscular therapy, palliative massage, pathology, polarity, pregnancy massage, reflexology, reiki, sports massage, therapeutic touch, touch for health.

SCHOOL STATEMENT: Mueller College provides an environment and curriculum that encourages exploration of consciousness, human potential and academic achievement. Our goal: qualified, conscious acupressure and massage practitioners.

#127 Pacific College of Oriental Medicine
7445 Mission Valley Rd.
San Diego, CA 92108
(800) 729-0941
www.ormed.edu

HOURS OF TRAINING: 112 to 1,000.

SCHOOL STATEMENT: Pacific College offers certificates in Oriental Body Therapy and Tui Na, and massage programs ranging from 112 to 1,000 hours.

#128 School of Healing Arts
1001 Garnet #200
San Diego, CA 92109
(619) 581-9429
www.SchoolOfHealingArts.com

HOURS OF TRAINING: 110, 500, 1,000.

DURATION OF COURSE: 110 hours 2-week intensive or 11 weeks. evenings/weekends; 1,000 hours approx. 2 years.

COST: 110 hours $713 including books; 1,000 hours $6,000.

YEAR FOUNDED: 1984.

ACCREDITATIONS/APPROVALS: approved for veterans benefits and vocational rehabilitation, approved for nursing CEU's.

GRADUATES PER YEAR (APPROX.): 250.

MODALITIES AND SUBJECTS: communication, counseling, food preparation, herbology, hypnotherapy, nutritional counseling, shiatsu, zen-touch, movement, Advanced programs: nutritional counselor, clinical massage therapist, fitness consultant, holistic health practitioner. Note: school teaches parasympathetic massage rather then swedish.

SCHOOL STATEMENT: We are dedicated to empowering and unifying the full potential of our lives… body, mind and spirit, fulfilling our dreams to embrace an inspired life.

#129 Vitality Training Center
243 N. Hwy 101, ste. 5
Solana Beach, CA 92075
(619) 259-9491

HOURS OF TRAINING: 100 to 1,200.

DURATION OF COURSE: 10 days to 18 months, day & evening & weekend programs available.

COST: $850 to $7,000.

FINANCIAL AID: work scholarship available.

YEAR FOUNDED: 1992.

GRADUATES PER YEAR (APPROX.): 60.

MODALITIES AND SUBJECTS: acupressure, advanced energetic, applied kinesiology, aromatherapy, body-mind, business & ethics, chair massage, chi gong, cranio-sacral therapy, deep tissue, equine sports massage, feldenkrais, healing touch, herbs & nutrition, hypnotherapy, infant massage, jin shin do, lymphatic drainage, movement therapy, myofascial release, neuromuscular therapy, pregnancy massage, reflexology, reiki, shiatsu, somatic therapy, spa therapist, sports massage & rehabilitation, tai chi, trigger point therapy, yoga teacher certification, yoga therapy.

SCHOOL STATEMENT: Service through heart-centered touch and education is our vision. Go beyond belief systems to "an open heart" and connect to healing wisdom and wholeness.

COLORADO

No State licensing

SCHOOLS:

#130 Academy of Healing Arts
592 Road 32
Clifton, CO 81520
(970) 434-4903

HOURS OF TRAINING: 810.

COST: $5,400.

YEAR FOUNDED: 1997.

GRADUATES PER YEAR (APPROX.): 15.

MODALITIES AND SUBJECTS: acupressure, balanced living, basic interactive skills, business management, ethics, hatha yoga, healing systems, intro. to tai chi, learning skills, life force & subtle energy, magnets & bodywork, mind-body health, nutrition & diet, pathology, practicum, referrals & specialties, reflexology, touch for health, wellness skills.

#131 Academy of Natural Therapy
123 Elm Ave.
Eaton, CO 80615
(970) 454-2224

HOURS OF TRAINING: 1,049 (in-class hours not specified).

DURATION OF COURSE: one year, day & evening programs available.

COST: $5,000 including books and student insurance. Payment plan without interest is available.

FINANCIAL AID: Scholarships or discounts, Veteran's Administration.

YEAR FOUNDED: 1989.

GRADUATES PER YEAR (APPROX.): 30.

MODALITIES AND SUBJECTS: acupressure, applied kinesiology, chair massage, hydrotherapy, infant massage, myofascial release, myotherapy, neuromuscular therapy, reflexology, shiatsu, sports massage.

SCHOOL STATEMENT: We are completely dedicated to producing the finest massage therapists anywhere. We keep the highest standard of instructors, facilities, training and instruction to insure success.

#132 Boulder School of Massage Therapy
6255 Longbow Dr.
Boulder, CO 80301
(303) 530-2100

HOURS OF TRAINING: 1,000.

DURATION OF COURSE: days 40 weeks, evenings 80 weeks, flexible schedules available.

COST: $8995 including books, linens, packets, insurance and fees.

FINANCIAL AID: Pell grants, Stafford loans, PLUS loans, VA benefits.

YEAR FOUNDED: 1975.

ACCREDITATIONS/APPROVALS: COMTA/approved, ACCSCT.

GRADUATES PER YEAR (APPROX.): 185.

MODALITIES AND SUBJECTS: applied kinesiology, anatomiken I and II, body-mind, career development I and II, chair massage, chi gong, client communication skills, clinical kinesiology, cranio-sacral therapy, equine sports massage, field placement I and II, hakomi bodywork, healing touch, hydrotherapy, infant massage, integrative therapeutic massage, lomilomi, lymphatic drainage, medical massage, movement I, II and III, myofascial release, myotherapy, neuromuscular therapy, normalization of soft tissue, nutrition, pathophysiology, polarity, postural integration, pregnancy massage, professional development, professional ethics, reflexology, reiki, shiatsu, structural kinesiology, therapeutic touch, trigger point therapies, watsu, yoga therapy, zero balancing.

SCHOOL STATEMENT: Comprehensive, experiential education in the art and science of massage therapy; seeking to balance professional expertise and personal growth in an environment that celebrates diversity.

#133 Center of Advanced Therapeutics
1221 S. Clarkson St., ste. 412
Denver, CO 80210
(303) 765-2201

HOURS OF TRAINING: 525 (in-class hours not specified).

DURATION OF COURSE: 9 months, day & evening & weekend programs available.

COST: $3,300. Payment plan without interest is available.

FINANCIAL AID: Reduced tuition for prior training.

YEAR FOUNDED: 1995.

MODALITIES AND SUBJECTS: connective tissue therapy, medical massage, myofascial release, neuromuscular therapy, polarity, shiatsu, sports massage, trigger point therapy.

SCHOOL STATEMENT: Our approach utilizes understanding of the body/mind to aid and speed healing. We provide the highest quality instruction in theory and practice of therapeutic massage.

#134 Collinson School of Therapeutics and Massage
2596 Palmer Park Blvd.,
Colorado Springs, CO 80909
(719) 473-0145

HOURS OF TRAINING: 1,000 (160 in-class hours).

DURATION OF COURSE: One four-hour evening class per week for 40 weeks plus 21 hours of study time each week.

COST: $3,300 includes books and in-class supplies.

YEAR FOUNDED: 1982.

GRADUATES PER YEAR (APPROX.): 25–30.

MODALITIES AND SUBJECTS: deep tissue massage, infant massage, kinesiology, pregnancy massage, stress & sports massage.

SCHOOL STATEMENT: We have the busy person in mind, teaching massage therapy with a minimum number of structured hours and a maximum of out of class hours.

#135 Colorado Institute of Massage Therapy
2601 East Vrain St.
Colorado Springs, CO 80909
(719) 634-7347

YEAR FOUNDED: 1985.

ACCREDITATIONS/APPROVALS: COMTA/approved.

#136 Colorado School of Healing Arts
7655 West Mississippi, suite 100
Lakewood, CO 80226
(303) 986-2320

HOURS OF TRAINING: 670 (565 in-class hours).

DURATION OF COURSE: 12 to 18 months, day and evening programs available.

COST: $4,850. Payment plan without interest is available.

FINANCIAL AID: Jefferson County and Adams County Employment & Training Services, US West, AT&T, Arapahoe County Employment Services, VA Dept. of Rehab., AFL/CIO, Mayor's Office for Employment & Training.

YEAR FOUNDED: 1986.

ACCREDITATIONS/APPROVALS: IMSTAC, ACCSCT.

GRADUATES PER YEAR (APPROX.): 200.

MODALITIES AND SUBJECTS: acupressure, AMMA, applied kinesiology, aromatherapy, body centered therapy, business, chair massage, chi gong, cranio-sacral therapy, diet & nutrition, healing touch, infant massage, integrative massage lab, massage clinical, massage level I & II & III, neuromuscular therapy, oriental medicine theory, palpation, polarity, reflexology, shiatsu, sports massage, trauma touch therapy™. Additional programs offered: Neuromuscular Massage Therapy Certification (300 hours, $2,235); Cranial Sacral Therapy Certification (530 hours, $4,090); Table Shiatsu Certification (500 hours, $3,695); Reflexology Certification (230 hours, $1,715); Sports Massage Certification (100 hours, $770); Trauma Touch Therapy™ Certification (100 hours, $770).

SCHOOL STATEMENT: The school emphasizes community, views the field as a service to humanity, and encourages students to link the training with their spiritual and professional goals.

#137 Colorado Springs Academy of Therapeutic Massage
3612 Galley Rd., suite A
Colorado Springs, CO 80909
(719) 597-0017 or 1-800-865-3414

HOURS OF TRAINING: 1,100 (in-class hours not specified).

DURATION OF COURSE: 8 months, day and evening programs available.

COST: $4,450 including books, ID, application and registration fee. Payment plan without interest is available.

FINANCIAL AID: Foundation Credit Corp.

YEAR FOUNDED: 1992.

GRADUATES PER YEAR (APPROX.): 80.

MODALITIES AND SUBJECTS: business, chair massage, deep tissue massage, myofascial release, neuromuscular therapy, nutrition, shiatsu, sports massage, student clinic internship, trigger point therapy.

SCHOOL STATEMENT: Curriculum emphasis is on clinical and rehabilitative massage. Video laser-disc human dissection and maniken system complement anatomy class.

#138 The Connecting Point School of Massage and Spa Therapies
Box 2101
Telluride, CO 81435
(Classroom: 104 Society Dr.)
(970) 728-6424

HOURS OF TRAINING: 500.

DURATION OF COURSE: 8 months (1 day & 2 evenings per week). or one year Saturdays.

COST: $4,000 including books, plus $25 application fee and $500 table. Payment plan without interest is available.

FINANCIAL AID: Discount for payment in full at start of course.

YEAR FOUNDED: 1993.

GRADUATES PER YEAR (APPROX.): 25.

MODALITIES AND SUBJECTS: acupressure, advanced techniques, aromatherapy, ayurveda, esalen, hydrotherapy, myofascial release, personal growth, reflexology, reiki, spa treatments, shiatsu, sports massage, trigger point therapy.

SCHOOL STATEMENT: Class size limited to 14 students, two teachers. Program emphasizes the process of change and growth in body, mind and spirit for students and clients.

#139 Cottonwood School of Massage Therapy
2620 S. Parker Rd. #300
Aurora, CO 80014
(303) 745-7725

HOURS OF TRAINING: 500.

DURATION OF COURSE: one year, day & evening programs available.

COST: $4,700, including books and table.

YEAR FOUNDED: 1992.

GRADUATES PER YEAR (APPROX.): 200.

MODALITIES AND SUBJECTS: advanced anatomy & pathology, aromatherapy, business, chair massage, cranio-sacral therapy, deep tissue massage, ethics, geriatric massage, lymphatic drainage, medical massage, neuromuscular therapy, ortho-bionomy, postural integration, pregnancy massage, reflexology, reiki, save your thumbs, shiatsu, sports massage, structural integration, student clinic, trigger point therapy.

SCHOOL STATEMENT: In an atmosphere of respect for the human body, our students learn both modern and time-honored massage therapy theories, skills and techniques.

#140 Crestone Healing Arts Center
P.O. Box 156
Crestone, CO 81131
(Classroom: 1689 Columbine Overlook)
(719) 256-4036

HOURS OF TRAINING: 520.

DURATION OF COURSE: 12 weeks, residential intensive.

COST: $5,300 including in-residence housing, fees and books.

YEAR FOUNDED: 1995.

GRADUATES PER YEAR (APPROX.): 20–30.

MODALITIES AND SUBJECTS: acupressure, business practice, chair massage, community massage practicum, CPR/first aid, emotional balancing techniques, esalen, group dynamics & special topics, herbology & massage, integrated massage, movement & chi enhancement, myotherapy, oriental healing philosophies, pregnancy massage, reflexology, reiki, shiatsu.

SCHOOL STATEMENT: The program immerses participants in an intense process of self-discovery, self-transformation, and self-healing through 12 weeks of concentrated in-residence massage training.

#141 Full Circle School of Massage Therapy
0210 Edwards Village Boulevard
Edwards, CO 81632
(303) 690-9002

Contact school for program information.

#142 Healing Arts Institute
4007 Automation Way
Fort Collins, CO 80525
(970) 223-9741 or 1-800-444-8244

HOURS OF TRAINING: 500 (C.M.T.) or 575 (BodyMind Therapist).

COST: 500 hours $4,000, 575 hours $4,648.

YEAR FOUNDED: 1991.

GRADUATES PER YEAR (APPROX.): 120.

MODALITIES AND SUBJECTS: C.M.T. program: applied kinesiology, body insight level I, II & III, business of self-employment, functional physiology, learning how you naturally learn, movement & body awareness, personal development, professional massage I, II & III, sports massage, student clinic. Also offered: Body-Mind Therapist, Body Insight Neuromuscular Practitioner, Certified Reflexologist, Sports Massage Classes, Continuing Education Courses.

SCHOOL STATEMENT: Being a fun and innovative school, our graduates display remarkable diversity and are encouraged to develop a style that is their own.

#143 Healing Spirits Massage Training Program
P.O. Box 7156
Boulder, CO 80306
(303) 776-7117 or 1-800-462-9908 ext. 61

HOURS OF TRAINING: 610 (500 in-class hours).

DURATION OF COURSE: one year, weekends plus 3 10-day intensives.

COST: $3,900.

FINANCIAL AID: work-study.

YEAR FOUNDED: 1997.

GRADUATES PER YEAR (APPROX.): 28.

MODALITIES AND SUBJECTS: aromatherapy, aston-patterning, body-mind, body psychology, body reading, breathwork, business skills, clinic, community placement, energy exploration, ethics & rapport, foundation massage, herbology, hydrotherapy, massage in motion, mentor program, movement & body awareness, neuro-muscular therapy, nutrition, pregnancy massage, reflexology, sounding, specific injury technique, strain counterstrain, table shiatsu, trigger point therapy, watsu aquatic bodywork.

SCHOOL STATEMENT: Healing Spirits honors the technical while maintaining spirit. We offer unique, intimate, supportive, quality education with heart, where personal discovery and individual style are encouraged.

#144 Heritage College of Health Careers, Inc.
#12 Lakeside Ln.
Denver, CO 80212
(303) 477-7240

HOURS OF TRAINING: 840.

DURATION OF COURSE: 9 to 10 months, day & evening & weekend programs available.

COST: $7,500 including books, supplies and insurance. Payment plan without interest is available.

FINANCIAL AID: Pell Grants.

YEAR FOUNDED: 1996.

ACCREDITATIONS/APPROVALS: ACCSCT.

GRADUATES PER YEAR (APPROX.): 50.

MODALITIES AND SUBJECTS: acupressure therapy, chair massage, CPR, ethics, integrative, internship, kinesiology, musculoskeletal, neuromuscular, nutrition, pathology, placement, shiatsu.

SCHOOL STATEMENT: The school emphasizes service to the community, ethics, encourage students to reach their professional goals.

#145 Massage Therapy Institute of Colorado
1441 York St., suite #301
Denver, CO 80206
(303) 329-6345

HOURS OF TRAINING: 1,051 (601 in-class hours).

DURATION OF COURSE: one year; day, evening & weekend programs available.

COST: $6,500 (includes books, massage table, supplies and insurance). Payment plan without interest is available.

FINANCIAL AID: Scholarships, Veteran's Administration, Colo. Rehab., JETS, Mayor's Office.

YEAR FOUNDED: 1986.

PREPARATION FOR OUT-OF-STATE LICENSING EXAM: Nebraska, Washington, Oregon.

GRADUATES PER YEAR (APPROX.): 130.

MODALITIES AND SUBJECTS: acupressure, alexander, AMMA, applied kinesiology, aromatherapy, aston-patterning, bioenergetics, body-mind, bowen technique, chair massage, chi gong, clinical practicum, cranio-sacral therapy, deep tissue, energy work, equine sports massage, feldenkrais, fisher method, geriatric massage, healing touch, heliotherapy, homeopathy, human engineering, hydrotherapy, infant massage, jin shin do, kinesiology I & II, lymphatic drainage, medical massage, movement, myofascial release, myotherapy, neuromuscular therapy, pathology, polarity, postur-

al integration, practice building, pregnancy massage, psychotherapy & bodywork, reflexology, reiki, rosen method, shiatsu, soft tissue manipulation, somatic therapy, sports massage, structural integration, therapeutic touch, touch for health, trager, trigger point therapy, tui na, watsu, yoga therapy.

SCHOOL STATEMENT: MTIC focuses on training several modalities of bodywork with a high degree of skill and expertise. Emphasis is on quality training provided through limited class size.

#146 Silver Sword Academy & Clinic of Massage Therapy & Spa Services
835 East 2nd Avenue, suite 85
Durango, CO 81301
(970) 247-5008

Contact school for program information.

CONNECTICUT

State Licensing 500 hours.

National Certification Exam accepted.

Board: (860) 509-7570

SCHOOL:

#147 Connecticut Center For Massage Therapy, Inc.
75 Kitts Lane
Newington, CT 06111
(860) 667-1886

25 Sylvan Road South
Westport, CT 06880
(203) 221-7325

HOURS OF TRAINING: 638; 44 credit hours.

DURATION OF COURSE: 19 months (five 12 week terms, separated by three-week breaks).

COST: $9,500.

FINANCIAL AID: Pell grants, Stafford Loans, PLUS loans, approved for veterans' benefits.

YEAR FOUNDED: 1982.

ACCREDITATIONS/APPROVALS: COMTA/Accredited, ACCSCT.

PREPARATION FOR OUT-OF-STATE LICENSING EXAM: contact school.

GRADUATES PER YEAR (APPROX.): 225.

MODALITIES AND SUBJECTS: acupressure, business practices, clinic/externship, energetic foundations, integrating acupressure, integratory seminar, kinesiology, palpation, pathology, professional foundations, standard first aid/CPR.

SCHOOL STATEMENT: Class size is limited to 20 students to maximize student/teacher interaction. Programs run mornings, afternoons, evenings and weekends. On-campus bookstore serves students and graduates.

DELAWARE

State Certification: 500 hours or 300 hours plus 2 years practice.

National Certification Exam accepted.

Board: (302) 739-4522, ext. 205

Delaware has long regulated massage as "adult entertainment" and has subjected the practice of massage to vice laws. The massage regulation law, enacted in 1994, creates an exemption to the adult entertainment law for persons who obtain certification to practice massage or bodywork in Delaware. Certification is voluntary, but those who practice without certification fall under the adult entertainment law.

The approved curriculum for certification is 50 hours anatomy, 50 hours physiology, 300 hours technique and theory and 100 hours electives.

SCHOOLS:

#148 Dawn Training Institute, Inc.
2400 West 4th St.
Wilmington, DE 19805
(302) 575-1322

Contact school for program information.

#149 Deep Muscle Therapy School
5317 Limestone Road
Wilmington, DE 19808
(302) 239-1613

HOURS OF TRAINING: 100 or 500.

DURATION OF COURSE: 100 hours 15 weeks, 500 hours approx. 12 months, day & evening & weekend programs available.

COST: $4,200 plus books approx. $300.

FINANCIAL AID: Work-study.

YEAR FOUNDED: 1996.

GRADUATES PER YEAR (APPROX.): 12.

MODALITIES AND SUBJECTS: alexander, applied kinesiology, aromatherapy, chair massage, feldenkrais, hydrotherapy, medical massage, movement therapy, myofascial release, myotherapy, neuromuscular therapy, pathology, rubenfeld synergy, therapeutic touch, touch for health, trigger point therapy.

SCHOOL STATEMENT: The school's emphasis in Basic is to give the students Swedish massage skills and in Advance the student learns how to treat musculoskeletal conditions.

#150 The Delaware School of Shiatsu &
Massage Therapy
5307 Limestone Rd., suite 103
Wilmington, DE 19808
(302) 234-7626

500-hours. Contact school for program information.

#151 Healing Touch, Inc.
939 South Governors Ave.
Dover, DE 19977
(302) 677-0178

Contact school for program information.

#152 Karen Carlson's International Academy of
Holistic Massage and Science
P.O. Box 3940
Greenville, DE 19807
(302) 777-7307

HOURS OF TRAINING: 1800 (500 in-class hours plus structured lab sessions).

DURATION OF COURSE: each level one year, Level I alternate Sundays, Level II alternate Saturdays.

COST: Level I $5,070, Level II $5,070 includes books & materials except table & uniform.

YEAR FOUNDED: 1977.

GRADUATES PER YEAR (APPROX.): 25–45.

MODALITIES AND SUBJECTS: allied health modalities, body mechanics, business development, chakra tuning, co-creative nature science, dowsing, ethics, fitness training, herbal & essence balancing, holistic healing, holistic reflexology®, hygiene, legalities, mediation, meridian massage, metabolic detoxification, therapeutic touch, touch for health, visualization.

SCHOOL STATEMENT: Levels I and II constitute a flexible track for compassionate individuals to progress through stages of personal healing to become a Holistic Natural Healing facilitator/practitioner.

#153 Owens Institute of Massage & Wholistic Sciences
2503 Sliverside Rd.
Wilmington, DE 19810
1-800-996-9367

Contact school for program information.

DISTRICT OF COLUMBIA

Licensing requirement: 500 hours.

National Certification Exam accepted.

Board: (202) 727-7823

SCHOOLS:

#154 Georgetown Bodyworks Healing Arts Institute
3000 Connecticut Avenue N.W. #102
Washington, DC 20008
(202) 328-7717
www.imagroup.com and www.learnmassage.com

1213 Thomas Avenue
Charlotte, NC 28205
(704) 335-0050

2450 Hawks Avenue
Ann Arbor, MI 48108
(734) 971-1950

2572 Oak Forest Drive
Holland, MI 49424
(616) 786-9753

HOURS OF TRAINING: 150 or 750 (50 or 250 in-class hours).

DURATION OF COURSE: 150 hours, 6 to 12 months; 750 hours, 18 to 24 months.

COST: 150 hours $2,195, 750 hours $4,995 both including table, bodyCushion, books, sheets and oil. Payment plan without interest is available.

FINANCIAL AID: Scholarships for single mothers.

YEAR FOUNDED: 1982.

GRADUATES PER YEAR (APPROX.): 150.

MODALITIES AND SUBJECTS: Canadian Deep Muscle Massage, Reach Therapy™, Bounce Therapy™.

SCHOOL STATEMENT: Loving, caring, **safe touch** should be part of American life. We are committed to teaching **safe structured touch** to everyone interested. Help us heal America.

#155 Potomac Massage Training Institute
4000 Albemarle St., NW, 5th floor
Washington, D.C. 20016
(202) 686-7046

HOURS OF TRAINING: 1,178 (515 in-class).

DURATION OF COURSE: 18 months part-time; day, evening and evening/weekend programs available.

COST: approx. $5,890 including books, CPR/first aid, professional massages.

FINANCIAL AID: scholarships, State rehabilitation agency funds.

YEAR FOUNDED: 1976.

ACCREDITATIONS/APPROVALS: COMTA/accredited.

GRADUATES PER YEAR (APPROX.): 100.

MODALITIES AND SUBJECTS: alexander, business & professional skills, chair massage, chi gong, clinic, communication, craniosacral therapy, deep tissue work, independent fieldwork, infant massage, kinesiology, massage practice, medical massage, neuromuscular therapy, polarity, pregnancy massage, reflexology, reiki, somatic therapy, sports massage, structural integration, study and homework, supervised fieldwork, trager.

SCHOOL STATEMENT: The massage program is holistic, recognizing each person's unique inner health and growth process, with anatomy, physiology, kinesiology and skill techniques forming the foundation.

FLORIDA

State Licensing: 500 hours.

National Certification Exam accepted.

Board: (850) 488-6021

APPROVED OUT-OF-STATE SCHOOLS:

Academy of Somatic Healing Arts (GA); Alexandria School (IN); Alternative Conjunction, The (PA); Atlanta School, Atlanta GA; Bancroft School (MA); Blue Cliff School (LA); Body Therapy Inst. (NC); Capelli Learning Center (GA); Finger Lakes School (NY); Georgia Inst. Of Therapeutic Massage; Lake Lanier School (GA); Medical Training College (LA); New Mexico Academy of Healing Arts; North Eastern Inst. (NH); Pennsylvania School of Muscle Therapy; Somerset School (NJ); Southeastern School (NC); Tennessee Institute of Healing Arts.

SCHOOLS:

#156 Academy of Career Training
3501 W. Vine St., suite 258
Kissimmee, FL 34741
(407) 943-8777

HOURS OF TRAINING: 500.

DURATION OF COURSE: 4½ months days or 9½ months evenings

COST: $2,795 includes 4 books.

YEAR FOUNDED: school 1995, massage program 1998.

MODALITIES AND SUBJECTS: business, HIV/AIDS, hydrotherapy, florida law & rules & history of massage, reflexology, sports massage, therapeutic stretching.

SCHOOL STATEMENT: Class size is kept small for individualized instruction and clinic operated to provide hands on training.

#157 Academy of Healing Arts Massage &
Facial Skin Care, Inc.
3141 South Military Trail
Lake Worth, FL 33463
(561) 965-5550 or 967-0899

HOURS OF TRAINING: 500 or 600.

DURATION OF COURSE: 500 hours 5 months, 600 hours 6 months; day and evening programs available.

COST: 500 hours $3,125, 600 hours $4,175.

FINANCIAL AID: Pell Grants, Direct Loan Stafford and Direct Loan unsubsidized.

ACCREDITATIONS/APPROVALS: approved for veterans' training,

ACCSCT.

YEAR FOUNDED: 1983.

GRADUATES PER YEAR (APPROX.): 125.

MODALITIES AND SUBJECTS: acupressure, aromatherapy, arthritis self-help, chair massage, client centered massage, connective tissue therapy, digestive massage, embodiment workshop, european body wraps, facial massage techniques, good business practices, healing touch, HIV/AIDS, hydrotherapy, joint movement, lymphatic drainage, myofascial release, myotherapy, nature of disease, neuromuscular therapy, nutritional health management, pathology, reflexology, reiki, shiatsu, soma therapy, sports massage, statutes/rules/history, touch for health, trigger point therapy. Also offered is 802 hour Beauty Therapy program, combining massage and skin care).

SCHOOL STATEMENT: AHA's goal is to offer education that prepares students for all the requirements and skills necessary to become licensed specialists with proper training and experience.

#158 Acupressure-Acupuncture Institute, Inc.
10506 N. Kendall Drive
Miami, FL 33176
(305) 595-9500
www.acupuncture.pair.com

HOURS OF TRAINING: 500 (in-class hours not specified).

DURATION OF COURSE: 6 months, evenings.

COST: $3,500. Payment plan without interest is available.

YEAR FOUNDED: 1983.

GRADUATES PER YEAR (APPROX.): 20.

MODALITIES AND SUBJECTS: basic massage therapy, clinical practicum, history of massage, HIV/AIDS, hydrotherapy, oriental bodywork, state rules.

SCHOOL STATEMENT: At the AAI we wish to transmit to our students both the knowledge necessary to heal and the Qi, the power, behind all healing.

#159 Alpha Institute of South Florida, Inc.
904 Park Ave.
Lake Park, FL 33403
(561) 845-1400

HOURS OF TRAINING: 500 (270-hour Facial Specialist also offered).

DURATION OF COURSE: 25 weeks, day and evening programs available.

COST: $3,329 including all books, sheet, shirt, CPR and insurance. Payment plan without interest is available.

YEAR FOUNDED: 1993.

GRADUATES PER YEAR (APPROX.): 100.

MODALITIES AND SUBJECTS: applied kinesiology, aromatherapy, body-mind, chair massage, cranio-sacral therapy, healing touch, infant massage, jin shin do, lymphatic drainage, myofascial release, myotherapy, neuromuscular therapy, pregnancy massage, reflexology, reiki, rolfing, somatic therapy, trager, trigger point therapy.

#160 Alpha School of Massage, Inc.
4642 San Juan Ave.
Jacksonville, FL 32210
(904) 389-9117

HOURS OF TRAINING: 501.

DURATION OF COURSE: 6 or 12 months, day & evening & weekend programs available.

COST: $3,100 (includes books and supplies). Payment plan without interest is available.

YEAR FOUNDED: 1993.

GRADUATES PER YEAR (APPROX.): 50.

MODALITIES AND SUBJECTS: acupressure, applied kinesiology, aromatherapy, chair massage, flexibility exercise, HIV education, hydrotherapy, infant massage, medical massage, myofascial release, neuromuscular therapy, pregnancy massage, psychology of massage, reflexology, shiatsu, sports massage, structural integration, trigger point therapy.

SCHOOL STATEMENT: We are dedicated to the ideals of holistic health and the role massage plays in the healing arts.

#161 Alpha School of Massage of the Treasure Coast
1599 SE Port St. Lucie Blvd.
Port St. Lucie, FL 34952
(561) 337-5533

Contact school for program information.

#162 America Duran Skin Care School
2100 Coral Way
Miami, FL 33145
(305) 642-4104

Contact the school for program information.

#163 American Institute of Massage Therapy, Inc.
2101 North Federal Highway
Ft. Lauderdale, FL 33305
(954) 568-6200 or (800) 752-2793
www.aimt.com

HOURS OF TRAINING: 600.

DURATION OF COURSE: 6 months full time, 12 months part-time; day, evening and weekend programs available.

COST: $4,500 including book package, shirt, water bottle, totebag, ring binder, one bottle of massage oil. Payment plan without interest is available.

FINANCIAL AID: Scholarships or discounts are available.

YEAR FOUNDED: 1983.

ACCREDITATIONS/APPROVALS: ACCET.

GRADUATES PER YEAR (APPROX.): 200.

MODALITIES AND SUBJECTS: aromatherapy, chair massage, colon therapy, colonic irrigation therapy (advanced program), communication skills, CPR, cranial sacral therapy, cryotherapy, deep tissue therapy, equine sports massage, ergonomics, field trips, geriatrics, HIV-AIDS, hydrotherapy, infant massage, manual lymphatic drainage, marketing & business practices, massage theory, medical massage, myofascial techniques, natural remedies, neuromuscular techniques, nutrition, pathology, personal development, practicum, radiological studies, range of motion, reflexology, rolfing, statutes & rules of massage, sports hydrotherapy, sports massage, stretching, structural integration, trager, trigger point therapy.

SCHOOL STATEMENT: AIMT provides high quality education, emphasizing the importance of perceiving the individual as a whole person and treating simultaneously health's physical and emotional aspects.

#164 Arlington School of Massage
1239 Rogero Rd.
Jacksonville, FL 32211
(904) 745-1688

Contact School for program information.

#165 Atlantic Academy
4427 Emerson St.
Jacksonville, FL 32207
(904) 398-2359

Atlantic Academy of Volusia County
225 North Causeway
New Smyrna Beach, FL 32169
(904) 424-9977

HOURS OF TRAINING: 500.

DURATION OF COURSE: 6 months (Jacksonville: day, evening and weekend programs; New Smyrna Beach: days).

COST: $3,100 including books, fees and materials. Payment plan without interest is available.

YEAR FOUNDED: Jacksonville 1991, New Smyrna Beach 1993.

GRADUATES PER YEAR (APPROX.): 50 at each location.

MODALITIES AND SUBJECTS: body-mind, bowen technique, chair massage, cranio-sacral therapy, infant massage, jin shin do, lymphatic drainage, medical massage, myofascial release, myotherapy, neuromuscular therapy, polarity, postural integration, pregnancy massage, reflexology, sports massage, structural integration, therapeutic touch, trigger point therapy.

SCHOOL STATEMENT: Specializing in the well-rounded therapist who wishes to become self-employed in medical or wellness centers.

#166 Bhakti Academe School of
Intuitive Massage & Healing
25410 US 19 N., suite 116
Clearwater, FL 34623
(813) 724-9727

HOURS OF TRAINING: 500.

DURATION OF COURSE: 6 months days, one year evenings.

COST: $2,500 plus $150 for books and $350 for table. Payment plan without interest is available.

YEAR FOUNDED: 1996.

GRADUATES PER YEAR (APPROX.): maximum of 48.

MODALITIES AND SUBJECTS: AIDS/HIV education, allied modalities, bhakti bodywork massage & energetic healing, hydrotherapy, massage law.

SCHOOL STATEMENT: Bhakti Academe's focus is love, spirituality, and intuitive massage and healing using group and individual body energy techniques. Bhakti means re-integration through love. (in Sanskrit).

#167 Boca Beauty Academy
8221 Glades Road
Boca Raton, FL 33434
(561) 487-1191

Contact school for program information.

#168 Boca Raton Institute
5499 North Federal Highway, suite A
Boca Raton, FL 33487
(407) 241-8105 or (800) 275-6764

HOURS OF TRAINING: 605.

DURATION OF COURSE: 6 months days, 7½ months evenings.

YEAR FOUNDED: 1983.

ACCREDITATIONS/APPROVALS: National Accrediting Commission of Cosmetology Arts and Sciences.

MODALITIES AND SUBJECTS: AIDS/HIV education, business principles & Florida law, clinics, cranio-sacral techniques, deep relaxation techniques, exercise physiology, hydrotherapy, kinesiology, neuromuscular therapy, reflexology, rolfing, shiatsu, somatic therapy, sports massage, stress management.

SCHOOL STATEMENT: The school offers a combined 905-hour skin care and massage program.

#169 Central Florida School of Massage Therapy
450 N. Lakemont Ave., suite A
Winter Park, FL 32792
(407) 673-6776

HOURS OF TRAINING: 525.

DURATION OF COURSE: 6 months days or one year evenings.

COST: $3,500 includes two books and school shirt. Payment plan without interest is available.

YEAR FOUNDED: 1996.

GRADUATES PER YEAR (APPROX.): 60.

MODALITIES AND SUBJECTS: AIDS/HIV education, allied modalities, chair massage, clinic, hydrotherapy, myofascial release, shiatsu, sports massage, statutes & rules, trigger point therapy. Advanced programs are offered in sports massage, spa theory & technique, energetic techniques, and medical massage.

SCHOOL STATEMENT: The school provides a comprehensive education in the art and science of Massage Therapy, balancing professional expertise with personal growth in a supportive environment.

#170 Coastal School of Massage Therapy, Inc.
434 Osceola Avenue
Jacksonville Beach, FL 32250
(904) 270-1700

HOURS OF TRAINING: 700 (512 in-class).

DURATION OF COURSE: 32 weeks, day and evening classes available.

COST: $4,375 plus $350 textbooks and $100 student liability insurance.

FINANCIAL AID: Employment Scholarships, Vocational Rehabilitation, Veteran's Administration.

YEAR FOUNDED: 1995.

GRADUATES PER YEAR (APPROX.): 35.

MODALITIES AND SUBJECTS: acupressure, AIDS education, aromatherapy, chair massage, cranio-sacral therapy, equine sports massage, Florida law, geriatric massage, health service management, hydrotherapy, infant massage, iridology, lymphatic drainage, myofascial release, natural wellness, neuromuscular therapy, oriental theory, pathology, polarity, pregnancy massage, reflexology, reiki, shiatsu, spa therapy, spiritual healing, sports massage ,structural integration, touch for health, yoga & tai chi chuan.

SCHOOL STATEMENT: The school produces well-trained, competent natural health care providers, who are prepared to practice therapeutic massage using a broad range of skills. Small class size.

#171 Community Technical and Adult Education
1014 SW 7th Road
Ocala, FL 34474

Contact school for program information.

#172 Core Institute
223 W. Carolina St.
Tallahassee, FL 32301
(850) 222-8673
www.coreinstitute.com

HOURS OF TRAINING: 500; revision to 750 hours planned.

DURATION OF COURSE: 6 months full-time, 12 months part-time, day and evening classes available.

COST: $4,500 (includes books).

FINANCIAL AID: VA benefits, job training program, vocational rehabilitation, private student loans from a local bank for qualified applicants.

YEAR FOUNDED: 1990.

ACCREDITATIONS/APPROVALS: COMTA/Accredited.

GRADUATES PER YEAR (APPROX.): 80.

MODALITIES AND SUBJECTS: applied anatomy, business, chair massage, communications, core body therapy (structural integration), core massage, HIV/AIDS, HIV/AIDS, hydrotherapy, law, medical massage (beginning and advanced), neuromuscular therapy, polarity, shiatsu, sports massage (beginning and advanced), thai massage, therapeutic touch, TMJ, trager, trigger point, wellness.

SCHOOL STATEMENT: community service is stressed.

#173 Daytona Institute of Massage Therapy
209 Dunlawton Ave., suite 18
Port Orange, FL 32119
(904) 788-5550

Contact school for program information.

#174 Educating Hands School of Massage
120 Southwest 8th St.
Miami, FL 33130
(305) 285-6991 or (800) 999-6991
www.massagetherapynetwork.com

HOURS OF TRAINING: 624.

DURATION OF COURSE: 6 months days, 8 or 11 months evenings.

COST: $4,980 includes books and supplies.

FINANCIAL AID: payment plans.

YEAR FOUNDED: 1981.

ACCREDITATIONS/APPROVALS: COMTA/approved.

GRADUATES PER YEAR (APPROX.): 120.

MODALITIES AND SUBJECTS: aromatherapy, body mechanics, business principles and development, chair massage, connective tissue massage, corrective exercise and movement, craniosacral, deep relaxation, deep tissue, guided imagery, heliotherapy, HIV/AIDS, hoshino therapy, hydrotherapy, infant massage, kinesiology and palpation, lymphatic drainage, meditation, neuromuscular therapy, pathology, polarity, reflexology, relaxation techniques, shiatsu, sports massage, stretching, student clinic, trager, understanding the client/practitioner relationship.

SCHOOL STATEMENT: Our program develops wholistic practitioners with sensitivity in their touch, creativity in their methods, and a dedication to personal growth.

#175 Emerald Coast Massage School
913-B North Beal Parkway
Fort Walton Beach, FL 32549
(850) 314-7714

HOURS OF TRAINING: 700 (500 in-class hours).

DURATION OF COURSE: 5 months full-time, 11 months part-time, day and evening programs available.

COST: $3,275 including all books, oil, bottles, cleaners. Payment plan without interest is available.

FINANCIAL AID: Scholarships or discounts, Veteran's Administration, State Vocational Rehab.

YEAR FOUNDED: 1994.

GRADUATES PER YEAR (APPROX.): 40.

MODALITIES AND SUBJECTS: acupressure, AIDS awareness, applied kinesiology, aromatherapy, business practices & development, chair massage, connective tissue, CPR, cranio-sacral therapy, equine sports massage, esalen, fitness, infant massage, joint mobilization, kinesiology, massage theory & practice, medical massage, meridian therapy, myofascial release, neuromuscular therapy, nutrition, PNF stretching, polarity, pregnancy massage, reflexology, reiki, shiatsu, sports massage, statutes & rules, therapeutic touch, trager, trigger point therapy, watsu, yoga therapy.

SCHOOL STATEMENT: Emerald Coast Massage School believes therapeutic massage is a viable alternative healing method for neuromuscular problems as well as general relaxation and stress relief.

#176 Erwin Technical School
2010 East Hillsborough Avenue
Tampa, FL 33610
(813) 231-1800 ext. 2441

HOURS OF TRAINING: 660.

COST: $800 including books.

YEAR FOUNDED: 1996.

GRADUATES PER YEAR (APPROX.): 30.

MODALITIES AND SUBJECTS: allied modalities, client-therapist relationship, deep swedish massage, entrepreneurship, first aid & CPR, florida massage law, foot reflexology, HIV/AIDS, hydrotherapy, hygiene, intuitive/eclectic style massage, massage history & theory, massage practicum, stress reduction, student clinic, wellness.

SCHOOL STATEMENT: The emphasis is on the art of touch - teaching students to give a quality, nourishing eclectic style massage based on awareness of self and client.

#177 Florida Academy of Massage
8695 College Parkway, suite 110
Fort Myers, FL 33919
(941) 489-2282 or 1-800-324-9543
www.floridaacademymassage.com

HOURS OF TRAINING: 540.

DURATION OF COURSE: 17 weeks days or 22 weeks evenings.

COST: $3,515 including school shirts, texts and workbooks.

FINANCIAL AID: Vocational Rehab, JTPA, Blind Services, Scholarships through FAPSC.

YEAR FOUNDED: 1992.

MODALITIES AND SUBJECTS: acupressure, AIDS/HIV education, aromatherapy, basic massage theory & clinical practice, bindegewebsmassage, bioenergetics, body mind, chair massage, cranio-sacral therapy, Florida state rules & history of massage, lymphatic drainage, myofascial release, neuromuscular therapy, pfrimmer deep muscle, postural integration, reflexology, reiki, shiatsu, sports massage, structural integration, theory & practice of hydrotherapy, touch for health, trigger point therapy, yoga therapy. Advanced trainings: contact school.

SCHOOL STATEMENT: Final term students perform virtually all the duties required in private practice under close supervision in an on-premises clinic, in the Student Clinic Practicum.

#178 Florida College of Natural Health
2001 W. Sample Rd., suite 100
Pompano Beach, FL 33064
(954) 975- 6400 or 1-800-541-9299

7925 NW 12th St., suite 201
Miami, FL 33126
(305) 597-9599 or 1-800-599-9599

887 E. Altamonte Dr.
Altamonte Springs, FL 32701
(407) 261-0319 or 1-800-393-7337

HOURS OF TRAINING: from 624 hours to A.S. degree in Natural Health.

DURATION OF COURSE: 5 months to 2 years (A.S.), day and evening programs available.

COST: $4,900 to $12,000.

FINANCIAL AID: Scholarships—FAPSC & special scholarships, Career College Association, Florida Gold Seal. Grants and loans—Pell grants, Stafford loans, PLUS loans.

YEAR FOUNDED: 1986.

ACCREDITATIONS/APPROVALS: ACCSCT, COMTA/Accredited.

GRADUATES PER YEAR (APPROX.): 900.

MODALITIES AND SUBJECTS: aromatherapy, chair massage, cranio-sacral therapy, equine sports massage, healing touch, infant massage, lymphatic drainage, myofascial release, neuromuscular therapy, reflexology, reiki, rolfing, sports massage, therapeutic touch, trager, trigger point therapy, yoga therapy. Programs: Therapeutic Massage (624 hours); Advanced Therapeutic Massage (900 hours); Therapeutic Massage & Skin Care (900 hours); Associate of Science, Natural Health (63.5 credits).

SCHOOL STATEMENT: Quality education combining courses in massage therapy, skin care and general education to offer short-term diploma programs or A.S. degrees.

#179 Florida Health Academy
10915 Bonita Beach Rd., suite 1161
Bonita Springs, FL 34135
(941) 495-8282

Florida Health Academy – Naples
261 Ninth St. South
Naples, FL 34102
(941) 263-9391

HOURS OF TRAINING: 540.

DURATION OF COURSE: 6, 9 or 12 months. Evening programs both locations, days Naples.

COST: $2,300 plus $225 books and supplies and uniform. Payment plan without interest is available.

FINANCIAL AID: JTPA.

YEAR FOUNDED: 1992.

GRADUATES PER YEAR (APPROX.): Naples 60, Bonita Springs 30.

MODALITIES AND SUBJECTS: acupressure, applied kinesiology, aromatherapy, business practices, chair massage cranio-sacral therapy, equine sports massage, Florida law, HIV/AIDS, hydrotherapy, infant massage, medical massage, neuromuscular therapy, pregnancy massage, reflexology, rolfing, shiatsu, sports massage, therapeutic touch, trigger point therapy, yoga therapy.

SCHOOL STATEMENT: FHA was established to provide the highest quality education through the integration of academics, clinical skills and experience.

#180 Florida School of Massage
6421 SW 13th Street
Gainesville, FL 32608
(352) 378-7891
www.massageonline.com

HOURS OF TRAINING: 705 to 1,000 (650 in-class hours).

DURATION OF COURSE: 6 months, days.

COST: $5,150 plus $100 application fee, $250 books and supplies, $400 to $600 table.

FINANCIAL AID: Work study (up to $600 applied to tuition for qualified students), Bureau of Blind Services, State Vocational Rehab., Fl. Dept. of Veteran's Affairs, Office for Social Security.

YEAR FOUNDED: 1973.

ACCREDITATIONS/APPROVALS: COMTA/Accredited.

PREPARATION FOR OUT-OF-STATE LICENSING EXAM: New York (additional training required).

GRADUATES PER YEAR (APPROX.): 150.

MODALITIES AND SUBJECTS: arthritis massage, awareness & communication skills, awareness & integrated massage, body-mind, business practices & ethics, carpal tunnel syndrome, chair massage, chi gong, community circle, connective tissue massage, CPR & first aid, directed independent study project, evaluation & treatment of knee injuries, evaluation & treatment of shoulder injuries, examination review, feldenkrais, florida massage laws & rules, foundations of bodywork & swedish massage, hydrotherapy, infant massage, kinesiology, living with AIDS, massage journals, myofascial release, neuromuscular therapy, ortho-bionomy, polarity, pregnancy massage, reflexology, shiatsu, sports massage, structural integration, trigger point therapy, tui na.

SCHOOL STATEMENT: FSM has 25 years of experience offering massage education as a vehicle for personal growth and empowerment, cultivating compassionate touch through a nurturing community experience.

#181 Florida's Therapeutic Massage School
1300 East Gadsden St.
Pensacola, FL 32501
(904) 433-8212

HOURS OF TRAINING: 700 (600 in-class hours, 100 hours clinic internship).

DURATION OF COURSE: 5½ months, day and evening programs available.

COST: $3,400 including required textbooks.

FINANCIAL AID: Veteran's Administration.

YEAR FOUNDED: 1992.

GRADUATES PER YEAR (APPROX): 150.

MODALITIES AND SUBJECTS: acupressure, AIDS/HIV education, applied kinesiology, aromatherapy, body-mind, business ethics & practices, chair massage, chi gong, clinic internship, communication skills, CPR, cranio-sacral therapy, deep tissue massage, feldenkrais, hakomi, healing touch, herbology, hospital internship, hydrotherapy, infant massage, kinesiology, lymphatic drainage, massage laws, medical massage, movement, myofascial release, neuromuscular therapy, nutrition, ortho-bionomy, pathology, polarity, postural integration, rebirthing, reflexology, sports massage, structural integration, therapeutic touch, trigger point therapy, tui na, watsu.

SCHOOL STATEMENT: Holistic curriculum: body, mind, emotions—whole person. FTMS is a place of learning, growth and healing

#182 Haney Vocational Technical Center
3016 Highway 77
Panama City, FL 32405
(850) 747-5500

Contact school for program information.

#183 HealthBuilders School of Therapeutic Massage, Inc.
2180 SR 3
St. Augustine, FL 32084
(904) 471-8828
www.oldcity.com/hb

HOURS OF TRAINING: 500.

DURATION OF COURSE: 26 weeks, day and evening programs available.

COST: $3,300 including books. Payment plan without interest is available.

YEAR FOUNDED: 1994.

GRADUATES PER YEAR (APPROX.): 25.

MODALITIES AND SUBJECTS: business practices & practice building, clinical practicum, deep tissue, HIV/AIDS education, hydrotherapy, mind-body integration, neuromuscular therapy, polarity, reflexology, shiatsu, statutes & rules & history.

SCHOOL STATEMENT: We provide the highest quality education, via highly qualified instructors, multimedia, and hands-on experience. Students receive the experience, knowledge and confidence to begin a career.

#184 Humanities Center School of Massage
4045 Park Blvd.
Pinellas Park, FL 33781
(813) 541-5200

HOURS OF TRAINING: 625 (in-class hours not specified).

DURATION OF COURSE: 6½ months days, 8 months evenings.

COST: $5,730 (includes books). Payment plan without interest is available.

FINANCIAL AID: Stafford loans, Pell grants.

YEAR FOUNDED: 1981.

ACCREDITATIONS/APPROVALS: COMTA/approved, ACCSCT.

GRADUATES PER YEAR (APPROX.): 200.

MODALITIES AND SUBJECTS: body mechanics, business practices, clinic internship, HIV/AIDS education, hydrotherapy, integrated relaxation methods, massage law, maniken anatomy, medical massage, neuromuscular therapies (trigger point, strain-counterstrain, muscle energy technique, myofascial release, pathology, postural analysis, clinic), range of motion, sexual ethics.

SCHOOL STATEMENT: small classes, emphasis on neuromuscular therapies, high technology / multi-media teaching.

#185 Lindsey Hopkins Technical Education Center
750 Northwest 20th St.
Miami, FL 33127
(305) 324-6070

HOURS OF TRAINING: 720 plus 90 hours of core curriculum.

DURATION OF COURSE: 9 months.

DAY/EVENING/WEEKEND: day and evening programs available

COST: under $800 tuition, $250 books and materials.

FINANCIAL AID: approved for veterans, JTPA, and other agencies. Call for specific information.

YEAR FOUNDED: around 1960.

GRADUATES PER YEAR (APPROX): 40–60.

MODALITIES AND SUBJECTS: allied modalities, aromatherapy, business practices & standards, chair massage, clinical practicum, CPR & first aid, employability skills, ethics, history of massage, HIV/blood-borne diseases, hydrotherapy, hygiene & sanitation

& safety, kinesiology, massage theory, statutes & rules, trigger point therapy.

SCHOOL STATEMENT: We provide students with the knowledge and palpatory skills to perform in a safe and ethical manner, in all settings in which Massage is provided.

#186 Loraine's Academy, Inc.
1012 58th St. N.
St. Petersburg, FL 33710
(813) 347-4247

HOURS OF TRAINING: 600 (in-class hours not specified).

DURATION OF COURSE: 5 months days, 7 months evenings.

COST: $4,850 including books.

FINANCIAL AID: Pell & FSEOG grants, subsidized/unsubsidized student loans, federal college work study programs.

YEAR FOUNDED: 1966.

ACCREDITATIONS/APPROVALS: NACCAS.

MODALITIES AND SUBJECTS: creative expression, HIV/AIDS, hydrotherapy, interpersonal skills, massage law, massage theory, myofascial technique, neuromuscular theory, oriental theory, postural analysis, sports massage, stress reduction, trigger point therapy.

SCHOOL STATEMENT: Small classes (12 or less), anatomy taught by physician, active student clinic, 100% pass rate on National Certification Exam, extraordinarily dedicated, educated and talented staff.

#187 Lotus Heart School of Massage
1403 Highland Ave.
Melbourne, FL 32935
(407) 757-3166

Contact School for program information.

#188 Magnolia Institute
618 NE First Street
Gainesville, FL 32601
(352) 373-4800

Contact school for program information.

#189 Orange Technical Education Centers
Westside Tech, 955 E. Story Road
Winter Garden, FL 34787
(407) 656-2851

Contact school for program information.

#190 Orlando Institute School of Massage Therapy
Casselberry Collection
3385 S. Hwy 17-92, suite 221
Casselberry, FL 32707
(407) 331-1101

HOURS OF TRAINING: 505.

DURATION OF COURSE: 24 weeks days, 36 weeks evenings.

COST: $3,500 (includes books). Payment plan without interest is available.

FINANCIAL AID: Scholarships or discounts are available.

YEAR FOUNDED: 1989.

GRADUATES PER YEAR (APPROX): 60.

MODALITIES AND SUBJECTS: acupressure, aromatherapy, business & law & ethics, chair massage, cranio-sacral therapy, energy assessment, HIV/AIDS, hydrotherapy, lymphatic drainage, massage theory & practicum, muscle testing, reflexology, shiatsu, sports massage, three in one concept.

SCHOOL STATEMENT: Orlando Institute views massage and the modalities as a cornerstone for preventative health care, and a valuable tool in restoring the body to good health.

#191 Pensacola Junior College
Massage Therapy Program
5555 W. Hwy. 98
Pensacola, FL 32507
(850) 484-2210 or 484-2229

HOURS OF TRAINING: 720.

DURATION OF COURSE: two semesters (approx. 8 months).

COST: $700 including books, fees, uniform and supplies.

FINANCIAL AID: Scholarships, Pell Grants, Veterans Administration, Social Security, Vocational Rehabilitation, JTPA, Workers Compensation, Work Study, and others.

YEAR FOUNDED: 1997.

ACCREDITATIONS/APPROVALS: Southern Association of Colleges and Schools.

GRADUATES PER YEAR (APPROX.): 45.

MODALITIES AND SUBJECTS: applied kinesiology, aromatherapy, body mechanics & movement, business management, chair massage, CPR, client/therapist relationship, communication dynamics, deep tissue, evaluation skills, ethics, first aid, flexibility exercises, HIV/AIDS awareness, hydrotherapy, infant massage, insurance billing, massage history, marketing skills, medical massage, myofascial release, neuromuscular therapy, nutrition, pathology, pregnancy massage, record keeping, shiatsu, sports massage, state laws & rules, supervised student clinic, trigger point therapy.

SCHOOL STATEMENT: Curriculum based around on-going student massage therapy clinic available to the public, low tuition fees (state funded Junior College), enrollment 3 times per year.

#192 Pensacola School of Massage Therapy
5080 Mobile Highway
Pensacola, FL 32506
(850) 456-6070

HOURS OF TRAINING: 700 (500 in-class hours).

DURATION OF COURSE: 5 months full-time, 11 months part-time, day and evening programs available.

COST: $3,275 including all books, oil, bottles, cleaners. Payment plan without interest is available.

FINANCIAL AID: Scholarships or discounts, Veteran's Administration, State Vocational Rehab.

YEAR FOUNDED: 1994.

GRADUATES PER YEAR (APPROX.): 40.

MODALITIES AND SUBJECTS: acupressure, AIDS awareness, applied kinesiology, aromatherapy, business practices & development, chair massage, connective tissue, CPR, cranio-sacral therapy, equine sports massage, esalen, fitness, infant massage, joint mobilization, kinesiology, massage theory & practice, medical massage, meridian therapy, myofascial release, neuromuscular therapy, nutrition, PNF stretching, polarity, pregnancy massage, reflexology, reiki, shiatsu, sports massage, statutes & rules, therapeutic touch, trager, trigger point therapy, watsu, yoga therapy.

SCHOOL STATEMENT: Pensacola School of Massage Therapy believes therapeutic massage is a viable alternative healing method for neuromuscular problems as well as general relaxation and stress relief.

#193 Port Charlotte School of Massage Therapy
    1057 Collingswood Blvd., Unit A
    Port Charlotte, FL 33953
    (813) 255-1966

HOURS OF TRAINING: 500 (in-class hours not specified).

DURATION OF COURSE: 6 months, days or evenings; part-time program also available.

COST: $3,200 tuition, $50 enrollment fee, $250 books. Payment plan without interest is available.

FINANCIAL AID: Workmen's Compensation, Veteran's Administration, Florida Dept. of Labor Blind Services.

YEAR FOUNDED: 1991.

MODALITIES AND SUBJECTS: AMMA, applied kinesiology, aromatherapy, berrywork, bindegewebsmassage, business, chair massage, cranio-sacral therapy, feldenkrais, infant massage, jin shin do, medical massage, myofascial release, neuromuscular therapy, polarity, positional release, postural integration, pregnancy massage, reflexology, shiatsu, sports massage, strain counterstrain.

SCHOOL STATEMENT: Our aim is to help each individual realize their potential in diverse areas of this profession, from stress reduction and relaxation to NMT and business.

#194 Ridge Technical Center
    7700 State Road 544
    Winter Haven, FL 33881
    (941) 422-6402 or (941) 299-2512

HOURS OF TRAINING: 850.

DURATION OF COURSE: 8 months days, evening program varies.

COST: approx. $1,250 including books, uniform shirts and cost of state exam.

FINANCIAL AID: Pell Grant, Workforce development.

ACCREDITATIONS/APPROVALS: Southern Association of Colleges and Schools, Council on Occupational Education.

GRADUATES PER YEAR (APPROX.): days, 24; evening varies.

MODALITIES AND SUBJECTS: allied modalities, basic business practices, health & safety practices, hydrotherapy, massage theory and practice, orientation, state rules and regulations. Additional bodywork modalities will be included in the program but details were not available at press time.

#195 Sarasota School of Massage Therapy
    1970 Main St.
    Sarasota, FL 34236
    (941) 957-0577

YEAR FOUNDED: 1980.

ACCREDITATIONS/APPROVALS: COMTA/approved, Southern Association of Colleges and Schools Commission on Occupational Educational Institutions, New York State Board of Regents, approved for veterans training.

#196 Sarasota School of Natural Healing Arts
    8216 S. Tamiami Trail
    Sarasota, FL 34238
    (941) 966-7117
    www.web-sarasota.com/ssnha

HOURS OF TRAINING: 525 (in-class hours not specified).

DURATION OF COURSE: 5 months, day and evening programs offered

COST: $4,735 includes book package.

YEAR FOUNDED: 1978.

GRADUATES PER YEAR (APPROX.): 70.

MODALITIES AND SUBJECTS: applied kinesiology, aromatherapy, chair massage, cranio-sacral therapy, healing touch, hydrotherapy, insurance & business, internship clinic, lymphatic drainage, massage law, medical massage, neuromuscular therapy, nutrition, polarity, reflexology, reiki, shiatsu, sports massage, therapeutic touch.

SCHOOL STATEMENT: The school is a transformational environment which prepares graduates to pass their state and national boards and embark upon successful careers as licensed massage therapists.

#197 School of Complementary Medicine
    100 East Broadway
    Oviedo, FL 32762
    (407) 366-8615

Contact school for program information.

#198 Seminar Network International, Inc.
    518 North Federal Highway
    Lake Worth, FL 33460
    (561) 582-5349 or (800) 882-0903

YEAR FOUNDED: 1987.

ACCREDITATIONS/APPROVALS: COMTA/approved, ACCET.

#199 Southeastern School of Neuromuscular and
    Massage Therapy, Inc.
    9088 Golfside Drive
    Jacksonville, FL 32256
    (904) 448-9499
    www.se-massage.com

HOURS OF TRAINING: 500.

DURATION OF COURSE: 6 months full-time, one year part-time, morning or evening classes.

COST: $5,300.

YEAR FOUNDED: 1992.

GRADUATES PER YEAR (APPROX.): 50 to 100.

MODALITIES AND SUBJECTS: business, clinical neuromuscular & structural bodywork (certification included in 500-hour program), ethics, hydrotherapy, laws & rules. Advanced program: 100-hour certification in Clinical Neuromuscular and Structural Bodywork by Kyle C. Wright (local instructors vary).

SCHOOL STATEMENT: Specializing in the training of the clinical therapist who typically works for or is referred to by physicians and other health care practitioners.

#200 South Technical Education Center
    Palm Beach County Schools, 1300 SW 30th Ave.
    Boynton Beach, FL 33426
    (561) 369-7000

Contact school for program information.

#201 Space Coast Massage & Allied Health Institute
    1333 Gateway Drive, ste. 1003
    Melbourne, FL 32901
    (407) 722-0061
    www.FLMASSAGE.COM

HOURS OF TRAINING: 500.

COST: $3,600.

YEAR FOUNDED: 1991.

MODALITIES AND SUBJECTS: allied modalities, business & marketing, chair massage, colon therapy, cranio-sacral therapy, ethics, florida law, HIV/AIDS, hydrotherapy, infant massage, myofascial release, neuromuscular therapy, nutrition, positional release, pregnancy massage, reflexology, shiatsu, sports massage.

SCHOOL STATEMENT: SCM&AHI also offers an Emergency Medical Technician (E.M.T.) and Paramedic Training Program. Call for a complimentary catalog.

#202 Suncoast School
4910 Cypress St.
Tampa, FL 33607
(813) 287-1099 or (813) 287-1050

HOURS OF TRAINING: 500 or 600.

DURATION OF COURSE: 6 months.

COST: 500 hours $4,275; 600 hours $5,275.

FINANCIAL AID: Pell grants, Stafford Loans, SLS/Plus loans.

YEAR FOUNDED: 1982.

ACCREDITATIONS/APPROVALS: COMTA/approved, ACCSCT, approved for full veterans' benefits, vocational rehabilitation.

PREPARATION FOR OUT-OF-STATE LICENSING EXAM: New York (by arrangement).

GRADUATES PER YEAR (APPROX.): 160.

MODALITIES AND SUBJECTS: acupressure, aromatherapy, bindegewebsmassage, body-mind, chair massage, community service (including student clinic, cancer clinic & special populations), CPR, creative and intuitive massage, Esalen, exercise physiology, Florida massage law, healing touch, health care practice building, helping relationship, history and theory of massage, HIV/AIDS, hydrotherapy, hygiene, introduction to instrumentation, musculoskeletal pathology, myofascial release, myotherapy, oriental modalities, pregnancy massage, sports massage, yoga therapy.

#203 Venice School of Massage Therapy, Inc.
10915 Bonita Beach Rd., #2121
Bonita Springs, FL 33923
(941) 495-0714

HOURS OF TRAINING: 500.

DURATION OF COURSE: 24 weeks full time, 36 weeks reduced load, 48 weeks half-time.

COST: $2,850. Payment plan without interest is available.

FINANCIAL AID: loans and grants, workforce council.

YEAR FOUNDED: 1988.

PREPARATION FOR OUT-OF-STATE LICENSING EXAM: New York.

MODALITIES AND SUBJECTS: acupressure, AMMA, applied kinesiology, aromatherapy, chair massage, equine sports massage, home birthing, infant massage, lymphatic drainage, medical massage, myofascial release, myotherapy, myotonology for fascial toning (face-lift massage), naturopathy seminar, neuromuscular therapy, oriental herbology, pregnancy massage, reflexology, shiatsu, sports massage, structural integration, trigger point therapy. Additional programs offered: Mini-massage program (40 hours), colon hydrotherapy (100 hours), exercise for rehabilitation (51 hours), advanced neuromuscular therapy (51 hours), understanding nutrition (100 hours), spa therapy (80 hours), management for establishments (80 hours), oriental medical shiatsu massage (105 hours).

SCHOOL STATEMENT: We work to give you a quality education, and good job placement, so you develop a higher level of income and a more enjoyable living.

#204 Wood Hygienic Inst., Inc.
P.O. Box 420580
Kissimmee, FL 34742
(407) 933-0009 or 839-3890

HOURS OF TRAINING: 500.

DURATION OF COURSE: 5 to 6 months days, 9 months evenings.

COST: $3,000.

FINANCIAL AID: veterans' benefits, payment plan.

YEAR FOUNDED: 1989.

GRADUATES PER YEAR (APPROX): 40.

MODALITIES AND SUBJECTS: aromatherapy, bronchial drainage, business marketing and management, chair massage, clinical terms and pathology, CPR/first aid, field trips, HIV/AIDS, hydrotherapy, infant massage, joint injury and mobilization, massage theory & practice, medical massage, myofascial release, neuromuscular therapy, palpation, positional release, postural integration, pregnancy massage, reflexology, sports massage, statutes and rules, structural integration, treatments for TMJ.

ADVANCED PROGRAMS: colonic irrigation course.

SCHOOL STATEMENT: Our orientation focuses on the importance of massage being taught on and in Orlando Regional Trauma Hospital premises. We are a medically oriented massage school.

GEORGIA

No State licensing.

SCHOOLS:

#205 Academy of Healing Arts
486 New Street
Macon, GA 31201
(912) 746-0025

Contact school for program information.

#206 Academy of Somatic Healing Arts
1924 Cliff Valley Way
Atlanta, GA 30329
(404) 315-0394

HOURS OF TRAINING: 700.

DURATION OF COURSE: 9 months full time, 13 months part time, courses offered days, evening and weekends.

COST: $7,075 includes application fee, class manuals and clinic shirt. Approximate additional expenses are texts $300, uniforms $125, linens $50, massage table $400 to $600 and CPR training $49 or free from Red Cross. Payment plan without interest is available.

FINANCIAL AID: 5% cash discount, approved by GA Dept. of Human Resources Division of Rehabilitative Services, GA Dept. of Labor, Veteran's Administration.

YEAR FOUNDED: 1991.

PREPARATION FOR OUT-OF-STATE LICENSING EXAM: Florida, Ohio.

GRADUATES PER YEAR (APPROX.): 90.

MODALITIES AND SUBJECTS: adjunctive modalities including hydrotherapy, heliotherapy, contrast therapy & natural healing techniques, body-mind, chi gong, clinical assessment & documentation, clinical practicum, clinical sports performance massage, community outreach, cranio-sacral therapy, hygiene & AIDS awareness, kinesiology, lymphatic drainage, medical terminology, myofascial release, neuromuscular therapy, practice building, pregnancy massage, rebirthing, reflexology, somatic nutrition, somatic therapy, trigger point therapy, visceral massage, zero-balancing.

SCHOOL STATEMENT: Emphasizing clinical/rehabilitation massage, we prepare Massage Therapists for participation in the field of wellness; dealing with the modern health challenges now facing humankind.

#207 Atlanta School of Massage
      2300 Peachford Rd., suite 3200
      Atlanta, GA 30338
      (770) 454-7167

HOURS OF TRAINING: 620 (in-class hours not specified).

DURATION OF COURSE: days 6 months or evenings for one year.

COST: $7,275.

FINANCIAL AID: Pell Grants, Stafford Loans, JPTA, Veteran's Administration.

YEAR FOUNDED: 1980.

ACCREDITATIONS/APPROVALS: COMTA/Accredited, ACCSCT.

PREPARATION FOR OUT-OF-STATE LICENSING EXAM: Florida.

GRADUATES PER YEAR (APPROX.): 225.

Certifications are offered in Integrated Massage & Deep Tissue Therapy or Clinical Massage or Wellness Massage & Spa Therapies (620 hours each).

MODALITIES AND SUBJECTS: acupressure, applied kinesiology, aromatherapy, body-mind, chair massage, exercise physiology, HIV/AIDS education, hygiene, myofascial release, neuromuscular therapy, pfrimmer deep muscle, polarity, postural integration, practice building skills, pregnancy massage, reflexology, shiatsu, spa therapies, sports massage, trigger point therapy.

SCHOOL STATEMENT: The Atlanta School of Massage programs emphasize integrating a variety of techniques with a refined ability to interact meaningfully with each client.

#208 Capelli Learning Center
      2581 Piedmont Road NE, suite C-1000
      Atlanta, GA 30324
      (404) 261-5271

HOURS OF TRAINING: 608.5.

COST: $4,850 plus $100 registration fee.

GRADUATES PER YEAR (APPROX.): 35.

MODALITIES AND SUBJECTS: acu-point theory, business, clinic, deep tissue massage techniques, ethics, florida law, HIV/AIDS education, hydrotherapy, metaphysics, nuat thai massage, oriental anatomy & physiology, oriental theory, reflexology.

SCHOOL STATEMENT: East meets west in a unique blend of oriental and western massage disciplines. 620-hour certification program in Swedish, Deep Tissue and Nuat Thai Massage.

#209 Georgia Institute of Therapeutic Massage, LLC
      2160 Central Ave.
      Augusta, GA 30904
      (706) 737-9291

HOURS OF TRAINING: 530.

DURATION OF COURSE: 10 months, day and evening programs available.

COST: $5,100 plus approx.$300 books and $500 to $600 table. Payment plan without interest is available.

FINANCIAL AID: Veteran's Administration.

YEAR FOUNDED: 1995.

PREPARATION FOR OUT-OF-STATE LICENSING EXAM: South Carolina, Florida.

GRADUATES PER YEAR (APPROX.): 25.

MODALITIES AND SUBJECTS: acupressure, business & law, chair massage, clinical practice, cranio-sacral therapy, deep tissue, healing touch, hydrotherapy, hygiene, integration of technique, neuromuscular therapy, pathology, polarity, reflexology, russian

massage, shiatsu.

SCHOOL STATEMENT: Swedish/Russian foundation is laid. Neuromuscular therapy treats pain. Acupressure/polarity add an energetic dimension. All are integrated. A&P, clinic and business complete the program.

#210 Lake Lanier School of Massage
      400 Brenau Ave.
      Gainesville, GA 30501
      (770) 287-0377

HOURS OF TRAINING: 550.

DURATION OF COURSE: 6 months, day & evening & occasional weekend programs available.

COST: $5,800 including application fee and books.

YEAR FOUNDED: 1993.

ACCREDITATIONS/APPROVALS: IMSTAC.

PREPARATION FOR OUT-OF-STATE LICENSING EXAM: Florida.

GRADUATES PER YEAR (APPROX.): 25.

MODALITIES AND SUBJECTS: AIDS awareness, applied kinesiology, aromatherapy, assault prevention, business & marketing, chair massage, cranio-sacral (intro), hydrotherapy, infant massage, massage law, massage theory, medical massage, myofascial release, neuromuscular therapy, nutrition & prevention, pathology, reflexology, russian massage, shiatsu, sports massage, stress management, student clinic - community events, therapeutic touch, touch for health, trigger point therapy.

SCHOOL STATEMENT: Our emphasis on sound physiological principles prepares graduates to work within the medical community. Small class size allows individual attention in a relaxed, fun setting!

#211 New Life Institute, Inc. School of
      Massage Excellence
      4330 Georgetown Square II, suite 500
      Atlanta, GA 30338
      (770) 457-2021

HOURS OF TRAINING: 630.

DURATION OF COURSE: 6 months days, 9 months evenings.

COST: $5,900 plus approx. $1,100 for fees, books and table.

FINANCIAL AID: loans from private lending institutions.

YEAR FOUNDED: 1994.

GRADUATES PER YEAR (APPROX.): 100.

MODALITIES AND SUBJECTS: anatomy drawing, aromatherapy, assessment, body-mind, business mastery, chair massage, chi gong, clinical pathology, clinical practicum, CPR & first aid, cranio-sacral therapy, deep tissue, documentation, energy healing, hydrotherapy, kinesiology, lymphatic drainage, mattes stretching, medical terminology, myofascial release, neuromuscular therapy, oriental medicine, polarity, reflexology, rehabilitation protocols, rolfing, shiatsu, stress management, tai chi, thai massage, touch for health, trager, yoga therapy.

SCHOOL STATEMENT: We train the therapist to be a health care professional. The core curriculum emphasizes anatomy, business, swedish, neuromuscular and chair massage.

HAWAII

State licensing: 570 hours

National Certification Exam not accepted.

Training at out-of-state schools may be accepted by Hawaii if the school is certified by AMTA or Rolf Institute.

Board: (808) 586-3000

SCHOOLS:

#212 Aisen Shiatsu School
1314 South King St., suite 601
Honolulu, HI 96814
(808) 596-7354

The school trains students in Shiatsu as preparation for licensure as Massage Therapists by the Hawaii Board of Massage. For program information, contact the school.

#213 All Hawaiian School of Massage
1750 Kalakaua Ave., suite 512
Honolulu, HI 96826
(808) 941-8101

Contact the school for program information.

#214 Aloha Kauai Massage Workshop
Box 622, Hanalei
Kauai, HI 96714
(808) 826-9990

HOURS OF TRAINING: 570 (150 basic, 420 apprenticeship).

GRADUATES PER YEAR (APPROX.): 10 to 16.

MODALITIES AND SUBJECTS: business practices, centering, deep tissue, esalen, hawaiian lomi lomi, PNF stretches, shiatsu, sports massage, yoga & corrective exercise therapy.

SCHOOL STATEMENT: Class size is kept small (10 to 16) with much individualized attention from the owners and teachers, Devaki and Kevin Holman.

#215 American Institute of Massage Therapy
407 Uluniu St. #204
Kailua, HI 96734
(808) 266-2468 (AIMT)

HOURS OF TRAINING: 570 hours (Level I – 150 hours, Level II – 110 hours, apprenticeship 310 hours).

COST: Level I – $1,750, Level II – $800 (books are included)

YEAR FOUNDED: 1984.

GRADUATES PER YEAR (APPROX.): 30.

MODALITIES AND SUBJECTS: acupressure, aromatherapy, craniosacral therapy, geriatric massage, healing touch, high touch, huna kane, integrative massage, lomi iwi, lomi lomi, meridian shiatsu, myofascial release, polarity, pregnancy massage, refelxology, sports massage, strain-counterstrain, touch for health.

SCHOOL STATEMENT: Hawaii's most holistic program - nurturing teaching environment, providing the vital steps to a successful massage therapy career and a balance between body, mind and soul.

#216 Big Island Academy of Massage
P.O. Box 691, Mountain View, HI 96771
Classroom: 211 Kinoole St, Hilo, HI 96720
(808) 935-1405 or 935-2596 (clinic)

HOURS OF TRAINING: 150 or 600 (150 or 420 in-class hours).

DURATION OF COURSE: 150 hours 3 months, 600 hours 12 to 18 months, day & evening & weekend programs available.

COST: 150 hours $1,500; 600 hours $3,500. Both include textbooks, handouts, oils, school shirts.

FINANCIAL AID: Discounts to Native Americans and Hawaiians, discounts for payment in full.

YEAR FOUNDED: 1992.

GRADUATES PER YEAR (APPROX.): 30.

MODALITIES AND SUBJECTS: acupressure, aromatherapy, applied kinesiology, body-mind, chair massage, clinical operations, cranio-sacral therapy, european massage, hawaiian huna, infant massage, kinesiology & pathology, lomilomi, lymphatic drainage, myofascial release, pregnancy massage, reflexology, reiki, masunaga shiatsu, sports massage & injury care, thai massage, touch for health, trigger point therapy.

SCHOOL STATEMENT: A quality and affordable pre-licensing program of eclectic techniques and routines to empower and prepare students for resort and clinical settings around the world.

#217 Hawaiian Islands School of Body Therapies
P.O. Box 390188
(Classroom: 78-6739 Alii Dr.)
Kailua-Kona, HI 96739
(808) 322-0048

HOURS OF TRAINING: 165, 645, 1,000.

DURATION OF COURSE: 165 hours 3 months, 645 hours one year, 1,000 hours 15 months.

COST: 165 hours $1,650; 645 hours $5,676; 1,000 hours $7,800 (all plus tax, books included).

YEAR FOUNDED: 1984.

ACCREDITATIONS/APPROVALS: State of Florida continuing education provider.

GRADUATES PER YEAR (APPROX.): 25.

MODALITIES AND SUBJECTS: aromatherapy, brain gym, business, clinical practicum, cranial-sacral therapy, exercise therapy, lomi lomi, geriatric massage, joint play, kinesiology and clinical anatomy, lymphatic drainage, neuromuscular therapy, pathology, polarity, principles of assessment and treatment, reflexology, reiki, shiatsu, sports massage, t'ai chi, thai massage, touch for health, yoga, zero balancing.

SCHOOL STATEMENT: The school teaches the Knight-Wind Method of restorative treatment therapies.

#218 Hawaii College of Health Science, Inc.
1750 Kalakaua Ave., suite 2404
Honolulu, HI 96826
(808) 941-8223

HOURS OF TRAINING: Phase I 150 or 180 hours, Phase II 200 and 420 hour programs.

DURATION OF COURSE: Phase I: 6 months evenings & weekends, Phase II self-paced.

COST: Phase I $1,750 (150 hours); Phase II $1,400 for 250 to 420 hours.

FINANCIAL AID: contact school.

YEAR FOUNDED: 1988.

GRADUATES PER YEAR (APPROX.): 80.

MODALITIES AND SUBJECTS: acupressure, clinical massage, counter strain, CPR, cranio-sacral therapy, deep tissue, foot reflexology, insurance billing, kinesiology, lomi lomi, lymphatic drainage, muscle energy (PNF), myofascial release, neurolinguistic programming, polarity, pregnancy massage, range of motion therapy, regional injury massage, reiki, shiatsu, sports massage, student clinic, thai massage, traditional chinese medicine with meridian theory, trigger point therapy. Specialization certifications are offered in oriental massage, myofascial release, medical massage, and a Physician's Assistant program.

SCHOOL STATEMENT: Physician directed. Licensing in massage

and acupuncture. Nineteen faculty include physicians, chiropractors, acupuncturists and Ph.D.s in addition to LMTs.

#219 Honolulu School of Massage, Inc.
1136 12th Ave., 2nd floor
Honolulu, HI 96816
(808) 733-0000

HOURS OF TRAINING: basic 180; professional 450 (total 630).

DURATION OF COURSE: basic 16 weeks; professional 8 months (combined program one year); day and evening/weekend programs available.

COST: basic $1,950; professional $4,600, includes books and handouts.

FINANCIAL AID: Veteran's Administration.

YEAR FOUNDED: 1981.

ACCREDITATIONS/APPROVALS: COMTA/approved.

GRADUATES PER YEAR (APPROX.): 100.

MODALITIES AND SUBJECTS: applied kinesiology, aromatherapy, body-mind, chair massage, CPR, cranio-sacral therapy, deep tissue, esalen, feldenkrais, first aid, hydrotherapy, lomilomi, lymphatic drainage, medical massage, neuroanatomy, pathology, polarity, practical myology, pregnancy massage, professionalism, reflexology, reiki, senior citizen massage, shiatsu, sports massage, student clinic, touch for health, trigger point therapy.

SCHOOL STATEMENT: The purpose of the Honolulu School of Massage is to provide the highest quality holistic education in the healing art and science of massage therapy.

#220 Institute of Body Therapeutics
P.O. Box 11634
Lahaina, HI 96761
(808) 667-5058

HOURS OF TRAINING: 600.

DURATION OF COURSE: 6–8 months, day & evening & weekend classes available.

COST: $3,000. Payment plan without interest is available.

YEAR FOUNDED: 1978.

GRADUATES PER YEAR (APPROX.): 20.

MODALITIES AND SUBJECTS: acupressure, body-mind, energy balancing, esalen, integrated body therapies, lomilomi, medical massage, myofascial release, myotherapy, neuromuscular therapy, reflexology, shiatsu, sports massage, structural kinesiology.

SCHOOL STATEMENT: The school can assist out-of-state trained therapists toward Hawaii licensure, and can tailor its program to the needs of individuals or small groups.

#221 Kalani Oceanside Retreat
RR2 Box 4500
Pahoa – Beach Road, HI 96778
(808) 965-7828 or 1-800-800-6886
www.kalani.com

HOURS OF TRAINING: 30 hours per week.

DURATION OF COURSE: 1 to 3 weeks.

COST: $600 to $1,140 per week, including study materials.

YEAR FOUNDED: 1980.

GRADUATES PER YEAR (APPROX.): 80.

MODALITIES AND SUBJECTS: acupressure, applied kinesiology, biokinetics, body awareness, body-mind, chi gong, esalen, feldenkrais, hakomi, Hawaiian spirituality, healing practices & hula, healing touch, injury care and prevention, kinesiology, lomilomi,

muscle sculpting, mythology, neuromuscular therapy, postural integration, rebirthing, reflexology, shiatsu, somatic therapy, spa technique, sports massage, structural integration, therapeutic touch, touch for health, wasser tanz, watsu, yoga therapy.

SCHOOL STATEMENT: Kalani's aloha spirit, pool/spa, thermal springs, delicious cuisine and comfortable environment are ideal for advancing and emerging natural health professionals and personal wellness vacations.

#222 Maui Academy of the Healing Arts
1993 South Kihei Rd., suite 210
Kihei, HI 96753
(808) 879-4266

HOURS OF TRAINING: 600 (450 in-class hours).

DURATION OF COURSE: 11 to 13 months, evenings and weekends.

COST: $3,864 plus $50 application fee and cost of books.

YEAR FOUNDED: 1988.

GRADUATES PER YEAR (APPROX.): 25–30.

MODALITIES AND SUBJECTS: body mechanics, business practices, communication skills, integrative mind/body techniques, jin shin do acupressure, laws & ethics, lomi lomi, lymphatic drainage, myofascial massage, pathology & treatment of injuries, polarity, reflexology, somatic exercise, sports massage, structural kinesiology, thai massage, thermal & hydrotherapy, trigger point therapy, zen shiatsu. Also offered: transformation lessons, psycho-energetics, AMNA, individualized studies and tailored instruction.

SCHOOL STATEMENT: This school offers a balanced blend of Eastern and Western modalities. Integrating this "cross training" philosophy is a keynote to training competent, compassionate massage therapists.

#223 Maui School of Therapeutic Massage
P.O. Box 1891
Makawao, HI 96768
(Classroom: 1043 Makawao Ave.)
(808) 572-2277 or 572-6996
www.maui.net/~massage

HOURS OF TRAINING: 600.

DURATION OF COURSE: 6 month to one year, day & evening & weekend programs available.

COST: $2,800.

FINANCIAL AID: Veteran's Administration, Department of Vocational Rehabilitation.

YEAR FOUNDED: 1995.

GRADUATES PER YEAR (APPROX.): 50.

MODALITIES AND SUBJECTS: acupressure, applied anatomy & assessment, aromatherapy, body-mind, chair massage, chi gong, clinical practice, cranio-sacral therapy, lomilomi, medical massage, myofascial release, myotherapy, neuromuscular therapy, polarity, pregnancy massage, reflexology, reiki, shiatsu, sports massage, treatment of common conditions, trigger point therapy.

SCHOOL STATEMENT: Our small, beautifully located school provides an excellent medical, therapeutic education with a holistic approach that fosters sensitivity and respect for the healing process.

#224 The Pacific Center for Bodywork and Awareness
P.O. Box 672
Kilauea, Kauai, HI 96754
(808) 828-6797
www.hawaiian.net/~gold/Presenc/

HOURS OF TRAINING: 50 to 600 (in-class hours not specified).

DURATION OF COURSE: 1 week to 5 months, day and weekend programs available.

COST: $675 to $3,800. Payment plan without interest is available.

FINANCIAL AID: scholarships, Vocational Rehabilitation – State of HI.

ACCREDITATIONS/APPROVALS: American Council of Hypnotist Examiners.

YEAR FOUNDED: 1991.

MODALITIES AND SUBJECTS: awareness oriented massage therapy, body-mind, communication skills for bodyworkers, hakomi bodywork, hypnotherapy counselor training, neuromuscular therapy, polarity, pregnancy massage, present centered awareness therapy, rebirthing, reflexology, somatic therapy, structural bodywork & awareness (structural integration), trigger point therapy, yoga therapy.

SCHOOL STATEMENT: We are dedicated to supporting students to become more present in their lives and with clients, in order to achieve greater health, happiness and freedom.

#225 Tao Massage School
P.O. Box 11130
Honolulu, HI 96828
(808) 947-4788 or 1-800-942-4788

Contact school for program information.

IDAHO

No State licensing.

SCHOOLS:

#226 The American Institute of Clinical Massage
W. 296 Sunset Ave. #10
Coeur d'Alene, ID 83815
(208) 765-9165

HOURS OF TRAINING: 600 (575 in-class hours).

DURATION OF COURSE: 12 months; day, evening and weekend programs available.

COST: $4,100 including books and materials. Payment plan without interest is available.

FINANCIAL AID: Local State Job Service Programs.

YEAR FOUNDED: 1996.

GRADUATES PER YEAR (APPROX.): 30.

MODALITIES AND SUBJECTS: acupressure, bodywork theory & practice, business, chair massage, chi gong, cranio-sacral therapy, equine sports massage, healing touch, kinesiology, myofascial release, pathology, oriental medicine, reiki, shiatsu, sports massage, student clinical practice, therapeutic touch, trager, trigger point therapy, watsu, yoga therapy.

SCHOOL STATEMENT: If a student has a strong desire to do bodywork, then someone is waiting for that student to learn the specific technique that will help.

#227 The Idaho Institute for Wholistic Studies
1412 W. Washington St.
Boise, ID 83702-5043
(208) 345-2704

ACCREDITATIONS/APPROVALS: IMSTAC.

#228 The Idaho School of Massage Therapy
5353 Franklin Rd.
Boise, ID 83705
(208) 343-1847

HOURS OF TRAINING: 155 to 500 (evenings and weekends).

YEAR FOUNDED: 1983.

MODALITIES AND SUBJECTS: Areas of specialization are Stress Management, Trigger point & Connective Tissue Therapy, Myofascial Release, Shiatsu, Tui Na, Reflexology, Sports Massage.

SCHOOL STATEMENT: ISMT's program allows students to emphasize Western or Eastern modalities while learning several styles of bodywork. This provides the community with versatile, caring practitioners.

#229 Moscow School of Massage
S. 600 Main
Moscow, ID 83843
(208) 882-7867

HOURS OF TRAINING: 536.

DURATION OF COURSE: 9 months (2 days per week and 2 Sat. per month).

COST: $4,500 plus $370 for texts, fees and educational skeleton. Payment plan without interest is available.

YEAR FOUNDED: 1994.

PREPARATION FOR OUT-OF-STATE LICENSING EXAM: Washington State.

GRADUATES PER YEAR (APPROX.): 24.

MODALITIES AND SUBJECTS: chair massage (intro), chi gong (qi gong self-massage), clinical & business management practices, clinical techniques, deep tissue, ethics, fundamentals of chinese medicine, geriatric massage (intro), hydrotherapy, infant massage (intro), kinesiology, law, lymphatic drainage (intro), medical terminology, myofascial release, pathology, polarity, pregnancy massage (intro), record-keeping, reflexology (intro), reiki, russian massage (intro), sports massage, trigger point therapy.

SCHOOL STATEMENT: MSM is dedicated to exceeding existing educational standards for massage therapists. The anatomical and clinical emphasis of our curriculum prepares students for successful massage careers.

#230 Twin Falls Institute of Holistic Studies
431 Blue Lakes Boulevard North
Twin Falls, ID 83301
(208) 733-9110

HOURS OF TRAINING: 108 basic, 500 total (ongoing advanced trainings of 32–48 hours each).

DURATION OF COURSE: Basic, 12 weekends; advanced classes mostly in the evenings.

COST: Basic $1,000, advanced classes $320 to $500 each.

YEAR FOUNDED: 1995.

GRADUATES PER YEAR (APPROX.): 12.

MODALITIES AND SUBJECTS: applied kinesiology, aromatherapy, hands-on training, history & theory of massage, introduction to body systems & terminology, myology, nutrition, pathology, professionalism & marketing & ethics, somatic therapy, watsu.

SCHOOL STATEMENT: Our purpose in providing education regarding holistic health is to bring awareness of old, new, and advanced concepts to enhance a healthier and happier lifestyle.

ILLINOIS

No State licensing.

SCHOOLS:

#231 Academy Massage Therapy
        425 – 17th St.
        Moline, IL 61265
        (309) 762-8231

HOURS OF TRAINING: 500 or 746 or 1107 (500 plus optional seminars).

DURATION OF COURSE: 500 hours 6 months, evenings.

COST: $7,399 includes application fee, tuition, books, table, lab fee, insurance. Payment plan without interest is available.

PREPARATION FOR OUT-OF-STATE LICENSING EXAM: Iowa.

MODALITIES AND SUBJECTS: acupressure, business practice, chair massage, chi gong, geriatric massage, healing touch, holistic health (chemistry, nutrition, herbology, homeopathy, aromatherapy), infant massage, massage for victims of abuse, pathology, pregnancy massage, psychology-sociology-sexuality-spirituality, reflexology, reiki, shiatsu, sports massage, theory & practice of massage, therapeutic touch, tai chi, theory of acupuncture & acupressure, touch for health, tui na, whole body massage, yoga therapy.

#232 Ancient Arts Training Center
        RR 1, Box 27-B
        Mt. Olive, IL 62069
        (217) 999-3607
        www.successmarketplace.com

HOURS OF TRAINING: 20 to 500, programs offered days or evenings & weekends.

COST: $300 to $3,000 including books and workbook.

FINANCIAL AID: discounts for couples or same family—health givers.

YEAR FOUNDED: 1995.

GRADUATES PER YEAR (APPROX.): 20.

MODALITIES AND SUBJECTS: acupressure, applied kinesiology, aromatherapy, body-mind, business management, canadian deep tissue massage, chair massage, deep tissue, ethics, feldenkrais, healing touch, pfrimmer deep muscle, reflexology, rolfing, shiatsu, therapeutic touch, trigger point therapy. Programs of 20 hours, 100 hours, 300 hours and 500 hours are offered.

SCHOOL STATEMENT: We believe you should study different forms and apply them into one full-body massage and learn to use your body and mind as a tool.

#233 Center for Therapeutic Massage & Wellness
        2704 Woodridge Dr.
        Woodridge, IL 60517
        (630) 960-9053

Contact school for program information.

#234 Chicago School of Massage Therapy
        2918 North Lincoln Ave.
        Chicago, IL 60657
        (773) 477-9444

HOURS OF TRAINING: 650 (515 in-class hours).

DURATION OF COURSE: 14 months, day and evening/weekend programs available.

COST: $7,000 includes books and other supplies. Payment plan without interest is available.

FINANCIAL AID: discounts are available.

YEAR FOUNDED: 1981.

ACCREDITATIONS/APPROVALS: COMTA/Accredited.

GRADUATES PER YEAR (APPROX.): 350.

MODALITIES AND SUBJECTS: acupressure/shiatsu, body mechanics and self-care, body mobilization techniques, chair massage, client management, clinical and community internship, communication skills, cryo—therapy, current trends and issues, directed independent study, energy approaches, first aid, history of massage, hospice work, hydrotherapy, hygiene, kinesiology, maniken or cadaver intensive, myofascial therapy, neuromuscular therapy certification, oriental medicine, palpation, pathology, pregnancy massage, professional ethics and credentialing, reflexology, sports injuries, sports massage, starting a practice, stress management, stretching, trigger point, zen shiatsu stretches.

SCHOOL STATEMENT: CSMT is dedicated to advancing the art and science of massage therapy through excellence in education, personal and professional development, and community service.

#235 The Clinic Massage Institute
        Hillcrest Shopping Center, 1041 S. Oakwood Ave.
        Geneseo, IL 61254
        (309) 944-5370

Contact school for program information.

#236 Edens Institute of Alternative Therapy
        114 E. DeYoung
        Marion, IL 62959
        (618) 993-2800 or 777-0116

HOURS OF TRAINING: 100 to 500 (in-class hours not specified).

COST: $8.00 per hour plus $150 for books and supplies. Payment plan without interest is available.

FINANCIAL AID: Scholarships or discounts, Illinois Disability, JTPA.

YEAR FOUNDED: 1993.

MODALITIES AND SUBJECTS: colon therapy, ear candling, herbology & wild edible plants, iridology, nutrition, reflexology.

#237 European Healing and Massage Therapy
        8707 Skokie Blvd #112
        Skokie, IL 60077
        (847) 673-7400

Contact school for program information.

#238 LifePath School of Massage Therapy
        7820 N. University, suite 110
        Peoria, IL 61614
        (309) 693-7284 or 1-888-2-LifePath

HOURS OF TRAINING: 700.

DURATION OF COURSE: 10 months, evenings and weekends.

COST: $7,000 ($200 discount for payment in full).

YEAR FOUNDED: 1992.

ACCREDITATIONS/APPROVALS: IMSTAC.

GRADUATES PER YEAR (APPROX.): 16 to 24.

MODALITIES AND SUBJECTS: aromatherapy, business ethics and professional practice, clinical experience, connective tissue massage, cross-fiber, deep tissue, hydrotherapy, joint mobilization and stretching, kinesiology, lymphatic drainage, nutrition, polarity, psychology for the bodyworker, reflexology, reiki, sports massage, St. John method neuromuscular therapy, trigger point, wellness concepts.

SCHOOL STATEMENT: We emphasize an integration of different modalities according to the client's needs, so that the whole person—body, mind and spirit can be therapeutically affected.

#239 Northern Prairie School of Therapeutic
Massage & Bodywork, Inc.
138 N. Fair St.
Sycamore, IL 60187
(815) 899-3382

HOURS OF TRAINING: 600 (475 in-class hours).

COST: $8,100 plus approximately $1,500 books and supplies.

YEAR FOUNDED: 1993.

ACCREDITATIONS/APPROVALS: IMSTAC.

GRADUATES PER YEAR (APPROX.): 50.

MODALITIES AND SUBJECTS: aromatherapy, assessment of problems & pathology, body mechanics I & II, business practices, complementary therapies, cranio-sacral therapy, fundamental bodywork techniques, guided imagery, herbal remedies, lymphatic massage, myofascial release, nutrition, optimal health practices, physical therapy modalities, psychology for bodyworkers, reflexology, shiatsu, special considerations, stretching, therapeutic touch.

#240 Redfern Training Systems School
of Massage Therapy
9 S. 531 Wilmette Ave.,
Darien, IL 60561
(630) 960-0844

Contact school for program information.

#241 Wellness & Massage Training Institute
618 Executive Dr.
Willowbrook, IL 60521
(630) 325-3773
www.wmti.com

HOURS OF TRAINING: 770 or 750.

DURATION OF COURSE: approximately three years, classes offered days, evenings or weekends.

COST: approximately $7,000 (varies with electives chosen). Payment plan without interest is available.

YEAR FOUNDED: 1989.

ACCREDITATIONS/APPROVALS: COMTA/Accredited.

GRADUATES PER YEAR (APPROX.): 75.

MODALITIES AND SUBJECTS: active assisted stretching, acupressure, kinesiology, aromatherapy, body/mind in perspective, bodywork and the adult child, bodywork and survivors of sex abuse, bodywork practitioner series, boundary issues for massage therapists, chair massage, clinical experience in oriental bodywork, CPR/first aid, cranio-sacral I, II and III, creating success through productive thinking, esalen massage techniques, ethical considerations in massage therapy, full circle, geriatric massage techniques, how to study effectively, infant massage, integrative studies in oriental bodywork, introduction to communication skills, introduction to chinese herbology, introduction to eastern philosophy, introduction to feng shui, introduction to nutrition or eastern nutrition, introduction to prescription medications, introduction to skin disease, introduction to stress management, introduction to wellness concepts, jin shin do (part I, part 2, intermediate and advanced), jin shin do acupressure facial, kinesiology, lymphatic drainage, massage practitioner series, movement and energy in massage, oriental medical theory I and II, ortho-bionomy (26 separate courses offered), positional release and massage, points and channels I and II, practicum in oriental studies, pregnancy massage, pressure sensitivity techniques, principles of structural massage, professional practice, readings in bodywork theory, re-

flexology I and II, self massage, shiatsu (basic, practicum, intermediate, advanced), special topics in oriental studies, special topics in wellness, sports massage (introductory and advanced), tai chi I, II, III & IV, the tao of touch, touch for health I and II, trigger point techniques, tui na (basic, practicum, intermediate, advanced, sports tui na, pediatric tui na).

SCHOOL STATEMENT: We are dedicated to providing the highest quality education in bodywork offering a well rounded course of study and employing experienced and dedicated faculty.

INDIANA

No State licensing.

SCHOOLS:

#242 Alexandria School of Scientific Therapeutics
P.O. Box 287, 809 S. Harrison St.
Alexandria, IN 46001
(756) 724-9152

HOURS OF TRAINING: 656.

DURATION OF COURSE: 41 weeks, days.

COST: $5,475.00 includes books, stationary items, lotions, sheets and towels. Payment plan without interest is available.

FINANCIAL AID: State.

ACCREDITATIONS/APPROVALS: COMTA/approved.

PREPARATION FOR OUT-OF-STATE LICENSING: most states.

YEAR FOUNDED: 1982.

GRADUATES PER YEAR (APPROX): 74.

MODALITIES AND SUBJECTS: chair massage, equine sports massage, infant massage, myofascial release, pfrimmer deep muscle therapy, reflexology, sports massage, yoga therapy, zero-balancing.

SCHOOL STATEMENT: We put the student first, to train good reputable people who have the knowledge to be the best they can be in the field.

#243 American Certified Massage School
1419 Tyler Ct.
Crown Point, IN 46307
1-888-662-2585 or (219) 662-8393

HOURS OF TRAINING: 662 (182 in-class hours).

DURATION OF COURSE: 30 weeks, day & evening programs available.

COST: $3,900 including books and insurance. Payment plan without interest is available.

FINANCIAL AID: Discount for prepayment.

YEAR FOUNDED: 1997.

GRADUATES PER YEAR (APPROX.): 24.

MODALITIES AND SUBJECTS: aromatherapy, infant massage, pregnancy massage, reflexology, sports massage, trigger point therapy.

SCHOOL STATEMENT: A.C.M.S. was created to provide massage education in a small class room environment, for people with a busy lifestyle.

#244 Health Enrichment Center, Inc.
Indiana Branch
6801 Lake Plaza Drive, Suite A102
Indianapolis, IN 46220
(317) 841-1414

See Listing for Health Enrichment Center, Inc. in Michigan.

#245 Healthy Lifestyle School of Massage Therapy
303 N. High St.
Muncie, IN 47305
(765) 281-9019

HOURS OF TRAINING: 1,200 (500 in-class hours).

DURATION OF COURSE: 41 weeks, day & evening/weekend programs available.

COST: $5,500 including four books. Payment plan without interest is available.

YEAR FOUNDED: 1997.

GRADUATES PER YEAR (APPROX.): 20.

MODALITIES AND SUBJECTS: chair massage, chi gong, cranio-sacral therapy, infant massage, medical massage, polarity, pregnancy massage, sports massage, yoga therapy.

SCHOOL STATEMENT: Focus is a healthy lifestyle of work, play, physical and mental exercises, diet and relaxation, while receiving all training necessary to have a massage business.

#246 Indiana College of Bodywork Modalities, Inc.
6990 Hillsdale Ct.
Indianapolis, IN 46250
((317) 841-3840 or 1-888-841-3840

HOURS OF TRAINING: 500 or 33 credits (medical massage), 500 or 33 credits (energy therapies), 750 or 50 credits (650 in-class hours)(therapeutic massage).

DURATION OF COURSE: each 10 months, day & evening & weekend programs available.

COST: 500 hours $3,700 plus $325 books, 750 hours $4,100 plus $400 books. Payment plan without interest is available.

FINANCIAL AID: Scholarships or discounts, Indiana Vocational Rehabilitation.

YEAR FOUNDED: 1997.

MODALITIES AND SUBJECTS: acupressure, applied kinesiology, aromatherapy, body-mind, chair massage, chi gong, cranio-sacral therapy, healing touch, infant massage, lymphatic drainage, medical massage, myofascial release, neuromuscular therapy, postural integration, pregnancy massage, reflexology, reiki, shiatsu, somatic therapy, sports massage, touch for health, trigger point therapy, yoga therapy.

#247 Institute of Mohr Integrated Bodywork
2200 Lake Ave., suite 290
Fort Wayne, IN 46805
(219) 424-4969

Contact school for program information.

#248 Lewis School & Clinic of Massage Therapy
3400 Michigan St.
Hobart, IN 46342
(219) 962-9640

ACCREDITATIONS/APPROVALS: COMTA/approved.

#249 Massage Therapy Clinic
118 E. Sixth St.
Bloomington, IN 47408
(812) 335-8361

HOURS OF TRAINING: 500.

DURATION OF COURSE: 15 weeks, day & evening programs available.

COST: $3,000 plus $75 for two books. Payment plan without interest is available.

FINANCIAL AID: 10% discount for ABMP members, Vocational Rehabilitation, other loans.

YEAR FOUNDED: 1995.

GRADUATES PER YEAR (APPROX.): 12–15.

MODALITIES AND SUBJECTS: applied kinesiology, business (ethics & plan), CPR, deep tissue, esalen, herbal nutrition, hydrotherapy & spa techniques, lymphatic drainage, medical massage, meditation techniques, meridian therapy, myofascial therapy, neuromuscular therapy, polarity, pregnancy massage, psychokinetic integrative technique, research project, science of relaxation, shiatsu, sports massage, tai chi, therapeutic touch, trigger point therapy.

SCHOOL STATEMENT: Teaching people to touch with compassion, skill and knowledge; celebrating self-discovery of healing abilities. Gain mastery of therapeutic knowledge for a successful career.

#250 Regional College of Massage Therapy, Inc.
5826 North Clinton
Fort Wayne, IN 46825
(219) 426-7268

Contact school for program information.

#251 Vibrant Life Resources School of Wholistic Health
6109 West Jefferson Blvd.
Fort Wayne, IN 46804
(219) 436-8807

Contact school for program information.

IOWA

STATE LICENSURE: 500 hours.

National Certification Exam accepted.

Board: (515) 281-6959

APPROVED OUT-OF-STATE SCHOOLS:

Academy of Massage Therapy (IL), Alternative Conjunction, The (PA) Asten Center of Natural Therapeutics (TX), Atlanta School of Massage, Bancroft School of Massage Therapy (MA), Blue Cliff School (LA), Boulder School of Massage Therapy, Cayce/Reilly School (VA), Chicago School of Massage Therapy, Clinic Massage Institute, The (IL) Colorado Institute of Massage Therapy, Deep Muscle Therapy Institute (PA), Desert Institute (AZ), Dr. Welbes' College (NE), Florida School of Massage, Gateway College (NE), Heartwood Institute (CA), Massage Therapy Institute of Colorado, Mueller College (CA), National Holistic Institute (CA), New Mexico School of Natural Therapeutics, North Eastern Institute (NH), Omaha School of Massage, Pennsylvania School of Deep Muscle Therapy, Phoenix Therapeutic Massage College, Sarasota School of Massage Therapy, Seattle Massage School, Sister Rosalind's School (MN), Somerset School (NJ), South Dakota School of Massage, Swedish Institute (NY), Utah College of Massage Therapy, Universal Center (NE).

SCHOOLS:

#252 Bio-Chi Institute
1925 Geneva
Sioux City, IA 51103
(712) 252-1157

Contact school for program information.

#253 Capri College of Massage Therapy
315 2nd Ave. SE
Cedar Rapids, IA 52401
(319) 354-1541 or 1-800-397-0612

425 E. 59th St.
Davenport, IA 52807
(319) 359-1306 or 1-800-728-1336

395 Main St. / P.O. Box 873
Dubuque, IA 52004
(319) 588-2379 or 1-800-728-0712

YEAR FOUNDED: school 1977; massage program 1994.

ACCREDITATIONS/APPROVALS: ACCSCT.

PREPARATION FOR OUT-OF-STATE LICENSING EXAM: may be available; contact school for specifics.

#254 Carlson College of Massage Therapy
11809 County Rd. x-28
Anamosa, IA 52205
(319) 462-3402

HOURS OF TRAINING: 1000 (625 in-class hours).

DURATION OF COURSE: 6 months, days.

COST: $5,000 includes textbooks, liability insurance and 2 clinic t-shirts.

YEAR FOUNDED: 1984.

ACCREDITATIONS/APPROVALS: COMTA/approved.

GRADUATES PER YEAR (APPROX.): 60.

MODALITIES AND SUBJECTS: acupressure, aromatherapy, benefits & contraindications, body movement & body mechanics, business practices, chair massage, clinic & outreach internship, herbology, hydrotherapy, lymphatic drainage, massage theory, techniques & practice, myofascial release, polarity, postural analysis & integration, pregnancy massage, professional ethics/boundaries, reflexology, shiatsu (intro.), specific deep tissue massage, sports massage (intro.), therapeutic touch, trigger point therapy.

SCHOOL STATEMENT: We offer a thorough comprehensive program located in a safe, beautiful country environment with walking trails, basketball and volleyball courts, fruit trees and herb gardens.

#255 College of Massage and the Healing Arts Center
2733 Douglas Ave.
Des Moines, IA 50310
(515) 277-2126

HOURS OF TRAINING: 500.

DURATION OF COURSE: 6 months, evenings & Saturdays.

COST: $5,500 includes portable massage table, accessories, books & clinic shirt.

FINANCIAL AID: Scholarships, some State and corporate funding.

YEAR FOUNDED: 1986.

GRADUATES PER YEAR (APPROX.): 30.

MODALITIES AND SUBJECTS: acupressure, alexander, applied kinesiology, aromatherapy, business practices & ethics, chair massage, chi gong, CPR & first aid, cranio-sacral therapy, healing touch, holistic massage introduction, infant massage, jin shin do, lymphatic drainage, myofascial release, newborn massage, oriental massage techniques intro., pregnancy massage, rebirthing, reflexology, reiki, russian massage, shiatsu, sports massage, student massage therapy clinic, thai massage, therapeutic touch, touch for health, western contemporary massage techniques, yoga therapy, zero-balancing.

SCHOOL STATEMENT: Positive learning environment, individual support and mentoring, creating exceptional holistic healers, strive to be living examples of what can happen with the benefits of massage.

#256 Dr. Welbes' College of Massage Therapy
P.O. Box 265
Hampton, IA 50441
(Classroom: 17 N. Federal)
(515) 456-2901

HOURS OF TRAINING: 600 (500 in-class hours).

DURATION OF COURSE: 63 days, taken weekends or two days per week.

COST: $$4,850 includes application fee, school shirt, laundry fee, insurance, texts, handouts. Payment plan without interest is available.

FINANCIAL AID: IA vocational rehabilitation, Job Training Program.

YEAR FOUNDED: 1993.

GRADUATES PER YEAR (APPROX): 8–10.

MODALITIES AND SUBJECTS: active isolated stretching, adjunct modalities, chair massage, clinical externship, CPR/first aid, ethics, health management & business, myotherapy, stress reduction, theory & practice of massage.

SCHOOL STATEMENT: Each student is important—highly individualized programs—small classes—emphasis on taking care of your hands and body while learning.

#257 Eastwind School of Holistic Healing
209 E. Washington St., suite 305
Iowa City, IA 52240
(319) 351-3262

HOURS OF TRAINING: 500.

COST: $5,000 plus approx $125 books.

YEAR FOUNDED: 1997.

GRADUATES PER YEAR (APPROX.): 20.

MODALITIES AND SUBJECTS: applied kinesiology, aromatherapy, bach flower essences, business practices & professional ethics, chinese herbalism, CPR & first aid, cranio-sacral approaches to bodywork, energy healing techniques levels I & II, oriental bodywork (shiatsu & acupressure), oriental theory (traditional chinese medicine), nutritional health, psychological aspects of bodywork, reiki I & II, relaxation meditation, sound & magnets in healing, special study, student clinic, western herbalism, western massage techniques.

SCHOOL STATEMENT: Eastwind is training practitioners for the future of healthcare. A broad-based, individually chosen program and small class size make students unique, competent, versatile practitioners.

#258 Institute of Therapeutic Massage & Wellness
3801 Marquette St.
(Medical Plaza Building, lower level)
Davenport, IA 52806
(319) 445-1055

Contact school for program information.

#259 Iowa College of Natural Health
1932 SW 3rd., suite 4
Ankeny, IA 50021
(515) 965-3991

524 Second St.
Webster City, IA 50595
(515) 832-3934

HOURS OF TRAINING: 500.

DURATION OF COURSE: 6 months days, 8 months evenings.

COST: $5,000 including books, uniforms, insurance and clinic fees.

FINANCIAL AID: Scholarships or discounts available.

YEAR FOUNDED: 1994.

GRADUATES PER YEAR (APPROX.): 40.

MODALITIES AND SUBJECTS: acupressure, aromatherapy, business, clinical internship, career placement, chair massage, infant massage, medical massage, myotherapy, pregnancy massage, reflexology, sports massage.

SCHOOL STATEMENT: Our objective is to provide the highest quality training available in all aspects of therapeutic massage, and to help students excel in their chosen career.

#260 Iowa Massage Institute
    3017 Indianola Road
    Des Moines, IA 50315
    (515) 287-4370 or 771-6330

HOURS OF TRAINING: 500.

DURATION OF COURSE: approx. 6 months, weekends.

COST: $4,500 including all fees, books and materials. Payment plan without interest is available.

FINANCIAL AID: Rehab. programs, employer funding.

YEAR FOUNDED: 1998.

GRADUATES PER YEAR (APPROX.): 20.

MODALITIES AND SUBJECTS: acupressure, aromatherapy, business practices, canine massage, chair massage, chi gong, clinical internship, cranio-sacral therapy, deep tissue, draping techniques, equine sports massage, ethics, infant massage, musculoskeletal pathology, myofascial release, pregnancy massage, reflexology, shiatsu, sports massage, trigger point therapy.

SCHOOL STATEMENT: Fundamental education in the art of massage therapy.

#261 Millennium College of Massage Therapy
    and Reflexology
    934 S. 17th
    Fort Dodge, IA 50501
    (515) 955-2296

HOURS OF TRAINING: 1,200 including internship hours and 200 hours of reflexology.

DURATION OF COURSE: 6 months.

COST: $5,000.

MODALITIES AND SUBJECTS: history of massage, Touch for Health, musculoskeletal pathology, reflexology, pregnancy massage, infant massage, acupressure, stress reduction, hydrotherapy, exercise and movement, professional ethics, business practices, first aid/CPR.

#262 Windemere School of Eastern Healing Arts
    P.O. Box 381
    Decorah, Iowa 52101
    Classroom: 211½ East Water Street
    1-800-874-0905 or (319)382-8495

Contact school for program information.

KANSAS

No State licensing.

SCHOOLS:

#263 BSMI Institute, LLC
    8665 W. 96th St., suite 300
    Overland Park, KS 66212
    (913) 649-3322

HOURS OF TRAINING: 500.

DURATION OF COURSE: self-paced, usually 15 to 18 months, mostly evenings & weekends.

COST: $4,750 plus $45 application fee.

YEAR FOUNDED: 1994.

PREPARATION FOR OUT-OF-STATE LICENSING EXAM: Iowa.

GRADUATES PER YEAR (APPROX.): 35.

MODALITIES AND SUBJECTS: acupressure, advanced massage, AMMA, applied kinesiology, aromatherapy, business of massage, chair massage, chi gong, clinical practice (student clinic), communicable diseases, cranio-sacral massage, geriatric massage, hydrotherapy, jin shin do, medical charting for massage, medical massage, pathology, polarity, pregnancy massage, reflexology, reiki, somatic therapy, so tai, sports massage I & II, touch for health I, II & III, traditional chinese medicine theory, traditional thai massage, trigger point therapy, tui na, UNTIE, working with the human energy field.

SCHOOL STATEMENT: Our curriculum reflects our belief that the best massage therapists have a broad range of skills and customize every massage to their client's needs.

#264 Johnson County Community College
    Massage Therapy Program
    12345 College Blvd. Box 67
    Overland Park, KS 66210
    (913) 469-4422
    www.johnco.cc.ks.us/conted/cpe

HOURS OF TRAINING: 500.

COST: $4,200.

YEAR FOUNDED: 1995.

GRADUATES PER YEAR (APPROX.): 20.

MODALITIES AND SUBJECTS: (Note: Anatomy & Physiology is a prerequisite) aromatherapy (intro), body mechanics, bodywork clinics, business practices, clinical bodywork, communicable diseases, cranio-sacral (intro), first aid & CPR, hydrotherapy, introduction to bodywork, kinesiology, myofascial (intro), nutrition, oriental bodywork & energy (intro), pathology, sports massage (intro).

#265 Kansas College of Chinese Medicine
    9235 E. Harry, Bldg. 100, suite 1A
    Wichita, KS 67207
    (316) 691-8822

HOURS OF TRAINING: 600 (480 in-class hours).

DURATION OF COURSE: two years, day & evening & weekend programs available.

COST: $5,000.

YEAR FOUNDED: 1996.

MODALITIES AND SUBJECTS: acupressure, chi gong.

SCHOOL STATEMENT: The school bridges Eastern and Western approaches to medicine that will provide solutions to today's problems. The curriculum prepares students for national certification.

#266 Kansas Massage Institute, Inc.
    4525 SW 21st
    Topeka, KS 66604
    (785) 273-4747

HOURS OF TRAINING: 350 or 600.

DURATION OF COURSE: 350 hours 5 months, 600 hours 9 months, evenings & some weekends.

COST: 350 hours $3,904, 600 hours $6,524 (students pay per individual class).

FINANCIAL AID: discounts are available.

YEAR FOUNDED: 1996.

GRADUATES PER YEAR (APPROX.): 10.

MODALITIES AND SUBJECTS: advanced deep tissue massage, advanced range of motion massage, anatomy & physiology I, II & III, applied kinesiology, aromatherapy, balance in harmony, body reflexology, business & law & ethics, chair massage, clinical nutrition, communicable diseases & hygiene, energy anatomy, foot/hand reflexology, herbology, hydrotherapy, infant massage, medical terminology, meridian therapy, pathology I & II, physiology of energy, polarity & body balancing, practical clinical I & II, prenatal massage, principles of the human aura, psychology, shiatsu, specialized massage, spinal touch therapy & clinical, sports injury, sports massage I & II, stress reduction & personal control, therapeutic clinical, therapeutic massage.

SCHOOL STATEMENT: The purpose of the Kansas Massage Institute is to train successful and professional practitioners, and to improve personal growth for each student.

#267 Paragon Natural Health Center
1027 A Washington Road
Newton, KS 67114
(316) 283-9570

Contact school for program information.

#268 Wichita Therapeutic Massage Group
and School, Inc.
535 N. Woodlawn, suite 340
Wichita, KS 67208

7700 E. Kellogg, Towne Square East
Wichita, KS 67207
(316) 682-9170 or 651-5016 or 651-5017

HOURS OF TRAINING: basic 100; additional trainings: iridology (basic 20, advanced 20), herbology (basic 20, advanced 20), aromatherapy (8), reflexology (20), deep tissue (50).

DURATION OF COURSE: Basic 6½ weeks, evenings & weekends.

COST: $800 ($8.00 per class hour). Payment plan without interest is available.

YEAR FOUNDED: 1993.

GRADUATES PER YEAR (APPROX.): 20–40.

MODALITIES AND SUBJECTS: acupressure, aromatherapy, chair massage, deep tissue, herbology, iridology, neuromuscular therapy, pregnancy massage, reflexology, shiatsu, sports massage.

KENTUCKY

No State licensing.

SCHOOLS:

#269 Kentucky Academy of Medical Massage
5016 Main St., Box 110
May's Lick, KY 41055
(606) 763-6334

Contact school for program information.

#270 The Louisville School of Massage
7410 New LaGrange Road, #320
Louisville, KY 40222
(502) 429-5765

HOURS OF TRAINING: 600 (550 in-class hours).

DURATION OF COURSE: 1 to 2 years day and evening programs available.

COST: $5,650. Payment plan without interest is available.

YEAR FOUNDED: 1986.

GRADUATES PER YEAR (APPROX.): 25.

MODALITIES AND SUBJECTS: acupressure, adjunct modalities, aromatherapy, business, chair massage, communication skills, community placement, cranio-sacral therapy, deep tissue massage, infant massage, jin shin do, lymphatic drainage, massage therapy I & II, medical massage, ,pathology, polarity, professional development, reflexology, reiki, sports massage, tai qi, trigger point therapy.

SCHOOL STATEMENT: LSM is dedicated to excellence in massage therapy. Our curriculum acknowledges and promotes the well-being of the whole person in body, mind and spirit.

LOUISIANA

State Licensing: 500 hours.

National Certification Exam accepted.

Board: (504) 658-8941

SCHOOLS:

#271 Blue Cliff School of Therapeutic Massage
1919 Veterans Blvd., suite 310
Kenner, LA 70062
(504) 471-0294

HOURS OF TRAINING: Massage 600; Oriental Bodywork 300; Advanced Sports Massage 135.

DURATION OF COURSE: Massage: 7½ to 8 months days, 13½ months evenings, 15½ months weekends; Oriental Bodywork 3 days per month for 12 months.

COST: Massage: $4,950 including application fee, registration fee, insurance, textbooks and materials. Oriental Bodywork $2,500 includes fees and insurance but not textbooks.

FINANCIAL AID: Dept. of Vocational Rehab., U.S. Dept. of Veterans Affairs.

YEAR FOUNDED: 1987.

ACCREDITATIONS/APPROVALS: COMTA/Accredited, ACCSCT.

PREPARATION FOR OUT-OF-STATE LICENSING EXAM: Florida.

GRADUATES PER YEAR (APPROX.): 150.

MODALITIES AND SUBJECTS: (Massage Program) acupressure, applied kinesiology, basic shiatsu, chi gong, CPR/first aid, chair massage, cranio-sacral therapy, community outreach, deep tissue massage, equine sports massage, ethics, HIV, healing touch, hydrotherapy, infant massage, laws & legislation, lymphatic drainage, marketing & professionalism, medical massage, myofascial release, neuromuscular therapy, pathophysiology, pregnancy massage, reflexology, somatic therapy, sports kinesiology I, sports massage I, sports shiatsu, supervised clinic, tai chi, therapeutic communication.

SCHOOL STATEMENT: Blue Cliff is dedicated to the personal and professional development of its students, the advancement of the profession, excellence in education, and community presence.

#272 Blue Cliff School of Therapeutic Massage
103 Calco Blvd.
Lafayette, LA 70503
(318) 269-0620

HOURS OF TRAINING: 600.

DURATION OF COURSE: 7½ months days, 12 months evenings/weekends.

COST: $4,950 including fees, books, insurance and materials.

FINANCIAL AID: Louisiana Rehabilitation Services.

YEAR FOUNDED: 1992.

PREPARATION FOR OUT-OF-STATE LICENSING EXAM: Florida.

GRADUATES PER YEAR (APPROX.): 40.

MODALITIES AND SUBJECTS: acupressure, applied kinesiology, basic shiatsu, CPR/first aid, chair massage, cranio-sacral therapy, community service project, deep tissue massage, HIV, healing touch, hydrotherapy, laws & legislation, marketing, neuromuscular therapy I & II, pathophysiology, reflexology, somatic therapy, sports kinesiology, sports massage, sports shiatsu, supervised clinical practice, tai chi & yoga, therapeutic communication.

SCHOOL STATEMENT: Blue Cliff is dedicated to the personal and professional development of its students, the advancement of the profession, excellence in education, and community presence.

#273 Blue Cliff School of Therapeutic Massage
3823 Gilbert Dr.
Shreveport, LA 71104
(318) 861-5959

HOURS OF TRAINING: 600.

DURATION OF COURSE: 7 months days, or 12 months evenings and one weekend per month.

COST: $4,950 including application fee, registration fee, insurance, textbooks and materials.

FINANCIAL AID: Louisiana Rehabilitation Services.

YEAR FOUNDED: 1995.

PREPARATION FOR OUT-OF-STATE LICENSING EXAM: Florida.

GRADUATES PER YEAR (APPROX.): 40.

MODALITIES AND SUBJECTS: acupressure, applied kinesiology, basic shiatsu, CPR/first aid, chair massage, cranio-sacral therapy, deep tissue massage, HIV, healing touch, hydrotherapy, laws & legislation, lymphatic drainage, marketing, myofascial release, neuromuscular therapy I & II, pathophysiology, reflexology, somatic therapy, sports kinesiology, sports massage, sports shiatsu, subtle energetic touch, supervised clinical practice, tai chi, therapeutic communication.

SCHOOL STATEMENT: Blue Cliff is dedicated to the personal and professional development of its students, the advancement of the profession, excellence in education, and community presence.

#274 Central LA School of Therapeutic Massage, Inc.
2901 Highway 28 East, suite C
Pineville, LA 71360
(318) 445-5433

HOURS OF TRAINING: 500.

COST: $3,730 plus $100 application fee.

YEAR FOUNDED: 1995.

MODALITIES AND SUBJECTS: business practices, clinical internship, CPR/first aid, deep tissue massage, kinesiology, neuromuscular therapy, reflexology, shiatsu, sports massage.

SCHOOL STATEMENT: The contents of this course meet and exceed the state of Louisiana and national requirements for licensure and certification. Convenient evening and weekend classes.

#275 In-Touch Bodyworks Institute, Inc.
2834 S. Sherwood Forest Blvd., C-1
Baton Rouge, LA 70816
(504) 293-8556

HOURS OF TRAINING: 600 (plus 40 hour externship).

DURATION OF COURSE: 5½ months days, 9 months evenings & weekends.

COST: $5,000 including books and school shirt. Payment plan without interest is available.

FINANCIAL AID: Student loans are available at a local bank.

YEAR FOUNDED: 1992.

GRADUATES PER YEAR (APPROX.): 15–25.

MODALITIES AND SUBJECTS: body mobilization techniques, business mastery, clinical practicum, connective tissue, CPR & first aid, deep tissue, hydrotherapy, law & ethics, myofascial release, neuromuscular therapy, polarity therapy, reflexology (body reflex systems), shiatsu, somatic chemistry, sports massage, therapeutic communication & processing.

SCHOOL STATEMENT: The school strives to produce massage therapists who are "in touch" with their skills, their ethical responsibilities, and their value as human beings.

#276 Louisiana Institute of Massage Therapy
1108 Lafitte St.
Lake Charles, LA 70601
(318) 474-9435
(Classroom: 1605 W. Common St., suite A)

HOURS OF TRAINING: 500.

DURATION OF COURSE: 12 months, weekends.

COST: $3,450 including books.

FINANCIAL AID: Job Training Partnership Act.

YEAR FOUNDED: 1990.

PREPARATION FOR OUT-OF-STATE LICENSING EXAM: Texas.

GRADUATES PER YEAR (APPROX.): 50.

MODALITIES AND SUBJECTS: adaptive massage, bindegewebsmassage, body mechanics, body mobilization techniques, chair massage, deep tissue, hydrotherapy, infant massage, myofascial release, myopractic, myotherapy, neuromuscular therapy, pregnancy massage, reflexology, sports massage, trigger point therapy, zahourek manniken muscle sculpting.

SCHOOL STATEMENT: In-hospital internship program, maniken muscle sculpting system, every other weekend classes, how to file insurance, boundary issues, problem solving by role playing, challenging and fun.

#277 Medical Training College
4528 Bennington Ave., suite 100
Baton Rouge, LA 70808
(504) 926-5820 or 926-8785

HOURS OF TRAINING: 674.

DURATION OF COURSE: 6 to 8 months; day and evening programs offered.

COST: $4,725.

FINANCIAL AID: Vocational rehabilitation, Veterans' Administration, bank financing.

YEAR FOUNDED: 1992.

GRADUATES PER YEAR (APPROX.): 50.

MODALITIES AND SUBJECTS: business/law, chair massage, connective tissue, health, hydrotherapy, infant massage, lymphatic drainage, myofascial release, neuromuscular therapy, nutrition, postural integration, pregnancy massage, reflexology, shiatsu, sports massage, technical alternatives, trigger point therapies, CPR/first aid, HIV/AIDS.

SCHOOL STATEMENT: Focus is on health care and community involvement.

MAINE

State Certification/registration.

National Certification Exam accepted.

Board: (207) 624-8624

SCHOOLS:

#278 Downeast School of Massage
      P.O. Box 24, 99 Moose Meadow Lane
      Waldoboro, ME 04572
      (207) 832-5531
      www.midcoast.com/~dsm

HOURS OF TRAINING:
      Program I: Sports massage 609
      Program II: Shiatsu 708
      Program III: Body/mind 603

DURATION OF COURSE: 11 months full time, 2 years part time; day & evening & weekend classes available.

COST: Sports $5,975, Shiatsu $6,869, Body/mind $5,850.

FINANCIAL AID: Scholarships are available.

YEAR FOUNDED: 1980.

ACCREDITATIONS/APPROVALS: COMTA/Accredited, military and veterans approved, approved for vocational rehabilitation.

GRADUATES PER YEAR (APPROX.): 60–80.

MODALITIES AND SUBJECTS: body-mind, business, chair massage, chronic pain, clinic, ethics, hydrotherapy, kinesiology, medical massage, movement analysis, myofascial release, neuromuscular therapy, nutrition, pathology, polarity, pregnancy massage, psychological aspects, reflexology, shiatsu, sports massage, tai chi, trauma, trigger point therapy, video mechanics.

SCHOOL STATEMENT: Our mission is to train individuals in the art and science of therapeutic massage for an entry level professional career, continuing education and personal growth.

#279 New Hampshire Institute for Therapeutic Arts
      39 Main St.
      Bridgeton, ME 04009
      (207) 647-3794

HOURS OF TRAINING: 750.

DURATION OF COURSE: 9 months, evenings & weekends.

COST: $5,600.

FINANCIAL AID: eligible institution for financial assistance from Canadian student aid.

YEAR FOUNDED: 1983.

ACCREDITATIONS/APPROVALS: COMTA/approved.

PREPARATION FOR OUT-OF-STATE LICENSING EXAM: As needed; have prepared for NY, FL, WA, OR.

GRADUATES PER YEAR (APPROX.): 24.

MODALITIES AND SUBJECTS: aromatherapy*, chair massage*, circulatory massage, cranio-sacral therapy, eastern techniques, eldersage* (geriatric), embryology, emergency procedures, equine sports massage*, ethics & professionalism, first aid & CPR, health service management, human sexuality, hydrotherapy, infant massage*, lymphatic drainage, medical massage, myofascial release, myotherapy, neuromuscular technique, nutrition, pathology, polarity, postural integration, pregnancy massage*, public health & hygiene, reflexology, shiatsu*, somatic therapy, sports massage, structural integration, touch for health, trigger point therapy, yoga therapy*. (*continuing education)

SCHOOL STATEMENT: Education offered in a fearless and non-competitive environment, partaking of both the traditional and evolutionary. Professional preparation allowing flexibility to enter numerous career opportunities.

#280 Polarity Realization Institute
      Portland, ME
      (978) 356-0980

HOURS OF TRAINING: 600-hour massage and bodywork training.

See listing for Polarity Realization Institute, Ipswich, MA.

MARYLAND

State Licensing requires 500 hours until 1/1/02 and 60 accredited college hours thereafter.

Board (Chiropractic Board): (410) 764-4726

SCHOOLS:

#281 Allegany College of Maryland
      1241 Willowbrook Rd.
      Cumberland, MD 21502
      (301) 784-5005

Contact School for program information.

#282 Ann Arundel Community College
      101 College Parkway
      Arnold, MD 21207
      (410) 647-7100

Contact school for program information.

#283 Baltimore School of Massage
      6401 Dogwood Rd.
      Baltimore, MD 21207
      (410) 944-8855

HOURS OF TRAINING: 500.

DURATION OF COURSE: 60 weeks, day and evening programs available.

COST: $4,750.

YEAR FOUNDED: 1981.

ACCREDITATIONS/APPROVALS: COMTA/approved, Maryland Higher Education Commission.

GRADUATES PER YEAR (APPROX.): 200.

MODALITIES AND SUBJECTS: contraindications, craniosacral therapy, deep muscle release work, deep tissue work, energy work, how to make a living successfully doing massage therapy, myofascial release, psycho-emotional release work, sensitivity training, sports massage, zero balancing.

SCHOOL STATEMENT: BSM offers comprehensive, challenging program, preparing massage therapists for employment. The courses are designed to focus on sensitivity and the transformational aspects of bodywork.

#284 Garrett County Community College
      P.O. Box 151
      McHenry, MD 21541
      (301) 387-3000

Contact school for program information.

MASSACHUSETTS

No State licensing.

SCHOOLS:

#285 Bancroft School of Massage Therapy
333 Shrewsbury St.
Worcester, MA 01604
(508) 757-7923

HOURS OF TRAINING: 826.

DURATION OF COURSE: 18 months days, 23 months evenings & weekends.

COST: $10,450.

FINANCIAL AID: Stafford Loans, PLUS loans.

YEAR FOUNDED: 1950.

ACCREDITATIONS/APPROVALS: COMTA/approved, Accrediting Commission of Career Schools/Colleges of Technology.

PREPARATION FOR OUT-OF-STATE LICENSING EXAM: Florida, Washington, New England states.

GRADUATES PER YEAR (APPROX.): 115–120.

MODALITIES AND SUBJECTS: active isolated stretching, business practices, chair massage, clinical massage, CPR, cranio-sacral therapy, equine sports massage, first aid, herbs, hydrotherapy, internship, medical massage, movement & palpation, myofascial release, neuromuscular therapy, oriental massage, reflexology, sports massage, yoga therapy.

SCHOOL STATEMENT: Bancroft's success comes from some very basic philosophical principles; integrity, honest, hard work, ethics, positive attitude, and a charitable heart.

#286 Central Mass School of Massage & Therapy
200 Main Street – Lower Level
Spencer, MA 01562
(508) 885-0306

HOURS OF TRAINING: 500.

DURATION OF COURSE: one year (day and evening classes offered plus Saturday seminars).

COST: $7,500.

YEAR FOUNDED: 1970.

MODALITIES AND SUBJECTS: body balancing, business administration, facial massage, general health, massage techniques & therapy, medical terminology, muscle therapy, nutrition, reflexology, reiki, sports massage & hydrotherapy, traction therapy.

SCHOOL STATEMENT: Students are taught the importance of the holistic health view of the body, and are prepared to play a significant role in the wellness movement.

#287 DoveStar Holistic Technology School
120 Court St
Plymouth, MA 02860
(508) 830-0068

HOURS OF TRAINING: 500 (in-class hours not specified).

DURATION OF COURSE: 6 months.

COST: $4,120.

#288 DoveStar Holistic Technology School
39 Pleasant St.
Attleboro, MA 02703
(508) 222-1683 or 1-888-222-5603

HOURS OF TRAINING: 500 (in-class hours not specified).

DURATION OF COURSE: 6 months.

COST: $4,120.

#289 Healing Touch Institute, Inc. School
of Muscle Therapy
27 Water Street, suite 405
Wakefield, MA 01880
(781) 246-2449

YEAR FOUNDED: 1992.

ACCREDITATIONS/APPROVALS: IMSTAC.

#290 Kripalu Center
P.O. Box 793
Lenox, MA 01240
(413) 448-3400

HOURS OF TRAINING: 200.

DURATION OF COURSE: 28 days (residential).

COST: $1,182 tuition plus room and board (ranging from $1,002 for dormitory to $3,634 for deluxe private room).

FINANCIAL AID: qualified for student loans.

YEAR FOUNDED: 1982.

GRADUATES PER YEAR (APPROX.): 100 to 150.

MODALITIES AND SUBJECTS: body dynamics, conscious communication, danskinetics, hara development, meditation, pranayama, t'ai chi, theory and techniques of Kripalu bodywork, yoga.

SCHOOL STATEMENT: Kripalu bodywork is an eclectic blend of swedish massage, energy balancing, yoga and meditative awareness. The school is a residential retreat center in the Berkshires.

#291 Massage Institute of New England, Inc.
22 McGrath Highway
Somerville, MA 02143
(617) 666-3700

HOURS OF TRAINING: 680 (plus 7-hour continuing education segments).

COST: $6,900.

YEAR FOUNDED: 1982.

ACCREDITATIONS/APPROVALS: COMTA/approved.

PREPARATION FOR OUT-OF-STATE LICENSING EXAM: The curriculum meets most states' criteria for licensing; contact school for information about individual states.

GRADUATES PER YEAR (APPROX.): 100.

MODALITIES AND SUBJECTS: western, scientific, eastern, energetic and emotional techniques. Continuing education ("Functional Body Series") offers continuing trainings in precise musculoskeletal techniques and esoteric energetic anatomy.

SCHOOL STATEMENT: A focus on the integration of body, mind, and spirit are integral within this holistic training program. Personal growth and burn-out prevention are emphasized.

#292 Muscular Therapy Institute
122 Rindge Ave.
Cambridge, MA 02140-2527
(617) 576-1300
www.mtti.com

HOURS OF TRAINING: 51.6 credit hours, 900 in-class hours.

DURATION OF COURSE: 1½ years (3 semester format) or 2 years (4 semesters), weekend programs available.

COST: approximately $13,797 including fees (3 semester) or $13,857 including fees (4 semester), including books and table. Payment plan without interest is available.

FINANCIAL AID: financial aid available if qualified (Federal Financial Aid Program)

YEAR FOUNDED: 1974

ACCREDITATIONS/APPROVALS: COMTA/approved, ACCET.

GRADUATES PER YEAR (APPROX.): 125.

MODALITIES AND SUBJECTS: approaches to holistic therapies, Benjamin system of muscular therapy, chair massage, clinical considerations and pathology, cranio-sacral therapy, foundations of massage, infant massage, lymphatic drainage, myofascial release, practice development, pregnancy massage, professional development, reflexology, reiki, skills and dynamics of therapeutic relationships, sports massage, trager, trigger point therapy, zero-balancing.

SCHOOL STATEMENT: The skill of massage and the art of healing.

#293 North Shore Institute of Massage
       120 Main St., P.O. Box 1639
       Gloucester, MA 01930
       (978) 282-3366

Contact school for program information.

#294 Polarity Realization Institute
       126 High St.,
       Ipswich, MA 01938
       (978) 356-0980

HOURS OF TRAINING: 180 or 600 (144 or 529 in-class hours).

DURATION OF COURSE: 180 hours 6 months; 600 hours 12 to 24 months; day, evening and weekend programs available.

COST: 180 hours $1,710; 600 hours $5,386.50 (plus required outside sessions). Payment plan without interest is available.

YEAR FOUNDED: 1981.

ACCREDITATIONS/APPROVALS: program approved by American Polarity Therapy Association, approved for nursing CEU's in Massachusetts and Maine, IMSTAC.

MODALITIES AND SUBJECTS: The five modules offered may be taken individually. Module 1 is Swedish massage, 180 hours; module 2 is polarity therapy certification, 160 hours; module 3 is advanced anatomy and physiology, 56 hours; module 4 is advanced massage and polarity electives, 148 hours; module 5 is advanced integration and evaluation, 56 hours. Classes: advanced aura and energetic anatomy, advanced chakra and energetic anatomy, advanced spinal and client evaluation, advanced vitality balancing, aromatherapy, body mechanics, business skills, chair massage, clinics, color and light, communication skills, cranio-sacral therapy, distance healing, eating disorders, hips and pelvic alignment, ice and heat, intuitive symbolic interpretation, myofascial release, polarity nutrition and yoga, psychosynthesis and body awareness, reflexology, running your subtle energies, sacral and sacroiliac, self-care and stretching, sexual abuse and transitions, sound therapy, sports massage.

SCHOOL STATEMENT: A combination of physical and energetic work. The modular program allows the student to begin a professional practice after completing the first 180 hours.

#295 Stillpoint Center
       P.O. Box 15
       60 Main St., P.O. Box 15
       Hatfield, MA 01038
       (413) 247-9322
       www.westmass.com/stillpoint

HOURS OF TRAINING: 919 (in-class hours not specified).

DURATION OF COURSE: 11 months full-time days, two years part-time evenings.

COST: $8,000. Payment plan without interest is available.

YEAR FOUNDED: 1980.

ACCREDITATIONS/APPROVALS: COMTA/approved, ACCSCT.

PREPARATION FOR OUT-OF-STATE LICENSING EXAM: NY and NH (additional coursework required; subject to enrollment minimums).

MODALITIES AND SUBJECTS: body awareness & mechanics, clinical preparation I & II, community clinical practicum externship, CPR/first aid, feldenkrais, hydrotherapy, integrative seminar, kinesiology, massage clinic, myology I & II, pathology, polarity, professional development I, II & III, professional worklife, reflexology, shiatsu, sports massage, therapeutic techniques, therapeutic touch, trigger point therapy.

SCHOOL STATEMENT: The programs we offer emphasize holism, massage with awareness and compassionate action.

MICHIGAN

No State licensing.

SCHOOLS:

#296 Ann Arbor Institute of Massage Therapy
       2835 Carpenter Rd.
       Ann Arbor, MI 48108
       (734) 677-4430

HOURS OF TRAINING: 620 (570 in-class hours).

DURATION OF COURSE: 11½ months, day & evening & weekend programs available.

COST: $6,000, including texts. Payment plan without interest is available.

YEAR FOUNDED: 1992

GRADUATES PER YEAR (APPROX.): 80

MODALITIES AND SUBJECTS: chair massage, maniken, myofascial release I, II & III, neuromuscular therapy I, II & III, reflexology, shiatsu, sports massage I & II, therapeutic massage, trigger point therapy.

SCHOOL STATEMENT: Our programs are founded on the most sound and ethical clinical and educational experience required to produce excellence in the field of massage therapy.

#297 Ann Arbor School of Massage and Bodywork
       1530 Northwood St.
       Ann Arbor, MI 48103
       (313) 662-1572

Contact school for program information.

#298 Blue Heron Academy of Clinical Massage Therapy
       2020 Raybrook SE, ste. 203
       Grand Rapids, MI 49546
       (616) 771-8094 or 285-9999

HOURS OF TRAINING: 600 (320 in-class hours), 1,000 (in-class hours not specified) and 2000 (in-class hours not specified).

DURATION OF COURSE: 6 months, evenings.

COST: 600 hour program $2,400 to $3,000.

YEAR FOUNDED: 1991.

GRADUATES PER YEAR (APPROX.): 60.

MODALITIES AND SUBJECTS: clinical massage therapy techniques, cranio-sacral therapy, medical massage, myofascial release, myotherapy, neuromuscular therapy, rehabilitation massage (frozen shoulder, low back pain, strain & sprain, range of motion),shiatsu, sports massage, therapeutic exercise, trigger point therapy.

SCHOOL STATEMENT: Training and hospital based internship in clinical massage therapy and physical rehabilitation of acute and chronic soft tissue and joint injuries.

#299 Career Development Center
5961 14th St. / P.O. Box 08067
Detroit, MI 48208
(313) 894-0610

Contact school for program information.

#300 Freedom Eagle Institute
684 Deer St.
Plymouth, MI 48170
(313) 207-0969 or 1-800-272-1247
www.freedomeagle.com

HOURS OF TRAINING: 600.

#301 Georgetown Bodyworks Healing Arts Institute
www.imagroup.com and www.learnmassage.com
2450 Hawks Avenue
Ann Arbor, MI 48108
(734) 971-1950

2572 Oak Forest Drive
Holland, MI 49424
(616) 786-9753

HOURS OF TRAINING: 150 or 750 (50 or 250 in-class hours).

DURATION OF COURSE: 150 hours, 6 to 12 months; 750 hours, 18 to 24 months.

COST: 150 hours $2,195, 750 hours $4,995 both including table, bodyCushion, books, sheets and oil. Payment plan without interest is available.

FINANCIAL AID: Scholarships for single mothers.

YEAR FOUNDED: 1982 (Georgetown Bodyworks, Washington DC).

MODALITIES AND SUBJECTS: Canadian Deep Muscle Massage, Reach Therapy™, Bounce Therapy™.

SCHOOL STATEMENT: Loving, caring, **safe touch** should be part of American life. We are committed to teaching **safe structured touch** to everyone interested. Help us heal America.

#302 Health Enrichment Center, Inc.
1820 N. Lapeer Road
Lapeer, MI 48446
(810) 667-9453

YEAR FOUNDED: 1985.

ACCREDITATIONS/APPROVALS: COMTA/approved.

#303 Institute of Natural Therapies
P.O. Box 222
Hancock, MI 49930
(906) 482-2222

HOURS OF TRAINING: 806 (500 in-class hours).

DURATION OF COURSE: 9 months, every other weekend.

COST: $3,950 includes all books. Payment plan without interest is available.

FINANCIAL AID: Scholarships or discounts, State of Michigan, Disabled Veterans.

YEAR FOUNDED: 1993.

GRADUATES PER YEAR (APPROX.): 12.

MODALITIES AND SUBJECTS: applied kinesiology, ashtanga yoga, business experience & ethics, cranio-sacral therapy, deep tissue, healing touch, myofascial release, neuromuscular therapy, structural integration, traditional chinese massage.

SCHOOL STATEMENT: We provide training designed for graduates to be superior in the market, and to become leaders and innovators in the future therapeutic massage field.

#304 Irene's Myomassology Institute
18911 Ten Mile Rd. #200
Southfield, MI 48075
(313) 569-HAND/4263
www.myomassology.com

HOURS OF TRAINING: 500.

DURATION OF COURSE: one year; day, evening & weekend classes available.

COST: $3793 including five required books.

FINANCIAL AID: payment plans.

YEAR FOUNDED: 1987.

GRADUATES PER YEAR (APPROX.): 200.

MODALITIES AND SUBJECTS: acupressure, anatomy coloring book, applied kinesiology, aromatherapy, bach flower remedies, basic and therapeutic massage, biomagnets, body mechanics, body-mind, business procedures, carpal tunnel, chair massage, chakra basics, chi gong, clinical experience, colon health, CPR, cranio-sacral therapy, crystal healing, energy balancing, ethics, first aid, herbology, hydrotherapy, infant massage, iridology, labor massage, leg exercises, lymphatic drainage, macrobiotics, meditation, myofascial release, neuro-linguistic programming, nuat thai, nutrition, paraffin therapy, pathology, pet massage, polarity, pregnancy massage, reflexology, reiki, response to emotional release, sanitary practices, shiatsu, side-lying massage, skin care, spiritual development, sports massage, stress management, stretching, structural and postural evaluation and treatment, therapeutic touch, three in one concepts series, touch for health, trigger points, yoga therapy.

SCHOOL STATEMENT: Irene utilizes forty years massage experience to promote natural healing. The institute provides a wonderful program in therapeutic bodywork and a discount supply store.

#305 Kalamazoo Center for the Healing Arts
3715 West Main
Kalamazoo, MI 49006-2842
(616) 373-0910
www.kcha.com

HOURS OF TRAINING: 520.

DURATION OF COURSE: 18 months, day & weekend programs available.

COST: $4,720.

FINANCIAL AID: contact school.

YEAR FOUNDED: 1986.

ACCREDITATIONS/APPROVALS: IMSTAC.

MODALITIES AND SUBJECTS: acupressure, advanced anatomy, aromatherapy, chair massage, cranio-sacral therapy, healing touch, infant massage, integrated bodywork therapies, lymphatic drainage, myofascial release, polarity, practicum, pregnancy massage, reflexology, sports massage, tai chi, the business of being a bodyworker, therapeutic touch.

SCHOOL STATEMENT: Focus is on inner growth as students become practitioners. Instruction is client-centered and the product of 12 years of running a large professional clinic.

#306 Kirtland Community College
10775 N. St. Helen Rd.
Roscommon, MI 48653
(517) 275-5121

Contact school for program information.

#307 Lakewood School of Therapeutic Massage
2950 Lapeer Rd.
Port Huron, MI 48060
(810) 987-3959

HOURS OF TRAINING: 700 (368 in-class hours).

DURATION OF COURSE: 9 months, day & evening & weekend programs available.

COST: $3,200 plus $200 books.

YEAR FOUNDED: 1997.

GRADUATES PER YEAR (APPROX.): 35–60.

MODALITIES AND SUBJECTS: acupressure, aromatherapy, assessment & techniques of therapeutic massage, bioenergetics, bodymind (body and mind together), chair massage, connective tissue approaches, cranio-sacral therapy, infant massage, muscles & meridians, myofascial release, neuromuscular therapy, polarity, postural integration, pregnancy massage, professional development & theory, reflexology, reiki, shiatsu, sports massage, touch for health, trager, trigger point therapy.

SCHOOL STATEMENT: Excellence in program content; balance in the Art and Science of Therapeutic Massage; Several Additional Bodywork Modalities; Holistic Emphasis; Personal Growth; Supportive Learning Environment.

#308 Lansing Community College
P.O. Box 40010
Lansing, MI 48901
(517) 483-1410

HOURS OF TRAINING: 500.

DURATION OF COURSE: variable, courses offered days, evenings, weekends.

COST: $1,150.

YEAR FOUNDED: 1977.

GRADUATES PER YEAR (APPROX): 35 to 40.

ACCREDITATIONS/APPROVALS: North Central Association of Colleges and Schools.

MODALITIES AND SUBJECTS: acupressure, business applications, consumer/health issues, healing touch, healthy lifestyles, human structural dynamics, massage practicum, medical massage, myotherapy, polarity I and II, reflexology, rolfing, self awareness/wellness, shiatsu, sports massage, stress management, touch for health, trigger point therapy.

#309 Michigan Institute of Massage Therapy
3518 Apple Valley Rd.
Okemos, MI 48864-3933
(At large school licensed to teach anywhere in MI)
(517) 347-2547

HOURS OF TRAINING: 150 to 1,100.

DURATION OF COURSE: 4 to 34 weeks.

COST: $1,500 to $6,000. Payment plan without interest is available.

YEAR FOUNDED: 1987 (workshops), 1998 (school).

MODALITIES AND SUBJECTS: body dynamics workshop, bookkeeping, deep tissue, ethics, hygiene, massage theory & movements, oriental massage, spa massage training, sports massage, wholistic massage. Program titles: Spa Massage Therapist, Advanced Bodywork Practitioner, Professional Massage.

#310 Michigan School of Myomassology, Inc.
3270 Greenfield Road
Berkley, MI 48072
(248) 542-7228

Contact school for program information.

#311 Stressage Massage Institute
16587 Wyoming
Detroit, MI 48221
(313) 864-8355

HOURS OF TRAINING: 300 or 600 (in-class hours not specified).

COST: 300 hours $1,695, 600 hours $3,618 (estimated).

YEAR FOUNDED: 1990.

GRADUATES PER YEAR (APPROX.): 30.

MODALITIES AND SUBJECTS: facial massage specialist certification, reflexology certification, spa modalities certification.

SCHOOL STATEMENT: SMI provides quality training in a relaxed interactive atmosphere. Our instructors are qualified in their specialty, their teaching skills, and ability to recognize students' individuality.

#312 Wellness Center, Inc.
1049 1st Capitol Drive
St. Charles, MO 63301
(314) 947-8242

Contact school for program information.

#313 Wellspring Institute:
School of Therapeutic Bodywork
20312 Chalon, St. Clair Shores, MI 48080
(810) 772-8520

HOURS OF TRAINING: 100, 300, 500, 1,000.

DURATION OF COURSE: 6 months to 2 years, evenings & weekends.

COST: 300 hours $3,000, 500 hours $4,200. Payment plan without interest is available.

FINANCIAL AID: Discounts available.

YEAR FOUNDED: 1981.

GRADUATES PER YEAR (APPROX): 15–20.

MODALITIES AND SUBJECTS: [Note: Swedish massage is not taught; the primary technique taught is "gentle deep tissue"]; acupressure, business practice, communications skills, craniosacral therapy, decalcification massage, elderly (geriatric) massage, emotional self-influencing, ethics, gentle deep tissue, herbal massage, hypnotherapy, massage with the dying & advanced cancer patients & abuse survivors, medical massage, pfrimmer, polarity, psychosomatics, reflexology, sports massage, therapeutic touch. Advanced programs: hypnosis, polarity therapy, medical massage, emotional release work, haelon personal & professional development program, independent study, research projects.

SCHOOL STATEMENT: We emphasize an emotional approach to massage, where students learn to work with client's emotional reaction to their touch. Hospital program staffed with school's graduates.

MINNESOTA

No State licensing.

SCHOOLS:

#314 Eagles Nest Institute
5096 Arnold Rd.
Duluth, MN 55803
(218) 724-3067

HOURS OF TRAINING: 200.

DURATION OF COURSE: 10 weeks mornings or 22 weeks evenings or 5-week summer intensive.

COST: $2,679 including 6 textbooks and all class materials.

FINANCIAL AID: Bank Loans available.

YEAR FOUNDED: 1989.

MODALITIES AND SUBJECTS: AIDS education, body awareness, body-mind, business, chair massage, clinical practice, CPR & first aid, deep tissue, esalen, functional histology, geriatric massage, healing touch, history of massage, infant massage, laws concerning massage, lymphatic drainage, medical massage, myofascial release, myotherapy, neuromuscular therapy, postural integration, pregnancy massage, professional standards & ethics, reiki, self-care techniques, somatic therapy, TMJ workshop, touch for health, trigger point therapy, yoga therapy.

SCHOOL STATEMENT: The program is designed to offer a solid fundamental, theoretical and skills base, with which a practitioner may start their own practice confidently and successfully.

#315 Minneapolis School of Massage and Bodywork, Inc.
220 Lowry Ave. NE
Minneapolis, MN 55418
(classroom: 2205 California St. NE)
(612) 788-8907

HOURS OF TRAINING: Massage Practitioner 202 hours, Sports Massage 527 hours, Comprehensive Massage Therapy 750

DURATION OF COURSE: Massage Practitioner 6 months, Sports Massage 10 months, Comprehensive 16 months, day and evening programs available.

COST: Massage Practitioner $1,864, Sports Massage $4,341.50, Comprehensive $6,026.50 (all prices include books). Payment plan without interest is available.

FINANCIAL AID: Minnesota State grants.

YEAR FOUNDED: 1975.

GRADUATES PER YEAR (APPROX): 300.

ACCREDITATIONS/APPROVALS: ACCSCT, IMSTAC.

MODALITIES AND SUBJECTS: acupressure, body wellness, business, chair massage, communications, esalen, infant massage, interfacing with health care professionals, pregnancy massage, shiatsu, special needs, sports massage, therapeutic massage courses, trigger point therapy.

#316 Northern Lights School of Massage Therapy
1313 S.E. Fifth St., ste. 209
Minneapolis, MN 55414
(612) 379-3822

HOURS OF TRAINING: 650 (600 in-class hours).

DURATION OF COURSE: one year full time, two years part time, day & evening & weekend programs available.

COST: approx. $6,500 including books, manuals, fees and AMTA membership.

YEAR FOUNDED: 1985.

ACCREDITATIONS/APPROVALS: COMTA/approved.

GRADUATES PER YEAR (APPROX.): 60.

MODALITIES AND SUBJECTS: acupressure, applied kinesiology, aromatherapy, body-mind, cranio-sacral therapy, feldenkrais, hakomi, healing touch, myofascial release, neuromuscular therapy, polarity, professional development, reflexology, reiki, science I & II, shiatsu, sports massage, trager, trigger point therapy.

SCHOOL STATEMENT: NLSMT is a non-profit corporation founded in 1985. NLSMT has become well known nationwide for its high standards, integrity and excellence in education.

#317 Saint Croix Center for the Healing Arts
3121 St. Croix Trail South / P.O. Box 354
Afton, MN 55001
(612) 436-6808

Contact school for program information.

#318 Sister Rosalind Gefre Schools
of Professional Massage
400 Selby Ave., suite G
St. Paul, MN 55102
(612) 228-0960 or (612) 698-9123

300 Elton Hills Drive
Rochester, MN 55901
(507) 286-8608

165 West Lind Court
Mankato, MN 56001
(507) 344-0220

HOURS OF TRAINING: 650.

DURATION OF COURSE: one year, day & evening programs available.

COST: $5,335. Payment plan without interest is available.

FINANCIAL AID: bank loans for qualified students.

YEAR FOUNDED: 1984.

ACCREDITATIONS/APPROVALS: IMSTAC, VA approved.

GRADUATES PER YEAR (APPROX.): 50.

MODALITIES AND SUBJECTS: acupressure, applied kinesiology, chair massage, esalen, healing touch, infant massage, lymphatic drainage, myofascial release, neuromuscular therapy, pregnancy massage, reflexology, shiatsu, sports massage, trigger point therapy. Additional programs: Reflexology (216 hours), On-Site Chair Technician (207 hours).

SCHOOL STATEMENT: The School is based on Christian principles of spiritual, psychological and physical well-being. Low student/teacher ratios, professional environment, highly skilled instructors.

#319 The Touch of Life School of Massage
574 Prairie Center Dr. suite 155
Eden Prairie, MN 55344
(612) 996-9655

Contact school for program information.

MISSISSIPPI

No State Licensing.

SCHOOLS:

#320 Blue Cliff School of Therapeutic Massage
942 E. Beach Blvd.
Gulfport, MS 39507
(228) 896-9727

HOURS OF TRAINING: 600.

DURATION OF COURSE: 7 months days or 13 months evenings.

COST: $4,950 including application fee, registration fee, insurance, textbooks and materials.

FINANCIAL AID: MS Dept. of Rehabilitation Services.

YEAR FOUNDED: 1997.

PREPARATION FOR OUT-OF-STATE LICENSING EXAM: Louisiana, Florida.

MODALITIES AND SUBJECTS: acupressure, applied kinesiology, basic shiatsu, chair massage, chi gong, CPR/first aid, cranio-sacral therapy, deep tissue, healing touch I, HIV, laws & legislation, marketing & professionalism, neuromuscular therapy I & II, pathophysiology, reflexology, somatic therapy, spa therapy, sports kinesiology, sports massage, supervised clinical practice, tai chi, therapeutic communication.

SCHOOL STATEMENT: Blue Cliff is dedicated to the personal and professional development of its students, the advancement of the profession, excellence in education, and community presence.

#321 The Natural Healing Arts School
of Massage Therapy
1360 Sunset Drive, suite #16
Grenada, MS 38901
(601)229-0010

HOURS OF TRAINING: 525.

DURATION OF COURSE: 6 months, day & evening & weekend programs available.

COST: $4,455 including books. Payment plan without interest is available.

YEAR FOUNDED: 1997.

MODALITIES AND SUBJECTS: acupressure, applied kinesiology, aromatherapy, business & marketing, chair massage, cranio-sacral therapy, healing touch, hydrotherapy, lymphatic drainage, medical massage, muscle massage connection, neuromuscular therapy, nutrition for health, oriental techniques, pathology, polarity, reflexology, rehabilitative techniques, reiki, shiatsu, sports massage, therapeutic touch.

SCHOOL STATEMENT: Program is structured to prepare graduates for professional careers as licensed massage therapists combining ancient and contemporary methods of health care emphasizing new medical theories.

MISSOURI

State licensing: 500 hours. See page 128.

SCHOOLS:

#322 Boyer School of Natural Therapy
5919 Hampton
St. Louis, MO 63109
(314) 832-4220
http://members.aol.com/aboyer1111/
BSNTHomePage.html

Contact school for program information.

#323 Kaleidoscope School of Massage
7645 Delmar Blvd.
St. Louis, MO 63130
(314) 862-7442

YEAR FOUNDED: 1994.

#324 Massage and Energy Connection
College of Application
7159 Manchester
Maplewood, MO 63143
(314) 647-0115

HOURS OF TRAINING: 100.

COST: $1,200 including books and insurance.

YEAR FOUNDED: 1993.

GRADUATES PER YEAR (APPROX.): 30.

MODALITIES AND SUBJECTS: basic & advanced massage, CPR, ki-atsu, kinetic integration series, oriental philosophy.

#325 Massage Therapy Training Institute
9140 Ward Parkway #100
Kansas City, MO 64114
(816) 523-9140

HOURS OF TRAINING: 500.

COST: $5,800.

ACCREDITATIONS/APPROVALS: IMSTAC.

YEAR FOUNDED: 1988.

GRADUATES PER YEAR (APPROX.): 25.

MODALITIES AND SUBJECTS: anatomy & physiology I, II & III, aromatherapy, basic counseling skills for wellness consultants, chair massage, chinese meridian therapy, color therapy, CPR & first aid, cranio-sacral balancing I & II, creating a successful practice, creating clarity in bodywork, defining sexuality & ethical issues, deep tissue bodywork, environmental influences on wellness, fibromyalgia & chronic pain syndrome, flower essence therapy, gender specific issues & wellness, herbalism I, II & III, hydrotherapy, infant massage instructor certification, iridology & massage, music & healing, myofascial release massage, neuro-myofascial release, nutrition & wellness consulting, pathophysiology, perinatal (pregnancy) massage, personal trainer training, polarity therapy, power of touch, practicum for wellness consultants, reflexology, shiatsu I & II, sooji chim hand therapy, sports massage I & II, stress management facilitation, stress management workshop, tai chi, therapeutic touch (basic & advanced), trigger point therapy, vibrational healing (intro), vibrational healing I. (Over 1,000 hours of total instruction are offered and courses may be taken individually in addition to the 500 hour program.)

SCHOOL STATEMENT: MTTI was founded in response to a heartfelt belief that nurturing touch could have a profoundly positive effect on our society and on individual wellness.

#326 National Institute for Muscle Therapy
144 Nostra Villa Dr.
Fenton, MO 63026
(314) 225-5503

HOURS OF TRAINING: 130 (in-class hours not specified).

COST: $1,200.

YEAR FOUNDED: 1977.

GRADUATES PER YEAR (APPROX.): 16.

MODALITIES AND SUBJECTS: basic massage theory, esalen, establishing your business, ethics, geriatric massage, self massage, sports injuries & applied remedies, sports massage.

#327 St. Charles School of Massage Therapy
519 S. Fifth
St. Charles, MO 63301
(314) 949-0232 or 949-0448
www.webusers.anet-stl.com

HOURS OF TRAINING: 500 (in-class hours not specified).

DURATION OF COURSE: 7 months; day, evenings, evening/weekends programs.

COST: $4,500 plus $199.42 books. Payment plan without interest is available.

YEAR FOUNDED: 1991, 500-hour program started 1997.

GRADUATES PER YEAR (APPROX.): 50.

MODALITIES AND SUBJECTS: chair massage, facial toning, foot reflexology, polarity, pranic healing, shiatsu, sports massage, touch for health, trager, trigger point therapy.

#328 Ozark Institute of Natural Therapies
1271 E. Montclair
Springfield, MO 65804
(417) 883-0300

HOURS OF TRAINING: 600.

DURATION OF COURSE: nine months.

YEAR FOUNDED: 1989.

SCHOOL CLOSED

MODALITIES AND SUBJECTS: ~~~~ terminology, pathological conditions, range ~~~ motion, palpation, prenatal massage, sports massage, reflexology, hydrotherapy, hygiene, business practices, ethical guidelines.

ADVANCED PROGRAMS: contact school.

CONTINUING EDUCATION: contact school.

MONTANA

No State licensing.

SCHOOLS:

#329 Asten Center
P.O. Box C – 121 W. Legion
Whitehall, MT 59759
(406) 287-5670 or 1-800-640-9009

HOURS OF TRAINING: 600.

COST: $6,245 including massage table, face cradle, arm cradle, bolster, school shirt, massage table travel bag, textbooks, AMTA student membership, one gallon massage lotion.

YEAR FOUNDED: 1990.

GRADUATES PER YEAR (APPROX.): 17.

MODALITIES AND SUBJECTS: business practices & ethics, clinical applications class (sprained ankle, carpal tunnel syndrome, whiplash, TMJ, sciatic pain, shoulder injuries, tennis elbow, spinal deviations, knee injuries, flat feet), externship practice, health & hygiene, hydrotherapy & cryotherapy, practice specific classes (pregnancy massage, massage for the elderly, infant massage, headaches), reflexology, sports massage, trigger point therapy.

SCHOOL STATEMENT: Emphasis is placed on thorough technical knowledge and massage skill levels in applying techniques of Swedish and Sports Massage. Small classes, personalized instruction. Quality education.

#330 Big Sky Somatic Institute
1802 11th Ave., suite A
Helena, MT 59601
(406) 442-8998

HOURS OF TRAINING: 130 to 1,000 (126 to 980 in-class hours).

DURATION OF COURSE: 4 to 18 months, Thurs.–Sun.

COST: Tuition is $8.00 per contact hour.

YEAR FOUNDED: 1996.

GRADUATES PER YEAR (APPROX.): 12.

MODALITIES AND SUBJECTS: bioenergetics, body-mind, chi gong, circulatory massage, esalen, integrative movement therapies, integrative somatics I & II, medical massage, micro-movement, muscle sculpting I, II & III, myofascial release, neuromuscular therapy, oriental theories & practice I & II, passive joint move-

ment, professional practice & business ethics, shiatsu, structural integration, tai chi, thai massage, trigger point therapy, tui na, tui na for sports injuries & for structural disorders & for common ailments, yoga.

SCHOOL STATEMENT: Massage is both an intuitive art and the skillful application of techniques. We provide tools for personal growth and a three centered approach to learning.

#331 Good Medicine Massage
404 E. 1st, suite C
Whitefish, MT 59937
(406) 862-3603

Contact school for program information.

#332 Rocky Mountain School of Massage
2215 Broadwater
Billings, MT 59102
(406) 652-2633

Contact school for program information.

#333 Starfire Massage School
9819 Waldo Rd.
Missoula, MT 59802
(406) 721-7519

HOURS OF TRAINING: 165, 500 or 600 (165, 470 or 550 in-class hours).

DURATION OF COURSE: 3 months, 9 months, 9 months.

COST: $1,500, $4,400, $4,900 includes books and IMA membership.

FINANCIAL AID: Discounts for prepayment.

YEAR FOUNDED: 1995.

GRADUATES PER YEAR (APPROX.): 20.

MODALITIES AND SUBJECTS: accessing patterns, acupressure I & II, aromatherapy, bodywork for spiritual emergence, breathwork, business practices, chair massage, CPR, creative self-care, ethics, eurodynamics energy balancing, hatha yoga, humans & hurts & healing, hydrotherapy, learning from the inside out, lymphatic drainage, meditation, opening to intuitive creativity, practicum, reiki I & II, shamanic journey, shiatsu, somatic therapy, sound healing, tai chi I & II, trigger point therapy, vibrational healing.

SCHOOL STATEMENT: Starfire unifies intuitive and scientific methods to create comprehensive professional bodywork certification programs. We support mental, emotional, physical and spiritual health empowering the healer within.

NEBRASKA

State Licensing: 1,000 hours.

National Certification Exam accepted.

Board: (402) 471-2117

APPROVED OUT-OF-STATE SCHOOLS:

Bio-Chi Institute, IA; Collinson School, Colorado Springs CO; Massage Therapy Institute, Denver CO; New Mexico Academy, Santa Fe NM

SCHOOLS:

#334 Gateway College of Massage Therapy
2607 Dakota Ave.
S. Sioux City, NE 68776
(402) 494-8390

HOURS OF TRAINING: 500 or 1,000 (350 or 750 in-class hours).

DURATION OF COURSE: 9 months or 12 months, day & evening &

weekend programs available.

COST: 500 hours $4,950, 1,000 hours $5,950, including all textbooks, 3 sets of sheets and towels, uniform shirt. Payment plan without interest is available.

FINANCIAL AID: Veteran's Administration.

YEAR FOUNDED: 1994.

GRADUATES PER YEAR (APPROX): 20.

MODALITIES AND SUBJECTS: anatomy & physiology (basic and advanced), chair massage, clinical externship, clinical practices, communications, health services management, infant massage, marketing, hydrotherapy, kinesiology, neuromuscular therapy, nutrition & wellness, pathology & hygiene, pregnancy massage, professional issues, public clinic, public service, reflexology, senior seminars, sports massage, trigger point therapy.

SCHOOL STATEMENT: Gateway College of MT teaches modalities which can be incorporated into adjunct medical treatments. The emphasis is on training therapists for medically related careers.

#335 Midwest School of Massage
2808 N. 75th St.
Omaha, NE 68134
(402) 398-3311

HOURS OF TRAINING: 1,000 (600 in-class hours).

DURATION OF COURSE: 9 months, day and evening programs available.

COST: $4,500 including books, lab fees, insurance one set of linens & lotions. Payment plan without interest is available.

YEAR FOUNDED: 1996.

MODALITIES AND SUBJECTS: Contact school.

SCHOOL STATEMENT: The school places strong emphasis on both academics and hands-on skills, stressing the integral relationship between structure and function in the human body.

#336 Myotherapy Institute
6020 S. 58th St.
Lincoln, NE 68516
(402) 421-7410

HOURS OF TRAINING: 1,000 to 1,500 (in-class hours not specified).

DURATION OF COURSE: 10 months or longer, day or evening programs available.

YEAR FOUNDED: 1993.

GRADUATES PER YEAR (APPROX.): 40.

MODALITIES AND SUBJECTS: acupressure, alexander technique, applied anatomy, aromatherapy, body-mind, business, chair massage, chi gong, cranio-sacral therapy, eastern techniques, equine sports massage, esalen, feldenkrais, hydrotherapy, hygiene, infant massage, kinesiology, kinetics seminar, massage clinic, massage practicum, medical massage, myofascial release, myotherapy, neuromuscular therapy, ortho-bionomy, pathology, polarity, postural integration, pregnancy massage, reflexology, shiatsu, spa training, sports massage, tai chi, trigger point therapy, yoga therapy.

#337 Omaha School of Massage Therapy
9748 Park Dr.
Omaha, NE 68127
(402) 331-3694
www.osmt.com

HOURS OF TRAINING: 1,000 (620 in-class).

DURATION OF COURSE: 9 months, day and evening programs available.

COST: $6,500 (includes books and fees). Payment plan without interest is available.

FINANCIAL AID: Pell Grants, Stafford Loans.

ACCREDITATIONS/APPROVALS: ACCSCT.

YEAR FOUNDED: 1991.

GRADUATES PER YEAR (APPROX.): 80.

MODALITIES AND SUBJECTS: acupressure, aromatherapy, business & health service management, chair massage, clinic practical, cranio-sacral therapy, exercise training, hydrotherapy, infant massage, kinesiology, neuromuscular therapy, ortho-bionomy, pathology, physiology, postural integration, pregnancy massage, professional issues & ethics, reflexology, reiki, wellness.

SCHOOL STATEMENT: It is our desire to promote natural and holistic health through massage, exercise and nutrition, also emphasizing high ethical standards and public awareness.

#338 Universal Center of Healing Arts
Non-Profit School of Massage Therapy
109 N. 50th Street
Omaha, NE 68132
(402) 556-4456

HOURS OF TRAINING: 500 to 1,000 (in-class hours not specified).

DURATION OF COURSE: 9 months to 2 years, Tu.+Sat. & evening+Sat. & weekend programs available.

COST: $3,000 to $6,000 including books $300 and registration fee $150.

FINANCIAL AID: Scholarships ranging from $500 to $2,000 are available.

YEAR FOUNDED: 1995.

GRADUATES PER YEAR (APPROX.): 36 maximum.

MODALITIES AND SUBJECTS: acupressure, AMMA, aromatherapy, board preparation study group, body-mind, business I, II & III, chair massage, community internship, community service or research project, healing touch, hydrotherapy, infant massage, introduction to internship, kinesiology, lymphatic drainage, massage theory, medical massage, myofascial release, myotherapy, neuromuscular therapy, pathology, polarity, pregnancy massage, reflexology, reiki, shiatsu, specialized massage, sports massage, therapeutic touch, touch for health, trigger point therapy, wellness.

SCHOOL STATEMENT: Descriptions by our graduates: "Caring", "Holistic", "Small and respectful classes", "Effective massage routine", "reviewed a variety of modalities", "solid preparation for nationals and state boards."

NEVADA

No State licensing.

SCHOOLS:

#339 Dahan Institute of Massage Studies
3430 E. Tropicana, suite 62
Las Vegas, NV 89121
(702) 434-1338

Contact school for program information.

#340 Massage Academy of Reno
1296 E. Plumb Lane, suite M
Reno, NV 89502
(702) 826-5584 or 1-888-826-5584

HOURS OF TRAINING: 700.

DURATION OF COURSE: 6 months, evenings.

COST: $3,000 plus $120 books.

YEAR FOUNDED: 1997.

GRADUATES PER YEAR (APPROX.): 20.

MODALITIES AND SUBJECTS: AIDS awareness, body mechanics, building a clientele, business record keeping, designing the massage, educational kinesiology, first aid & CPR, getting ready to touch, history of massage, hygiene & sanitation & safety, indications & contraindications, kinesiology, marketing strategy, massage & the law, medical terminology, passive movement, passive stretching, pathology, practicum, professional development, professional ethics, resume writing, special populations, the scientific art of massage, wellness education.

#341 Nevada Career Institute
3025 E. Desert Inn Rd.
Las Vegas, NV 89121
(702) 893-3300

HOURS OF TRAINING: 540 (in-class hours not specified).

DURATION OF COURSE: 27 weeks, day & evening programs offered.

COST: $5,600 including books, uniform, lab supplies. Payment plan without interest is available.

FINANCIAL AID: Scholarships or discounts, Pell Grants, Student Loans.

YEAR FOUNDED: 1992.

ACCREDITATIONS/APPROVALS: ACCET, CEU's for nurses.

GRADUATES PER YEAR (APPROX.): 100.

MODALITIES AND SUBJECTS: acupressure, aromatherapy, business administration & job preparation, clinic & equipment & products, chair massage, CPR/first aid, healing touch, history & advancement of therapeutic massage, infant massage, kinesiology, law & ethics, lymphatic drainage, massage for nursing & health care, medical massage, pathology, polarity, pregnancy massage, reiki, safety & sanitation, shiatsu, specialized massage, sports massage, therapeutic exercises & physical fitness, therapeutic touch, trigger point therapy, yoga therapy.

#342 Northwest Massage School
7310 Smoke Ranch Rd., suite A
Las Vegas, NV 89128
(702) 254-7577

Contact school for program information.

#343 Physicians Institute of Therapeutic Massage
1140 Almond Tree Ln. #312
Las Vegas, NV 89104
(702) 369-5472

600-hour program. Contact school for program information.

#344 Ralston School of Massage
c/o Washoe Medical Center
77 Pringle Way, Reno, NV 89520-0109
(702) 328-5450

HOURS OF TRAINING: 560.

DURATION OF COURSE: 6 months to 2 years, day and evening programs available.

COST: $3,976.08 includes tuition, books, CPR, liability insurance.

YEAR FOUNDED: 1988.

GRADUATES PER YEAR (APPROX.): 50.

MODALITIES AND SUBJECTS: acupressure, TouchPro chair massage, hydrotherapy, strain counterstrain, stretching, sports massage, trigger point therapy.

SCHOOL STATEMENT: Ralston School of Massage strives to develop each student's individual abilities to facilitate an effective, well-planned, balanced and compassionate massage.

NEW HAMPSHIRE

New Hampshire: Graduates receive comprehensive instruction in human anatomy and physiology, pathology, different massage techniques and practices, ethics, law, hygiene, first aid, and therapeutic skills.

State Licensing: 750 hours.

National Certification Exam accepted.

  Board: (603) 271-4594

SCHOOLS:

#345 DoveStar Holistic Technology School
50 Whitehall Road
Hooksett, NH 03106-2104
(603) 669-9497 or (603) 669-5104

HOURS OF TRAINING: 750.

DURATION OF COURSE: average 12 months; varies with individual students' schedules; day and weekend programs available.

COST: $6,750.

FINANCIAL AID: work-study available.

YEAR FOUNDED: 1973.

ACCREDITATIONS/APPROVALS: American Council of Hypnotist Examiners.

GRADUATES PER YEAR (APPROX.): 70.

MODALITIES AND SUBJECTS: acupressure, alchemical hypnotherapy, alchemical synergy, colon hydrotherapy, kriya massage, reiki, reiki-alchemia, sports massage.

SCHOOL STATEMENT: Flexible program tailored to each student. Primary focus is on sensitivity and integration of physical, emotional release, and energy work for optimum benefits.

#346 New England Academy of Therapeutic Sciences
402 Amherst St.
Nashua, NH 03063
(603) 886-8433
www.neats.com

HOURS OF TRAINING: massage 950 (800 in-class); equine massage 1,400 (600 in-class); day and evening/weekend programs available.

COST: $7,250 includes books.

YEAR FOUNDED: 1992.

GRADUATES PER YEAR (APPROX): 60.

MODALITIES AND SUBJECTS: acupressure, biomechanics, breathwork, business practices, chair massage, circulatory massage, cranio-sacral therapy*, equine sports massage*, ethics, exercise physiology, first aid/CPR, homeopathy, hydrotherapy, lymphatic drainage, medical massage, myofascial release*, nutrition, pathology, polarity, practicum, public health and hygiene, reflexology, reflex point therapy, reiki, shiatsu, sports massage, trigger point therapy, tui na, yoga therapy. (*continuing education)

#347 New Hampshire Community Tech. College
505 Amherst St.
Nashua, NH 03061
(603) 882-7022
www.nashua.tec.nh.us

HOURS OF TRAINING: 825 (700 in-class hours).

DURATION OF COURSE: 1 to 2 years, day & evening & weekend programs available.

COST: $4,800 includes books and materials. Payment plan without interest is available.

FINANCIAL AID: Federal financial aid eligible program (Title IV).

YEAR FOUNDED: 1996.

PREPARATION FOR OUT-OF-STATE LICENSING EXAM: Program meets most states' requirements; contact school for specifics.

GRADUATES PER YEAR (APPROX.): 40.

MODALITIES AND SUBJECTS: acupressure, applied kinesiology, aromatherapy, deep tissue, esalen, hypnotherapy, jin shin do, kinesiology, medical massage, myofascial release, myotherapy, neuromuscular therapy, pathology, pregnancy massage, reflexology, russian massage, shiatsu, sports massage, trigger point therapy.

SCHOOL STATEMENT: Program strives to produce well-rounded, knowledgeable massage therapists with a balance of medical sciences and somatic arts.

#348 New Hampshire Community Technical College – Claremont
One College Drive
Claremont, NH 03743
(603) 542-7744 or 1-800-0658
www.nhctcs.tec.nh.us/

HOURS OF TRAINING: 850 hours (725 in-class hours plus 125 practical internship).

COST: $110 per credit (approx. $4,000 total).

YEAR FOUNDED: college 1968; massage program 1996.

GRADUATES PER YEAR (APPROX.): 12–20.

MODALITIES AND SUBJECTS: clinical evaluation & treatment, deep tissue massage, esalen, ethics & rules & business management, hydrotherapy, internship, kinesiology, pathology, pregnancy massage, reflexology, self-care & stress management, shiatsu, sports massage.

SCHOOL STATEMENT: The Massage Therapy Certificate program is designed with an emphasis on the biological sciences. Completion prepares the student for the NH and National Certification exams.

#349 New Hampshire Institute for Therapeutic Arts
153 Lowell Rd.
Hudson, NH 03051
(603) 882-3022

HOURS OF TRAINING: 750.

DURATION OF COURSE: 9 months, evenings & weekends.

COST: $5,600.

FINANCIAL AID: eligible institution for financial assistance from Canadian student aid.

YEAR FOUNDED: 1983.

ACCREDITATIONS/APPROVALS: COMTA/approved.

PREPARATION FOR OUT-OF-STATE LICENSING EXAM: As needed; have prepared for NY, FL, WA, OR.

GRADUATES PER YEAR (APPROX.): 36.

MODALITIES AND SUBJECTS: aromatherapy*, chair massage*, circulatory massage, cranio-sacral therapy, eastern techniques, eldersage* (geriatric), embryology, emergency procedures, equine sports massage*, ethics & professionalism, first aid & CPR, health service management, human sexuality, hydrotherapy, infant massage*, lymphatic drainage, medical massage, myofascial release, myotherapy, neuromuscular technique, nutrition, pathology, polarity, postural integration, pregnancy massage*, public health & hygiene, reflexology, shiatsu*, somatic therapy, sports massage, structural integration, touch for health,

trigger point therapy, yoga therapy*. (*continuing education)

SCHOOL STATEMENT: Education offered in a fearless and non-competitive environment, partaking of both the traditional and evolutionary. Professional preparation allowing flexibility to enter numerous career opportunities.

#350 North Eastern Institute of Whole Health, Inc.
School of Massage Therapy
22 Bridge St.
Manchester, NH 03101
(603) 623-5018

HOURS OF TRAINING: 750 (690 in-class hours).

DURATION OF COURSE: one year; programs available days, evenings, day & Saturday, evening & Saturday.

COST: $5,800 includes all books and handouts, t-shirt and supplies.

FINANCIAL AID: Veteran's Administration, NH Job Training Council.

YEAR FOUNDED: 1993.

GRADUATES PER YEAR (APPROX): 125.

MODALITIES AND SUBJECTS: acupressure, aromatherapy, business practices & marketing, chair massage, CPR, cranio-sacral therapy, equine massage, esalen massage, geriatric massage, history and theory of massage, hydrotherapy, hygiene, infant massage, lomilomi, lymphatic drainage, massage practicum, neuromuscular therapy, NLP, physical & emotional rebalancing, polarity, pregnancy massage, reflexology, rules & professionalism & ethics, shiatsu, sports massage, trigger point & pressure point therapy.

SCHOOL STATEMENT: For a healthier life, our philosophy is training massage therapists who heal the body, mind, and spirit through traditional and modern eastern and western modalities.

NEW JERSEY

No State licensing

SCHOOLS:

#351 Academy of Massage Therapy
401 S. Van Brunt Street, suite 204
Englewood, NJ 07631
(201) 568-3220

HOURS OF TRAINING: 50 to 769 hours.

DURATION OF COURSE: 6 days to one year, day & evening & weekend programs available.

COST: $595 to $6,350. Payment plan without interest is available.

YEAR FOUNDED: 1992.

GRADUATES PER YEAR (APPROX.): 75.

MODALITIES AND SUBJECTS: AMMA, body wisdom, business & marketing & management, chair massage, chi gong, clinic, community service, energetic healing, jin shin jitsu, medical massage, myology, NCE review, neurology, pain management, pathology, pregnancy massage, reflexology, reiki, shiatsu, sports massage, thai massage.

SCHOOL STATEMENT: Academy of Massage Therapy is as committed to your career as you are; great teachers, unique choice of programs, easy payment plans and excellent placement!

#352 Academy of Natural Health Sciences
102 Green Street
Woodbridge, NJ 07095
(732) 634-2155

Contact school for program information.

#353 Body, Mind & Spirit Learning Alliance
917-2 No. Main St.
Toms River, NJ 08753
(732) 349-7153

HOURS OF TRAINING: 550 (in-class hours not specified).

DURATION OF COURSE: one year, evenings & weekends.

COST: $4,800 includes books. Payment plan without interest is available.

YEAR FOUNDED: 1996.

GRADUATES PER YEAR (APPROX.): 8.

MODALITIES AND SUBJECTS: aromatherapy, business skills & independent practice, cranio-sacral therapy, five element theory, medical massage, neuromuscular therapy, reflexology, reiki, shiatsu, sports massage, trager, yoga.

SCHOOL STATEMENT: Our goal is to provide students with a thorough knowledge of massage techniques and an understanding of how the human body is affected by bodywork.

#354 Center for Therapeutic Massage School
963 Holmdel Road
Holmdel, NJ 07733
(908) 332-0333

Contact school for program information.

#355 The Center for Transpersonal Body/Mind Studies
51 Upland Ave.
Metuchen, NJ 08840
(732) 548-8579

HOURS OF TRAINING: 300 (200 hours in-class).

DURATION OF COURSE: 12 months, evenings and weekends.

COST: $2,450 includes text and additional courseware.

YEAR FOUNDED: 1970. Payment plan without interest is available.

ACCREDITATIONS/APPROVALS: approved for independent college credit, approved by Holistic Nurses Assn.

GRADUATES PER YEAR (APPROX.): 40.

MODALITIES AND SUBJECTS: acupressure, aromatherapy, bioenergetics, body-centered processing skills, body-mind, cranio-sacral therapy, cross-cultural massage and healing methods, folk healing, gestalt therapy, healing touch, medical intuition, medical massage, myofascial release, polarity, reflexology, shamanism, somatics, therapeutic touch, trager, transpersonal bodywork and psychology.

SCHOOL STATEMENT: Our faculty consists of a group of dedicated, experienced and innovative leaders, teachers, therapists and healers in the field of body-mind therapies.

#356 Garden State Center For Holistic Health Care
1203 Route 70 West
Lakewood, NJ 08701
(732) 364-0882

HOURS OF TRAINING: 675 (600 in-class hours).

DURATION OF COURSE: 6 months full-time or 12 months part-time.

COST: $5,195 including books and registration. Payment plan without interest is available.

FINANCIAL AID: Discounts for previous training or experience.

YEAR FOUNDED: 1992.

GRADUATES PER YEAR (APPROX.): 30.

MODALITIES AND SUBJECTS: acupressure, business management, chair massage, CPR, cranio-sacral therapy, crystal therapy, energy therapies, externship, infant massage, medical massage, myofascial release, myology, neurology, neuromuscular therapy, oriental bodywork, pathology, polarity, pregnancy massage, reflexology, reiki, sports massage, stress management, swedish theory & principles, therapeutic touch, trager, vedic massage, yoga therapy.

SCHOOL STATEMENT: Students learn the holistic approach in an environment which inspires self-confidence, enthusiasm and rapid learning. Safe and effective techniques, high standard of professional ethics.

#357 Healing Hands Institute for Massage Therapy
41 Bergenline Ave.
Westwood, NJ 07675
(201) 722-0099
www.HealingHandsInstitute.com

HOURS OF TRAINING: 600 or 1,000 (600 in-class).

DURATION OF COURSE: 6, 12 or 24 months, day and evening programs available.

COST: 600 hours $5,540, 1,000 hours $8,600(includes books). Payment plan without interest is available.

FINANCIAL AID: NJ State Workforce, Veteran's Administration.

YEAR FOUNDED: 1990.

ACCREDITATIONS/APPROVALS: COMTA/Accredited.

PREPARATION FOR OUT-OF-STATE LICENSING EXAM: New York.

GRADUATES PER YEAR (APPROX.): 120.

MODALITIES AND SUBJECTS: acupressure, applied kinesiology, aromatherapy, art of touch and biomechanics, body integration, business management, chair massage, chinese massage, deep tissue, hydrotherapy, medical massage, myofascial release, neuromuscular therapy, pathology, practicum, pregnancy massage, professional ethics, rebirthing, reflexology, shiatsu, sports massage.

SCHOOL STATEMENT: The mission of Healing Hands is to provide an education in the science of massage therapy with emphasis on the highest academic and practice standards.

#358 Healing Hands School of Massage
515 White Horse Pike
Haddon Heights, NJ 08035
(609) 546-7471

See listing for Healing Hands School of Massage, Philadelphia, PA.

#359 Health Choices Center for the Healing Arts
170 Township Line Rd., bldg. B
Belle Mead, NJ 08540
(908) 359-3995

HOURS OF TRAINING: 600 (526 in-class hours).

DURATION OF COURSE: one year, day & evening programs available.

COST: $5,885 plus $380 for books.

FINANCIAL AID: JPTA, WDP, DVA.

YEAR FOUNDED: 1978.

GRADUATES PER YEAR (APPROX.): 60.

MODALITIES AND SUBJECTS: acupressure, aromatherapy, body-mind, business skills, chair massage, infant massage, neuromuscular therapy, polarity, shiatsu, sports massage, yoga therapy.

SCHOOL STATEMENT: "Let us teach your hands to do your heart's work." Spirit, Mind, Body approach. We teach an integrated massage of Swedish, Shiatsu, Polarity, and Neuromuscular.

#360 Helma Corp. Institute of Massage Therapy
853 Garrison Ave.
Teaneck, NJ 07666
(201) 836-8176

HOURS OF TRAINING: 550 (includes 220 hours of supervised clinic practice)

DURATION OF COURSE: 7-9 months, 5 evening per week plus half-day Sunday

COST: $3,525 (includes required texts)

YEAR FOUNDED: 1984

GRADUATES PER YEAR (APPROX.): 50 to 75

MODALITIES AND SUBJECTS: business and marketing, chair massage, clinic practicum, CPR, geriatric massage, hydrotherapy, kinesiology, pathology, pregnancy massage, reflexology, shiatsu, sports massage

#361 Institute For Therapeutic Massage, Inc.
125 Wanaque Ave.
Pompton Lakes, NJ 07442
(973) 839-6131

HOURS OF TRAINING: 500 (in-class hours not specified)

DURATION OF COURSE: 9 months, day and evening programs available

COST: $4,200 including books and supplies. Payment plan without interest is available.

YEAR FOUNDED: 1994

GRADUATES PER YEAR (APPROX.): 70

MODALITIES AND SUBJECTS: applied energetic techniques, aromatherapy, business & ethics, chair massage, geriatric massage, intro. to oriental bodywork, massage for survivors of abuse, medical massage, myotherapy, pathology, pregnancy massage, reflexology, reiki, shiatsu, sports massage, trigger point therapy.

SCHOOL STATEMENT: We are committed to training competent, qualified, professional massage therapists, dedicated to a field where one person can make a difference in many other lives.

#362 JSG School of Massage Therapy at Loving Hands
676 Winters Ave.
Paramus, NJ 07652
(201) 265-3523

HOURS OF TRAINING: 550

DURATION OF COURSE: 6 months, evenings & weekends.

COST: $5,500 including books, materials and student insurance. Payment plan without interest is available.

FINANCIAL AID: Discount with early registration.

YEAR FOUNDED: 1997.

GRADUATES PER YEAR (APPROX.): 20.

MODALITIES AND SUBJECTS: acupressure, applied kinesiology, aromatherapy, business practices & ethics, chair massage, CPR, cranio-sacral therapy, geriatric massage, hydrotherapy, infant massage, kinesiology, lymphatic drainage, massage theory & practice, medical massage, myofascial release, NCE exam review, pregnancy massage, reflexology, reiki, shiatsu, sports massage, therapeutic touch, trager, trigger point therapy.

SCHOOL STATEMENT: The school is oriented for health professionals, especially nurses, and emphasizes the medical setting. Advanced standing is available giving credit for previous education and training.

#363 Kinley Institute for Massage and Related Studies
668 Raritan Road
Clark, NJ 07066
(732) 382-2434

Contact school for program information.

#364 Morris Institute of Natural Therapeutics
3108 Rt. 10 West
Denville, NJ 07834
(973) 989-8939
www.aromatherapy4u.com

HOURS OF TRAINING: 520 (in-class hours not specified).

DURATION OF COURSE: 25 weeks (6 months), day & evening & weekend programs available.

COST: $3,295 includes textbooks and handouts. Payment plan without interest is available.

YEAR FOUNDED: 1963.

GRADUATES PER YEAR (APPROX.): 75 (massage) 300 for related courses.

MODALITIES AND SUBJECTS: aromatherapy, business skills, chair massage, hygiene, insurance, legislation, professional ethics, reflexology, shiatsu, sports massage, touch for health.

SCHOOL STATEMENT: We strive to educate people in the natural healing modalities to maintain proper balance, mentally, physically and spiritually by channeling attitudes toward positive horizons.

#365 North Jersey Massage Training Center
3699 Rt. 46
Parsippany, NJ 07054
(973) 263-2229 or 402-1222

HOURS OF TRAINING: 500.

DURATION OF COURSE: 6 months; day, evening and weekend programs offered.

COST: $5,700, includes texts (discount for pre-payment).

YEAR FOUNDED: 1980.

MODALITIES AND SUBJECTS: barefoot shiatsu, chair massage, deep tissue, energetic bodywork, geriatric massage, neuromuscular therapy, pregnancy massage, spa techniques, tai chi, yoga.

SCHOOL STATEMENT: Our program combines Eastern energetic bodywork, traditional Barefoot Shiatsu, with advanced western modalities, i.e., neuromuscular and deep tissue techniques.

#366 Somerset School of Massage Therapy
120 Centennial Ave.
Piscataway, NJ
(732) 356-0787
www.massagecareer.com

HOURS OF TRAINING: 575.

DURATION OF COURSE: 6 months full time or 12 months part time, day and evening programs available.

COST: $5,385 (includes books). Payment plan without interest is available.

FINANCIAL AID: approved for veterans' benefits, some state funding programs.

YEAR FOUNDED: 1987.

ACCREDITATIONS/APPROVALS: COMTA/Accredited.

PREPARATION FOR OUT-OF-STATE LICENSING EXAM: Florida, Iowa.

MODALITIES AND SUBJECTS: acupressure, business & ethics, chair massage, chi gong, CPR/fist aid, cranio-sacral therapy, deep tissue massage, HIV/AIDS awareness, hydrotherapy, infant massage, myofascial release, neuromuscular therapy, pregnancy massage, reflexology, reiki, somatic therapy, sports massage, student clinic internship, tai chi, zero-balancing.

SCHOOL STATEMENT: We graduate massage therapists who are therapeutic and nurturing, anatomically specific and intuitive, with the business skills necessary for success in today's job market.

#367 Swedish American Massage Institute (SAMI)
       120 Maple Ave.
       Red Bank, NJ 07701
       (732) 530-1188

HOURS OF TRAINING: 500, day, evening and weekend classes plus optional workshops available.

COST: $4,965 includes books and materials.

FINANCIAL AID: scholarships, NJ Comm. for the Blind, NJ Dept. of Rehab.

YEAR FOUNDED: 1991.

GRADUATES PER YEAR (APPROX.): 36.

MODALITIES AND SUBJECTS: acupressure, applied kinesiology, aromatherapy, chair massage, lymphatic drainage, medical massage, myofascial release, pregnancy massage, reflexology, sports massage, therapeutic touch, trigger point therapy.

SCHOOL STATEMENT: Modules may be taken consecutively or spread out over two years to accommodate the busy adult student's scheduling and financial needs.

#368 Therapeutic Massage Training Center
       177 Weston Ave.
       Chatham, NJ 07928
       (Classroom: New Providence Chiropractic)
       (973) 635-4655

HOURS OF TRAINING: 500 (in-class hours not specified).

DURATION OF COURSE: 8 months (September to the following May).

COST: $4,125 including required books. Payment plan without interest is available.

YEAR FOUNDED: 1986.

GRADUATES PER YEAR (APPROX.): 12 (class size limited to maximum 12 students).

MODALITIES AND SUBJECTS: clinical massage, sports massage, reflexology.

NEW MEXICO

State Licensing: 650 hours

National Certification Exam accepted

  Board: (505) 476-7090

SCHOOLS:

#369 Crystal Mountain Apprenticeship in the
       Healing Arts
       118 Dartmouth SE
       Albuquerque, NM 87106
       (505) 268-4411

HOURS OF TRAINING: 700 (in-class hours not specified).

DURATION OF COURSE: 6 months, day and evening programs are available.

COST: $4,500 (includes books). Payment plan without interest is available.

FINANCIAL AID: work-study, loans, Vocational Rehabilitation, Human Resources Development Institute.

YEAR FOUNDED: 1988.

GRADUATES PER YEAR (APPROX.): 96.

MODALITIES AND SUBJECTS: abuse issues, applied kinesiology, aromatherapy, body-centered healing, body-mind, business skills, chair massage, clinical internship, CPR/first aid, cranio-sacral therapy, deep tissue massage, esalen, healing touch, herbology, hydrotherapy, interviewing techniques, kinesiology, lomi ha'a mauli-ola, lomilomi, movement re-education, neuromuscular therapy, nutrition, pathology, polarity, polar-reflexology, postural integration, pregnancy massage, process work, professional ethics, reflexology, shiatsu, sports massage, therapeutic exercise, trager, trigger point therapy, visceral manipulation therapy.

SCHOOL STATEMENT: Our mission is to provide quality education and to respectfully facilitate personal growth and healing through the integration of body, mind and spirit.

#370 Eastern New Mexico School of Massage Therapy
       P.O. Box 2142
       Clovis, NM 88101
       (505) 763-0551

HOURS OF TRAINING: 660.

DURATION OF COURSE: 10 months, weekends.

COST: $4,150 includes $150 book fee.

YEAR FOUNDED: 1997.

GRADUATES PER YEAR (APPROX.): 14.

MODALITIES AND SUBJECTS: biomechanics & postural analysis, business practices & ethics, chair massage, contraindications, cranio-sacral therapy, herbology, hydrotherapy, infant massage, lymphatic drainage, myofascial release, neuromuscular therapy, nutrition, polarity, pregnancy massage, reflexology, shiatsu, sports massage, trigger point therapy, yoga.

SCHOOL STATEMENT: Quality education and career development prepare graduates to become innovators in the field of massage therapy and bodywork.

#371 The Medicine Wheel
       1243 B West Apache
       Farmington, NM 87401
       (888)-327-1914
       www.acrnet.com/medicinewheel

HOURS OF TRAINING: LMT 735 (660 in-class); AOS 1,200 (1,020 in-class).

DURATION OF COURSE: LMT 8 months, evenings and weekends; AOS 20 months, days, evenings & weekends.

COST: LMT $5,000; AOS $9,000.

FINANCIAL AID: student loans, Veteran's Administration, Department of Vocational Rehabilitation.

ACCREDITATIONS/APPROVALS: IMSTAC.

YEAR FOUNDED: 1992.

GRADUATES PER YEAR (APPROX): 10.

MODALITIES AND SUBJECTS: aromatherapy, business practicum, chinese massage I & II (tui na), client relationship & stress management, counseling skills, cranio-sacral therapy I & II, diet & nutrition I & II, ethics, first aid & CPR, herbology I & II, hydrotherapy, legal issues, lymphatic drainage, mind-body connection, muscle bio-feedback, neuromuscular therapy I & II, polarity I & II, report writing & assessment, research paper, shiatsu I & II, therapeutic touch I & II, therapeutic yoga, TMJ work, traditional chinese medical theory.

SCHOOL STATEMENT: Emphasis is on tui-na and traditional chinese medical theory, in conjunction with the mind-body connection.

#372 Mesilla Valley School of Therapeutic Arts
       P.O. Box 1227, Mesilla, NM 88046
       Classroom: 741 N. Alameda, suite 15, Las Crusas,
       NM 88005
       (505) 527-1239

HOURS OF TRAINING: 700.

COST: $3,500 plus approx $200 books.

YEAR FOUNDED: 1987.

GRADUATES PER YEAR (APPROX.): 20.

MODALITIES AND SUBJECTS: acupressure, assessment, deep relaxation techniques, holistic health & hygiene, hydrotherapy, kinesiology, lymphatic massage, muscle energy techniques, myofascial release, pathology, practice development, professional ethics, reflexology, SOAP note charting, special populations, therapeutic movement, therapeutic touch, trigger point therapy.

SCHOOL STATEMENT: This ten-month program provides quality, eclectic massage education ranging from deep relaxation techniques to dealing with pain problems that require networking with other health professionals.

#373 **Muscle Therapy Center**
1711 North Jefferson
Hobbs, NM 88240
(505) 393-3425

HOURS OF TRAINING: 650.

COST: $3,500.

YEAR FOUNDED: 1994.

GRADUATES PER YEAR (APPROX.): 12.

MODALITIES AND SUBJECTS: connective tissue work, deep tissue, first aid & CPR, geriatric massage, human health & hygiene, hydrotherapy, kinesiology, lymphatic drainage, pediatric massage, practice development, pregnancy massage, professional ethics, reflexology, shiatsu, sports massage, therapeutic exercise, trigger point therapy.

#374 **New Mexico Academy of Healing Arts**
P.O. Box 932
Santa Fe, NM 87504
(505) 982-6271
www.nmhealingarts.org

HOURS OF TRAINING: 650 (502 in-class), 1,000 (896 in-class).

DURATION OF COURSE: 650-hours 6 months days or 12 months evenings; 1000-hour course nine months days.

COST: 650-hours $6,000; 1,000 hours $8,000.

FINANCIAL AID: Scholarships or discounts are available.

YEAR FOUNDED: 1981.

ACCREDITATIONS/APPROVALS: COMTA/approved, APTA.

GRADUATES PER YEAR (APPROX.): 125.

MODALITIES AND SUBJECTS: AMMA, anatomy with Manikens, aromatherapy, biosonics, body mechanics, chair massage, communication skills I & II, community meeting, cranio-sacral therapy, deep tissue, feldenkrais, first aid & CPR, medical massage, medicinal herbs, meditation, ortho-bionomy, polarity, pregnancy massage, professional development & ethics, reflexology, self-care, shiatsu, sports massage, student clinic, trigger point therapy, yoga therapy. Advanced programs: Associate Polarity Practitioner, Registered Polarity Practitioner, shiatsu, advanced sports/clinical massage.

SCHOOL STATEMENT: Through a cutting-edge curriculum and an organic approach to education, we graduate artistic and resourceful therapists into the dynamic healing arts profession every year.

#375 **New Mexico College of Natural Healing**
Box 211
Silver City, NM 88062
(Classroom: 3030 Pinos Altos Road)
(505) 538-0050 or 1-888-813-8311

HOURS OF TRAINING: 780.

DURATION OF COURSE: 9 months days or 18 months evenings & weekends.

COST: $5,500 plus $500 for text, insurance, supplies and two required massages.

FINANCIAL AID: Scholarships or discounts available.

YEAR FOUNDED: 1996.

GRADUATES PER YEAR (APPROX.): 20.

MODALITIES AND SUBJECTS: acupressure, advanced massage, authentic movement, bioenergetics, body movement, business & practice management, chi gong, clinical internship, clinical pathology, confidentiality, connective tissue, designing the massage or bodywork session, effects & benefits & contraindications, face & scalp massage, first aid & CPR, gestalt, getting ready to touch, heliotherapy, herbology, history of massage & bodywork, hydrotherapy, hygiene & sanitation & safety, infant massage, intuitive bodywork, kinesiology, lymphatic drainage, nutrition east, pregnancy massage, professional & legal issues, range of motion, reflexology, shiatsu, special populations, spinal release, structural integration, therapeutic exercises & techniques, traditional chinese medicine, trigger point therapy, voice therapy, wellness education.

SCHOOL STATEMENT: Come explore the magic of finding emotional and physical balance in your heart through movement, understanding, sensory awareness, vocalization, group discussion and touch.

#376 **New Mexico School of Natural Therapeutics**
202 Morningside SE
Albuquerque, NM 87108
(505) 268-6870 or 1-800-654-1675
www.nmsnt.org.nathealth

HOURS OF TRAINING: 750

YEAR FOUNDED: 1974.

ACCREDITATIONS/APPROVALS: COMTA/approved, NM Division of vocational rehabilitation.

PREPARATION FOR OUT-OF-STATE LICENSING EXAM: can be arranged; contact school for specifics.

GRADUATES PER YEAR (APPROX.): 100.

MODALITIES AND SUBJECTS: body-mind counseling skills, business procedures & professional ethics, deep tissue, first aid & CPR & hygiene, flower remedies, herbology, HIV education & alternative treatments, homeopathy, hydrotherapy, infant massage, internship & clinical practice, neuromuscular therapy, nutrition, philosophy of nature care, polarity, postural analysis, pregnancy massage, reflexology, shiatsu, sports massage, swedish gymnastics, tai chi & table posture.

SCHOOL STATEMENT: The school emphasizes energy work and holistic approaches. Core faculty have 10 to 18 years teaching experience at this school.

#377 **The Scherer Institute of Natural Healing**
935 Alto St.
Santa Fe, NM 87501
(505) 982-8398
www.newmexiconet.com/scher.htm

P.O. Box 2118 / 1337-H Gusdorf Rd.
Taos, NM 87571
(505) 751-3143

HOURS OF TRAINING: 750.

DURATION OF COURSE: 6 months full-time (days) or 11 months part-time (evenings/weekends).

COST: $6,250 including books.

FINANCIAL AID: scholarships and work-study.

YEAR FOUNDED: 1979.

ACCREDITATIONS/APPROVALS: COMTA/approved (Santa Fe only).

PREPARATION FOR OUT-OF-STATE LICENSING EXAM: program meets most states' requirements — contact school with specific inquiries.

GRADUATES PER YEAR (APPROX.): 80.

MODALITIES AND SUBJECTS: body-mind, business, chair massage, connective tissue, cranio-sacral therapy, hakomi bodywork, herbal medicine, hydrotherapy, infant massage, intuitive massage, medical massage, myofascial release, naturopathic principles & techniques, nurturing & therapeutic massage, orthobionomy, pathology, pregnancy massage, professional development, reflexology, shiatsu, somatic therapy, touch for health, trigger point therapy, watsu.

SCHOOL STATEMENT: We teach a grounded physiological and technical foundation in theory and practice while encouraging the development of sensitivity and presence. We support our graduates' success.

#378 Taos School of Massage
P.O. Box 208
Arroyo Seco, NM 87514
(classroom 1017 Dea Lane, Taos)
(505) 758-2725

HOURS OF TRAINING: 650.

DURATION OF COURSE: 7 to 12 months.

COST: $4,800.

FINANCIAL AID: Scholarships or discounts available.

YEAR FOUNDED: 1994.

GRADUATES PER YEAR (APPROX.): 7–12.

MODALITIES AND SUBJECTS: acupressure, applied kinesiology, body-centered facilitation, body-mind clearing, body reading, chair massage, chinese 5-element theory, deep connective tissue, herbology & nutrition, internal organ massage, lymphatic reflex point massage, mediation work, meridian massage, muscle testing, neuromuscular therapy, pregnancy massage, reality engineering, reflexology, shiatsu, sports massage, touch for health, trigger point therapy, tui na, yoga therapy.

SCHOOL STATEMENT: To train healers in BodyMind Clearing—a system combining Deep Tissue Massage, Applied Kinesiology, and Body Centered Facilitation Skills, within the Self-expression Model of Healing.

#379 Universal Therapeutic Massage Institute, Inc.
3410 Aztec Rd. NE
Albuquerque, NM 87107
(505) 888-0020 or 1-800-557-0020

HOURS OF TRAINING: 670 (520 in-class hours).

DURATION OF COURSE: 6 months, day and evening programs available.

COST: $3,850 plus tax (includes books). Payment plan without interest is available.

YEAR FOUNDED: 1993.

GRADUATES PER YEAR (APPROX.): 100.

MODALITIES AND SUBJECTS: applied kinesiology, aromatherapy, business, chair massage, chi gong, clinic internship, CPR & first aid, cranio-sacral therapy, ethics, exercise, hydrotherapy, infant massage, interview techniques, joint mobilization, lymphatic drainage, massage theory & history, medical massage, myofas-

cial therapy, neuromuscular therapy, palpation, polarity, pregnancy massage, range of motion, reflexology, relaxation, shiatsu, sports massage, stress management, touch for health, trigger point therapy, zero-balancing.

SCHOOL STATEMENT: small class size for personal attention.

#380 White Mountain School of Applied Healing
1204 Mechem #10
Ruidoso, NM 88345
(505) 258-3046

HOURS OF TRAINING: 654 (in-class hours not specified).

DURATION OF COURSE: one year, weekends.

COST: $3,800 including books and lab fee.

YEAR FOUNDED: 1997.

GRADUATES PER YEAR (APPROX.): 10.

MODALITIES AND SUBJECTS: acupressure, applied kinesiology, aromatherapy, body-mind, business, chair massage, deep tissue, herbal medicine, infant massage, lymphatic drainage, massage in a doctor's office, medical massage, myofascial release, neuromuscular therapy, postural integration, public relations, reflexology, reiki, shiatsu, sports massage, structural integration, tai chi, trigger point therapy.

SCHOOL STATEMENT: Healing of Body, Mind and Spirit with a strong medical background. Working with student's individual talents.

NEW YORK

State Licensing: 605 hours.

National Certification Exam not accepted.

  Board: (518) 474-3817 or 474-3866

APPROVED OUT-OF-STATE SCHOOLS:

Connecticut Center for Massage Therapy, Pennsylvania School of Muscle Therapy, Sarasota School of Massage Therapy.

SCHOOLS:

#381 Finger Lakes School of Massage
1251 Trumansburg Road
Ithaca, NY 14850
(607) 272-9024
www.flsm.com

HOURS OF TRAINING: 850.

DURATION OF COURSE: 5½ months full-time, 2 years weekends + advanced workshops.

COST: $7,100 includes required books and study guides.

FINANCIAL AID: Veteran's Administration, VESID, JTPA.

YEAR FOUNDED: 1993.

PREPARATION FOR OUT-OF-STATE LICENSING EXAM: Florida and Hawaii.

GRADUATES PER YEAR (APPROX.): 140.

MODALITIES AND SUBJECTS: aromatherapy, business practices, chair massage, communication skills, connective tissue therapy, directed independent study, energy palpation, hydrotherapy, infant massage, kinesiology, massage practicum with disabled adults & children & people with AIDS & senior citizens, medical massage, neuromuscular therapy, polarity, pregnancy massage, reflexology, shiatsu, sports massage, structural integration, trager, trigger point therapy, yoga therapy.

SCHOOL STATEMENT: Our primary goal is to offer a high-quality massage education in a caring, mutually respectful environment, promoting health, acceptance, personal inquiry and compassion.

**#382 The New Center College For Wholistic Health
Education & Research
School for Massage Therapy**
6801 Jericho Turnpike, suite 300
Syosset, NY 11791-4413
(516) 364-0808 or 1-800-922-7337
www.newcenter.edu

HOURS OF TRAINING: 1,230 / 63 credits (Associate in Occupational Studies).

DURATION OF COURSE: 16 months (4 trimesters), courses offered days and evenings.

COST: $250 per credit (plus texts, supplies and massage table approximately $1,300).

FINANCIAL AID: Federal Pell grants, Stafford Loans, SLS/Plus, Veteran's Administration, Vocational Rehabilitation, Tuition Assistance Program.

YEAR FOUNDED: 1981.

ACCREDITATIONS/APPROVALS: NY Board of Regents, NY Dept. of Education, ACCET, COMTA/Accredited.

GRADUATES PER YEAR (APPROX.): 400.

MODALITIES AND SUBJECTS: AMMA therapy basic technique I & II and applied technique I & II, anatomy & physiology I & II, aromatherapy, bindegewebsmassage, chair massage, chi gong, craniosacral therapy, ethics & professional development I & II, european technique I & II and applied technique, infant massage, kinesiology, massage therapy clinic I & II, myofascial release, myology I & II, neurology, neuromuscular therapy, oriental anatomy & physiology I & II, oriental clinical assessment, ortho-bionomy, pathology I & II, pregnancy massage, public health, reflexology, shiatsu, sports massage, t'ai chi chuan I, II, III & IV, tui na.

SCHOOL STATEMENT: The mission of The New Center College is to transform health care in the United States and improve the quality of life of Americans.

#383 New York Institute of Massage
P.O. Box 645
Buffalo, NY 14231
(716) 633-0355 or 1-800-884-6946 (NYIM)

HOURS OF TRAINING: 735 (675 in-class).

DURATION OF COURSE: 30 weeks, morning, afternoon and evening programs available.

COST: $6,750.

FINANCIAL AID: GI bill, JTPA, VESID, VVTA, TRA, DWF, Commission of the Blind.

YEAR FOUNDED: 1994.

GRADUATES PER YEAR (APPROX.): 110.

MODALITIES AND SUBJECTS: business management, community service (20 hours), CPR & first aid, exercise physiology, health and hygiene, hydrotherapy, infection control, myology, neurology, neuromuscular therapy, NY massage law, oriental massage, pathology, sports massage, student clinic (40 hours).

#384 Onondaga School of Therapeutic Massage
220 Walton St.
Syracuse, NY 13202
(315) 424-1159

HOURS OF TRAINING: 800 (in-class hours not specified).

DURATION OF COURSE: 6 months full-time, 12 months part-time; day, evening & weekend programs available.

COST: $7,350 includes books and fees.

FINANCIAL AID: Scholarships or discounts are available.

YEAR FOUNDED: 1997.

GRADUATES PER YEAR (APPROX.): 100.

MODALITIES AND SUBJECTS: applied kinesiology, chair massage, hydrotherapy, infant massage, medical massage, pregnancy massage, shiatsu, soft tissue, sports massage.

**#385 Swedish Institute, Inc.
School of Massage Therapy**
226 West 26th St., Fifth Floor
New York, NY 10001
(212) 924-5900

HOURS OF TRAINING: 694.

DURATION OF COURSE: 12 months.

DAY/EVENING/WEEKEND: day and evening programs available.

COST: $7,035 plus approximately $500 for books and uniforms.

FINANCIAL AID: Stafford Loans, Unsubsidized Stafford Loans, Parent Plus Loans, Pell grants; contact school financial aid officer for information regarding eligibility.

YEAR FOUNDED: 1916.

GRADUATES PER YEAR (APPROX): 600.

ACCREDITATIONS/APPROVALS: COMTA/approved, Career College Association, New York Bureau of Veterans Education, Commission for the Blind and Visually Handicapped, New York Department of Vocational Education for Individuals with Disabilities, Department of Immigration and Naturalization.

PREPARATION FOR OUT-OF-STATE LICENSING EXAM: can be arranged — contact school.

MODALITIES AND SUBJECTS: arthrology, business practices seminar, clinical internship program, CPR, deep tissue, first aid, joint kinesiology, manipulation, medical massage, pathology, shiatsu.

SCHOOL STATEMENT: Students work in a medically-oriented clinic, treating patients referred by their doctors.

NORTH CAROLINA

No State licensing.

SCHOOLS:

#386 Body Therapy Institute at South Wind Farm
300 South Wind Road
Siler City, NC 27344
(919) 663-3111 or 1-888-4500

HOURS OF TRAINING: 650 (605 in-class).

DURATION OF COURSE: 8 months days or 12 months evenings & weekends.

COST: $6,850 includes books.

FINANCIAL AID: work-study.

YEAR FOUNDED: 1983.

ACCREDITATIONS/APPROVALS: Licensed by NC Comm. Coll. System, COMTA/approved.

PREPARATION FOR OUT-OF-STATE LICENSING EXAM: Florida.

GRADUATES PER YEAR (APPROX.): 64.

MODALITIES AND SUBJECTS: alexander, aromatherapy, body-mind, business & marketing, chair massage, community service project, cranio-sacral therapy, hakomi, hydrotherapy, myofascial release, optimal body mechanics, oriental bodywork, personal integration, polarity, professional ethics & laws, reflexology, shiatsu, somatic psychology, somatic therapy, sports massage, structural integration, supervised clinical practicum, trager, yoga therapy. Advanced programs: orthopedic massage, teacher training.

SCHOOL STATEMENT: Combining Eastern and Western bodywork approaches in a model that supports healing and integration of the whole person—at our 150-acre country campus.

#387 Carolina School of Massage Therapy
103 W. Weaver St
Carrboro, NC 27510
(919) 933-2212

YEAR FOUNDED: 1987.

ACCREDITATIONS/APPROVALS: COMTA/approved.

#388 Forsyth Technical Community College
2100 Silas Creek Parkway
Winston-Salem, NC 27103

HOURS OF TRAINING: 590 (520 in-class).

DURATION OF COURSE: 42 weeks days, one year mornings or evenings.

COST: $2,500 including books.

GRADUATES PER YEAR (APPROX.): 25.

MODALITIES AND SUBJECTS: aromatherapy, business, chair massage, chi gong, CPR, deep tissue, hands on anatomy, infant massage, myofascial release, neuromuscular therapy, polarity, pregnancy massage, sports massage, therapeutic touch, trigger point therapy.

SCHOOL STATEMENT: At FTCC we take pride in offering top quality education at a low price. Our goal is for our students to succeed!

#389 Gaston College
201 Highway 321 South
Dallas, NC 28034-1499
(704) 922-6379

Contact school for program information.

#390 Georgetown Bodyworks Healing Arts Institute
1213 Thomas Avenue
Charlotte, NC 28205
(704) 335-0050
www.imagroup.com and www.learnmassage.com

HOURS OF TRAINING: 150 or 750 (50 or 250 in-class hours).

DURATION OF COURSE: 150 hours, 6 to 12 months; 750 hours, 18 to 24 months.

COST: 150 hours $2,195, 750 hours $4,995 both including table, bodyCushion, books, sheets and oil. Payment plan without interest is available.

FINANCIAL AID: Scholarships for single mothers.

YEAR FOUNDED: 1982 (Georgetown Bodyworks, Washington DC).

MODALITIES AND SUBJECTS: Canadian Deep Muscle Massage, Reach Therapy™, Bounce Therapy™.

SCHOOL STATEMENT: Loving, caring, **safe touch** should be part of American life. We are committed to teaching **safe structured touch** to everyone interested. Help us heal America.

#391 Gloria's Asthenic Therapy School
101 McFayden Dr.
Fayetteville, NC 28314
(910) 487-5115 or 609-9562 (pager)

HOURS OF TRAINING: 500.

DURATION OF COURSE: 19 weeks, evenings & Saturdays.

COST: $3,500.

FINANCIAL AID: Scholarships or discounts available.

YEAR FOUNDED: 1998.

MODALITIES AND SUBJECTS: acupressure, advanced massage & bodywork, aromatherapy, berrywork, business & marketing, chair massage, CPR, deep tissue, HIV/AIDS, hygiene & posture, law & ethics, massage as a healing practice, pathology, reflexology, sports massage.

The Institute Of Integrative Health
143 Woodview Road
Rutherfordton, NC 28139
(828) 287-0955
www.blueridge.net/~wholeyou

Information received after deadline; contact school for details.

#392 North Carolina School of Natural Healing
Rm. 510 – 20 Battery Park Ave.
Asheville, NC 28801
(704) 252-7096

HOURS OF TRAINING: 625 (also offered: 500-hour Enlightenment and Energy Healing)

DURATION OF COURSE: 9½ months, evening & weekend programs available.

COST: $5,200 plus $425 books. Payment plan without interest is available.

FINANCIAL AID: Scholarships or discounts for hardship.

YEAR FOUNDED: 1991.

GRADUATES PER YEAR (APPROX.): 22.

MODALITIES AND SUBJECTS: acupressure, aromatherapy, business practices & professionalism, chi gong, clinical pathology, connective tissue massage & structural rebalancing, cranio-sacral therapy, esalen, joint mobilization, massage & bodywork theory & assessment & practice, movement awareness & reeducation, myofascial release, neuromuscular therapy, polarity, reiki, shiatsu, structural integration, trager, trigger point therapy, yoga therapy.

SCHOOL STATEMENT: Spiritual and energetical orientation to grounded technical training. Meditation, mindfulness, clairvoyance and clairsentience integrated into a standard core curriculum.

#393 North Carolina School of the Healing Arts
400 Oberlin Rd., suite 140
Raleigh, NC 27605
(919) 821-1444

HOURS OF TRAINING: 10 to 2,000 (10 to 1,000 in-class hours).

DURATION OF COURSE: one weekend to several years, day & evening & weekend programs available.

COST: 10 hours $165.00; 30 hours $1,400; 125 hours $1,750; 400 hours $5,600; 525 hours $6,850; 1,000 hours $12,000; 2,000 hours $22,000. Prices include workbooks, classroom supplies.

YEAR FOUNDED: 1992.

GRADUATES PER YEAR (APPROX.): 10.

MODALITIES AND SUBJECTS: acupressure, applied kinesiology, aromatherapy, bioenergetics, bio-magnets, body-mind, chair massage, dowsing, geriatric massage, herbology, holistic massage, hypnotherapy, infant massage, lymphatic drainage, medical massage, naturopathic massage, neuromuscular therapy, pregnancy massage, reflexology, reiki, structural integration, yoga therapy.

SCHOOL STATEMENT: Our standard is based on twenty years of successful practice. Each individual has their own innate blueprint. Prevention is the key focus, maintenance a requirement.

#394 Sandhills Community College, Continuing Ed. Dept.
2200 Airport Road
Pinehurst, NC 28374
(910) 695-3766

HOURS OF TRAINING: 650.

DURATION OF COURSE: 3 semesters, 3 evenings per week.

COST: $3,000 includes books.

YEAR FOUNDED: 1998.

MODALITIES AND SUBJECTS: acupressure, applied kinesiology, aromatherapy, body electric massage, body-mind, chair massage, cranio-sacral therapy, healing touch, herbs, hydrotherapy, infant massage, medical massage with Einsteinian approach, myomassology techniques (19), polarity, pregnancy massage, reflexology, reiki, shiatsu, sports massage, therapeutic touch, touch for health, trigger point therapy.

#395 The Southeastern School of Neuromuscular and Massage Therapy, Inc.
4 Woodlawn Green, suite 200
Charlotte, NC 28217
(704) 527-3104
www.se-massage.com

HOURS OF TRAINING: 500.

DURATION OF COURSE: 6 months full-time or one year part-time. Morning, evening and weekend programs available.

COST: $5,300.

YEAR FOUNDED: 1994.

GRADUATES PER YEAR (APPROX.): 100–150.

MODALITIES AND SUBJECTS: business, clinical neuromuscular & structural bodywork (certification included in 500-hour program), ethics, hydrotherapy, laws & rules. Advanced program: 100 hour certification in Clinical Neuromuscular and Structural Bodywork by Kyle C. Wright (local instructors vary).

SCHOOL STATEMENT: Specializing in the training of the clinical therapist who typically works for or is referred to by physicians and other health care practitioners.

#396 Therapeutic Massage Training Institute
726 East Blvd.
Charlotte, NC 28203
(704) 338-9660

HOURS OF TRAINING: 600.

DURATION OF COURSE: 13 months, evenings & weekends.

COST: $5,435. Payment plan without interest is available.

FINANCIAL AID: NC State Vocational Rehab.

YEAR FOUNDED: 1986.

GRADUATES PER YEAR (APPROX.): 32.

MODALITIES AND SUBJECTS: acupressure, aromatherapy, bindegewebsmassage, business & marketing, chair massage, deep tissue, ethics, infant massage, kinesiology, lymphatic drainage, medical massage, movement therapy, myofascial release, nutrition, polarity, reflexology, sports massage, treatment & evaluation.

SCHOOL STATEMENT: We provide a supportive professional environment where students strengthen awareness and sensitivity while learning the scientific and technical application of therapeutic massage.

NORTH DAKOTA

State licensing requires 500 hours.

National Certification Exam not accepted.

Board: (701) 225-3906

The Board recommends AMTA-approved schools and offers reciprocity only to AMTA members.

SCHOOL:

#397 Sister Rosalind Gefre Schools of Professional Massage
Fargo, ND

For information about this school, please contact Sister Rosalind's Rochester, MN school at 300 Elton Hills Drive, Rochester, MN 55901 (507) 286-8608.

OHIO

State Licensing: 600 hours over at least 12 months.

National Certification Exam not accepted.

Board: (614) 466-3934

APPROVED OUT-OF-STATE SCHOOLS

Academy of Somatic Healing Arts, GA; Atlanta School of Massage, GA; Blue Cliff School, LA; Boulder School of Massage Therapy, Boulder, CO; Brenneke School of Massage, Seattle, WA; Chicago School of Massage Therapy, Chicago, IL; Desert Institute of the Healing Arts, Tucson, AZ; Desert Resorts School, CA; Florida Institute, Oviedo, FL (formerly Reese Institute); Hawaiian Islands School, HI; Health Enrichment Center, Lapeer, MI; Massage Therapy Institute of Colorado; New Center, Syosset, NY; New Mexico Academy of Healing Arts, Santa Fe, NM; Swedish Institute, New York, NY; Utah College of Massage Therapy, UT; Utting School of Massage, WA.

SCHOOLS:

#398 American Institute of Massotherapy
212 Jefferson St.
Tiffin, OH 44883
(419) 448-1355
www.tiffinohio.com/aim/

Contact school for program information.

#399 Central Ohio School of Massage
1120 Morse Rd., suite 250
Columbus, OH 43229
(614) 841-1122 or (800) 466-5676

HOURS OF TRAINING: 670.

DURATION OF COURSE: 18 months.

DAY/EVENING/WEEKEND: day and evening programs available.

COST: $5,850 plus application fee.

FINANCIAL AID: payment plan.

YEAR FOUNDED: 1964.

ACCREDITATIONS/APPROVALS: COMTA/approved.

MODALITIES AND SUBJECTS: pathology, ethics, business practices, patient approach, uses of heat and cold, restorative exercises

ADVANCED PROGRAMS: 170-hour MyoFascial Therapist program.

#400 Cincinnati School of Medical Massage
11250 Cornell Park Dr., #203
Cincinnati, OH 45242
(513) 469-6300

Contact school for program information.

#401 Cleveland School of Massage/Advanced Bodywork Institute
10683 Ravenna Road
Twinsburg, OH 44087
(330) 405-1933

HOURS OF TRAINING: 100+.

DURATION OF COURSE: 4 months, one day per week.

COST: $2,400 including book and course materials. Payment plan without interest is available.

YEAR FOUNDED: 1996.

GRADUATES PER YEAR (APPROX.): 54.

MODALITIES AND SUBJECTS: business skills, polarity, reflexology. This program is for those who wish to do general massage as a career, not massage therapy; this is not a state licensing program. The Advanced Bodywork Institute is for already licensed massage therapists, and teaches counter strain, M.E.T., myofascial release, myotherapy, neuromuscular therapy, ortho-bionomy, polarity, reflexology, reiki, structural integration, trigger point therapy.

SCHOOL STATEMENT: To empower people with the gift of healing self and others through education, in a supportive environment that encourages self-growth.

#402 Columbus Academy of Medical Massage
4207 E. Broad St., ste A
(classroom 3600 Main St., Hilliard)
Columbus, OH 43213-1200
(614) 777-1161

HOURS OF TRAINING: 136 or 650.

DURATION OF COURSE: 17 weeks or 12 months, day and evening programs available.

COST: 136 hours $1,750; 650 hours $6,050 including lab shirt, liability insurance, all required texts. Payment Plan without interest is available.

FINANCIAL AID: Scholarships or discounts available.

YEAR FOUNDED: 1994.

GRADUATES PER YEAR (APPROX.): 25.

MODALITIES AND SUBJECTS: acupressure, AMMA, applied kinesiology, applied muscle anatomy, aromatherapy, business principles, canine & feline massage, clinical practice, equine sports massage, ethics, hygiene, infant massage, massage theory, massage practical, medical massage, myofascial release, neuromuscular therapy, pregnancy massage, reflexology, sports massage, touch for health, trigger point therapy.

SCHOOL STATEMENT: The Academy's mission: provide superior education utilizing varied approach that instills empathy and integrity; promote individual development in the ever-expanding field of massage therapy.

#403 Columbus State Community College
550 E. Spring St.
Columbus, OH 43216
(614) 227-5353

Contact school for program information.

#404 Dayton School of Medical Massage
4457 Far Hills Ave
Dayton, OH 45429
(937) 294-6994

Contact school for program information.

#405 EHOVE Adult Career Center – Massage Therapy Program
316 West Mason Rd.
Milan, OH 44846
(419) 627-9665 or 499-4663

HOURS OF TRAINING: 600.

DURATION OF COURSE: 18 months, day and evening programs available.

COST: $6,000 plus approx. $350 for books, application fee, uniform and misc.

FINANCIAL AID: Contact school.

YEAR FOUNDED: 1997.

MODALITIES AND SUBJECTS: business, chair massage, ethics, first aid & CPR, massage theory & practicum, myofascial release, neuromuscular therapy.

#406 Hocking College
3301 Hocking Parkway
Nelsonville, OH 45764
(740) 753-3591 or (800) 282-4163

Contact school for program information.

#407 Massage Away School of Therapy
6685 Doubletree Avenue
Columbus, OH 43229
(614) 825-MAST (6278)

HOURS OF TRAINING: 710.

DURATION OF COURSE: 40 weeks, 18 months or 24 months, day & evening & weekend classes available.

COST: $6,000. Payment plan without interest is available.

FINANCIAL AID: Early tuition payment discount.

YEAR FOUNDED: 1994.

GRADUATES PER YEAR (APPROX.): 52.

MODALITIES AND SUBJECTS: business, chi gong, communication, cranio-sacral therapy, ergonomics for massage therapists, ethics, geriatric massage, infant massage, massage theory, myofascial release, neuromuscular therapy, reflexology, shiatsu, SOAP charting, sports massage, student clinic, working with HIV+ persons, yoga therapy.

SCHOOL STATEMENT: MAST's mission is to teach, nurture and develop massage therapists in their own individual style, art and energy through basic and continuing education.

#408 Midwestern College of Massotherapy
Office: 3857 East Broad St.
Classroom: 3589 E. Main St.
Columbus, OH 43213
(614) 231-1973

Not a state-approved school; graduates are not eligible for state licensing exam.

#409 National Institute of Massotherapy
2110 Copley Rd.
Akron, OH 44320
(330) 867-1996

National Institute of Massotherapy
(Cleveland Branch)
12684 Rockside Rd.
Garfield Hts., OH 44125
(216) 662-6955

HOURS OF TRAINING: 740.

DURATION OF COURSE: one year full-time two years part-time; day and evening programs, all programs meet some weekends.

COST: $7,450.

FINANCIAL AID: scholarships, veterans benefits, retraining programs.

YEAR FOUNDED: 1991.

GRADUATES PER YEAR (APPROX.): 120.

MODALITIES AND SUBJECTS: alexander technique, aromatherapy, business, chair massage, cranio-sacral therapy, feldenkrais, hydrotherapy, infant massage, lymphatic drainage, neuromuscular therapy certification, neurolymphatic reflexes, ortho-bionomy certification, polarity certification, postural integration, pregnancy massage, reflexology, reiki, shiatsu, sports massage, therapeutic touch, touch for health.

SCHOOL STATEMENT: NIM is dedicated to helping students achieve proficiency in therapeutic skills and developing the personal awareness necessary for a successful practice in bodywork.

#410 North Central Technical College
2441 Kenwood Circle
Mansfield, OH 44901
(419) 755-4800

Contact school for program information.

#411 Northeast Ohio College of Massotherapy
3507 Canfield Rd.
Youngstown, OH 44511
(330) 793-7562

Contact school for program information.

#412 Northwest Academy of Massotherapy, Inc.
1910 Indian Wood Circle, suite 301
Maumee, OH 43537
(419) 893-6464

HOURS OF TRAINING: 640.

DURATION OF COURSE: 18 months, day and evening programs available.

COST: approx. $6,500.

YEAR FOUNDED: 1995.

GRADUATES PER YEAR (APPROX.): 40 to 60.

MODALITIES AND SUBJECTS: business principles, chair massage*, massage practical & clinical, massage theory, medical terminology, myofascial release*, neuromuscular therapy*, reflexology, sports massage*. (*continuing education)

SCHOOL STATEMENT: Furnish professional knowledge to achieve therapeutic massage skills, develop communication skills, and personal awareness, all to function independently as successful career in massage therapy.

Ohio Academy of Holistic Health, Inc.
3033 Dayton-Xenia Rd.
Dayton, OH 45434
1-800-833-8122 or (937) 427-0506

Information received after deadline; contact school for details.

#413 Self-Health, Inc. School of Medical Massage
P.O. Box 474
130 Cook Road
Lebanon, OH 45036
(513) 932-8712

HOURS OF TRAINING: approximately 726.

DURATION OF COURSE: 18 months evenings or 12 months days.

COST: $6,425 includes book & lab fees & some supplies.

YEAR FOUNDED: 1980.

ACCREDITATIONS/APPROVALS: COMTA/approved.

GRADUATES PER YEAR (APPROX.): 75.

MODALITIES AND SUBJECTS: business practices & Ohio state law, cadaver study class, death & dying, dural membrane/tube release, functional symmetry, half-day clinical with Dr. Heather Morgan, M.D., indications & contraindications, integument pathology, intra-interpersonal dynamics, myofascial therapy, neuromuscular pain & assessment, palpatory & verbal assessment skills, polarity, structural & functional analysis and assessment, symptomology, therapeutic touch.

SCHOOL STATEMENT: SHI is a private, professional, career-oriented school with a tradition of humanistic education committed to the professional development of individuals entering the healthcare profession.

#414 Tri-State College of Massotherapy
Woodworth Prof. Ctr., 9159 Market St., ste. 43
North Lima, OH 44452
(330) 629-9998

Contact school for program information.

#415 The Youngstown College of Massotherapy, Inc.
14 Highland Ave.
Struthers, OH 44471
(330) 755-1406 or 1-800-454-1406

HOURS OF TRAINING: 605 (in-class hours not specified).

DURATION OF COURSE: 18 months, day & evening & weekend programs available.

COST: $6,300. Payment Plan without interest is available.

FINANCIAL AID: Discount for prepayment.

YEAR FOUNDED: 1995.

ACCREDITATIONS/APPROVALS: Approved for Veterans' Training.

GRADUATES PER YEAR (APPROX.): 60.

MODALITIES AND SUBJECTS: aromatherapy, chair massage, clinical, CPR, cranio-sacral therapy, equine sports massage, healing touch, massage theory & practicum, medical massage, neuromuscular therapy, postural integration, reflexology, sports massage, trigger point therapy.

OKLAHOMA

No State licensing.

SCHOOLS:

#416 Central State Massage Academy
8440 N.W. Expressway, One Market Square
Oklahoma City, OK 73162
(405) 722-4560

HOURS OF TRAINING: 600 (300 in-class hours).

DURATION OF COURSE: 30 weeks, evenings and weekends.

COST: $1,981 including supply kit and textbook.

YEAR FOUNDED: 1995.

MODALITIES AND SUBJECTS: acupressure, aromatherapy, business practices, chair massage, contraindications, day spa treatments, hydrotherapy, hygiene, infant massage, pregnancy massage, professional ethics, reflexology, sports massage.

SCHOOL STATEMENT: This program covers the basics of massage therapy, with emphasis on anatomy and physiology. Students are encouraged to create their own style.

#417 Massage Therapy Institute of Oklahoma
9433 East 51st St., suite H
Tulsa, OK 74145
(918) 622-6644

HOURS OF TRAINING: 250 (200 in-class) or 500 (400 in-class).

DURATION OF COURSE: 250 hours 16 weeks, 500 hours 32 weeks, days and evening programs available.

COST: 250 hours $2,000, 500 hours $4,000. Payment plan without interest is available.

FINANCIAL AID: Scholarships or discounts available.

YEAR FOUNDED: 1992.

GRADUATES PER YEAR (APPROX.): 36.

MODALITIES AND SUBJECTS: acupressure, body-mind, body psychology, business & ethics, chair massage, chronic pain massage, clinical practicum I & II, connective tissue & deep tissue techniques, cranio-sacral therapy, first aid/CPR, geriatric massage, hydrotherapy, hygiene, massage for specific conditions, medical & clinical terminology, medical massage, myofascial release, neuromuscular therapy, passive joint movement, passive stretching, pathology, postural integration, practice management, pregnancy massage, range of motion, reflexology, shiatsu, spa standards, sports massage, structural integration, subtle bodywork, trigger point therapy.

SCHOOL STATEMENT: We provide quality education to achieve professional competency in Therapeutic Massage and Bodywork. We are committed to public education, community service, and high standards.

#418 The Oklahoma School of Natural Healing
       1660 E. 71st St., suite 2-0
       Tulsa, OK 74136
       (918) 496-9401

HOURS OF TRAINING: technician 250 (140 in-class), therapist 650 (420 in-class), master therapist 1,000 (in-class hours not specified).

DURATION OF COURSE: technician 3½ month plus practicum, therapist 10 months plus practicum, master therapist 2 years plus practicum.

COST: technician $1,950.15, therapist $4,436.95, master therapist $7,854.95. All courses include equipment, massage table, wall charts and oil.

FINANCIAL AID: job training partnership act, vocational rehabilitation.

YEAR FOUNDED: 1980.

GRADUATES PER YEAR (APPROX.): 30.

MODALITIES AND SUBJECTS: acupressure, business skills and ethics, carpal tunnel massage, chair massage, cranio-sacral therapy, deep tissue therapies, heliotherapy, herbology, hydrotherapy, lymphatic drainage, myofascial release, nutrition, orthobionomy, polarity, reflexology, total body modification.

SCHOOL STATEMENT: We educate you to listen to the tissues of the body and appropriately respond, providing the ultimate experience of massage for your clients and yourself.

#419 Praxis College
       808 NW 88th St.
       Oklahoma City, OK 73114
       (405) 949-2244

HOURS OF TRAINING: 500 or 1,200.

DURATION OF COURSE: 500 hours 6 months; 1,200 hours two years, evenings.

COST: 500 hours $500, 1,200 hours $3,000. Payment plan without interest is available.

FINANCIAL AID: scholarships and discounts available.

YEAR FOUNDED: founded 1976, state licensed 1987.

MODALITIES AND SUBJECTS: apprenticeship, aromatherapy, bath attendant, business, chair massage, energy field massage, ethics, externship, human relations, hydrotherapy, Knieppism, massage for the childbearing year, non-traditional medicine, nutrition, oriental massage, origins of the profession, pain control, pharmacology and pathology, physical assessment, pregnancy, infant and geriatric massage, psychotherapeutic massage, re-

flexology, skilled touch, sports massage, supervised practice, techniques of healthy living.

SCHOOL STATEMENT: The program is taught in part at medical school, with clinical rotation at major hospitals. Masters program and reflexology certification are available.

OREGON

State Licensing: 330 hours.

National Certification Exam not accepted.

  Board: (503) 378-2070

APPROVED OUT-OF-STATE SCHOOLS:

Brenneke School, Seattle WA; Brian Utting School, Seattle WA; Cedar Mountain Center, WA; Colorado Springs Academy, CO; Crystal Mountain, NM; Florida School of Massage, FL; Hawaiian Islands School, Kailua-Kona HI; Health Enrichment Center, Lapeer MI; Heartwood Institute, Garberville CA; Massage Therapy Institute, Denver CO; Mueller College, San Diego CA; New Hampshire Institute, NH; New Mexico Academy, Santa Fe NM; New Mexico School, Albuquerque NM; Richmond Academy of Massage, Richmond VA; Scherer Institute, NM; Seattle Massage School, Seattle WA.

SCHOOLS:

#420 Ashland Massage Institute
       P.O. Box 1233
       Ashland, OR 97520
       (541) 482-5134

HOURS OF TRAINING: 550.

DURATION OF COURSE: nine months, evenings and some weekends.

COST: $4,185 tuition & application fee, $245 books, $400 for table if student does not own one.

FINANCIAL AID: Approved for Veterans Training, some student financing available.

YEAR FOUNDED: 1988.

GRADUATES PER YEAR (APPROX.): 20.

MODALITIES AND SUBJECTS: assessment skills for massage therapists, business & ethics, counterstrain technique, hydrotherapy, introduction to deep tissue, kinesiology, massage for specific conditions, myofascial trigger point therapy, neuromuscular activation, oriental bodywork, pathology, polarity, practical review, shiatsu, supervised clinic.

SCHOOL STATEMENT: Quality training emphasizes Swedish proficiency, western and energetic techniques, solid sciences foundation, and competent professional entry. Communications-focused fall retreat. Movement and stillness themes throughout.

#421 Cascade Institute of Massage & Body Therapies
       1250 Charnelton St.
       Eugene, OR 97401
       (503) 687-8101

HOURS OF TRAINING: 565.

DURATION OF COURSE: one year, three or four evenings per week plus occasional Saturdays.

COST: $4,640.

FINANCIAL AID: discount for pre-payment, Veteran's Administration, Dislocated workers.

YEAR FOUNDED: 1989.

PREPARATION FOR OUT-OF-STATE LICENSING EXAM: Washington.

GRADUATES PER YEAR (APPROX.): 35-40.

MODALITIES AND SUBJECTS: acupressure, advanced swedish, AMMA, breema, cadaver lab for the LMT, chair massage, community outreach, deep tissue, ethics, hydrotherapy, introduction to posture dynamics, kinesiology, massage clinic, myofascial release, pain assessment, pregnancy massage, professional development, PNF, reflexology, trigger point therapy.

#422 Central Oregon Community College
Massage Therapy Program
2600 NW College Way
Bend, OR 97701
(541) 383-7280 or 383-7418

HOURS OF TRAINING: 520, 1040 or 95 Credits (A.A.S. Degree in Massage).

DURATION OF COURSE: 520 hours 9 months, 1040 hours 18 months, A.A.S. degree 18 months; day and evening programs available.

COST: $3,950 per year. Payment plan without interest is available.

FINANCIAL AID: Scholarships through the College.

YEAR FOUNDED: 1996.

GRADUATES PER YEAR (APPROX.): 40.

MODALITIES AND SUBJECTS: acupressure, advanced treatment I, II & III, applied accounting A, B & C, applied kinesiology, aromatherapy, body-mind, business communication, chair massage, clinic, cranio-sacral therapy, english composition, entrepreneurship, feldenkrais, first aid, general education courses, health & fitness for life, human anatomy & function I & II, hydrotherapy, infant massage, internships, interpersonal communication, kinesiology I, II & III, library skills, massage & ethics, medical massage, pathology, physical education, postural integration, pregnancy massage, reflexology, shiatsu, small business management A, B, &C, sports massage, technical writing, trigger point therapy, watsu.

SCHOOL STATEMENT: We train students to blend the art of massage with the science of the body and to complement health care providers as professionals.

#423 Central Oregon School of Massage
86-A SW Century Dr.
Bend, OR 97702
(541) 382-3292

HOURS OF TRAINING: 680 or 550.

COST: $5,400 or $4,500.

YEAR FOUNDED: 1997.

GRADUATES PER YEAR (APPROX.): 30.

MODALITIES AND SUBJECTS: chair massage, communications & business, hydrotherapy, introductions to different modalities, kinesiology, pathology, student clinic. Many workshops also offered.

#424 East-West College of the Healing Arts
4531 S.E. Belmont St.
Portland, OR 97215
(503) 231-1500 or (800) 635-9141
www.ewcha.com

HOURS OF TRAINING: 529 or 661.

DURATION OF COURSE: 9 to 18 months, day and evening programs available.

COST: 529 hours $5,500, 661 hours $6,700. Payment plan without interest is available, discount or massage table included for prepayment in full.

FINANCIAL AID: EWC private scholarships available.

YEAR FOUNDED: 1972 (Midway School); 1981 East-West College.

ACCREDITATIONS/APPROVALS: COMTA/approved, Veterans Administration, U.S. Dept. of Immigration and Naturalization, Oregon State Vocational Rehabilitation Division, Oregon Commission for the Blind, Job Training Partnership Act.

PREPARATION FOR OUT-OF-STATE LICENSING EXAM: All states except New York and Nebraska.

GRADUATES PER YEAR (APPROX.): 230.

MODALITIES AND SUBJECTS: chair massage, clinic practices, cranio-sacral therapy, deep tissue, hydrotherapy, infant massage, insurance billing, kinesiology, lymphatic drainage, massage & kinesiology & movement, massage for common injuries, myofascial release, neuromuscular therapy, pathology, polarity, pregnancy massage, reflexology, shiatsu, side-lying massage, sports massage, trigger point therapy.

#425 Lane Community College
1059 Willamette St.
Eugene, OR 974011
(541) 726-2207

Contact the school for program information.

#426 Oregon Coast School of Massage
1845 SW Hwy. 101, suite 2
Lincoln City, OR 97367
(541) 994-2728

HOURS OF TRAINING: 500 (approx. 450 to 475 in-class hours).

DURATION OF COURSE: 12 to 18 months, day and evening-weekend programs available.

FINANCIAL AID: Vocational Rehabilitation.

YEAR FOUNDED: 1997.

GRADUATES PER YEAR (APPROX.): 10–15.

MODALITIES AND SUBJECTS: advanced integrated kinesiology, berrywork, body mechanics, business & ethics, chair massage, clinic (contact with public), clinic & on-site work, communication & sensitivity training, deep tissue, hydrotherapy, infant massage, lymphatic drainage, myofascial release, nutrition, polarity, postural integration, reflexology, self-care for therapist, shiatsu, spa treatments, sports massage, structural integration, tai chi, tui na, yoga therapy.

SCHOOL STATEMENT: Small classes, one on one training as needed, emphasis on personal growth and quality, healing education. Located on the beautiful Oregon coast.

#427 Oregon School of Massage
9500 SW Barbur Blvd., suite 100
Portland, OR 97219
(503) 244-3420 or (800) 844-3420

HOURS OF TRAINING: 555.

DURATION OF COURSE: minimum of one year; students proceed at their own pace; day, evening & weekend programs available.

COST: $6,435 including books and miscellaneous expenses. Payment plan without interest is available.

FINANCIAL AID: discounts for early payment.

YEAR FOUNDED: 1984.

PREPARATION FOR OUT-OF-STATE LICENSING EXAM: Washington.

GRADUATES PER YEAR (APPROX.): 140.

MODALITIES AND SUBJECTS: chair massage, deep tissue massage, foot reflexology, hakomi integrative somatics, hydrotherapy, kinesiology, nutrition, pathology, polarity, pregnancy massage, professional development, reiki, shiatsu, side-lying massage, sports massage, student practicum clinic, the psychology of touch. Advanced programs: shiatsu certification, deep tissue massage.

SCHOOL STATEMENT: Program includes emphasis on psycho-spiritual and communication dimensions of bodywork.

#428 Rogue Community College
3345 Redwood Highway
Grants Pass, OR 97527
College: (503) 471-3500

HOURS OF TRAINING: 500.

DURATION OF COURSE: 9 months, days.

COST: $2,000.

FINANCIAL AID: Scholarships through RCC Foundation, student loans.

YEAR FOUNDED: 1990.

GRADUATES PER YEAR (APPROX.): 15.

MODALITIES AND SUBJECTS: business practices for massage therapists, CWE: massage, esalen, hydrotherapy, integrated studies massage, massage exam review, oriental massage (acupressure), pathology for massage practices, reflexology, shiatsu.

SCHOOL STATEMENT: This program prepares students for employment as massage therapists and provides supplemental training for persons previously or currently employed in a health science occupation.

#429 Salem School of Massage
420 Mill St. SE
Salem, OR 97301
(503)585-8912

HOURS OF TRAINING: 607 (535 in-class hours).

DURATION OF COURSE: One year, evenings.

COST: $5,700 including books. Payment plan without interest is available.

FINANCIAL AID: Mid-Willamette Jobs Council, Vocational Rehabilitation.

YEAR FOUNDED: 1990.

GRADUATES PER YEAR (APPROX.): 50.

MODALITIES AND SUBJECTS: aromatherapy, berrywork, chair massage, deep tissue, herbology, infant massage, kinesiology, lymphatic drainage, medical terminology, myofascial release, pathology, polarity, reflexology, reiki, shiatsu, sports massage.

SCHOOL STATEMENT: Salem School of Massage educates individuals in the process of becoming Oregon Licensed Massage Technicians, by providing excellent skills, tools and information.

PENNSYLVANIA

No State licensing

SCHOOLS:

#430 Academy of Medical Arts and Business
2301 Academy Drive
Harrisburg, PA 17112
(717) 545-4747
www.acadcampus.com

HOURS OF TRAINING: 740 (490 in-class hours).

DURATION OF COURSE: 30 weeks days or 32 weeks evenings.

COST: $5,860 including books, table package, 1 gallon gel, 2 polo shirts, NCE fee. Payment plan without interest is available.

FINANCIAL AID: Scholarships or discounts, Federal grants and Student Loans.

YEAR FOUNDED: 1980.

ACCREDITATIONS/APPROVALS: ACCSCT.

GRADUATES PER YEAR (APPROX.): 200.

MODALITIES AND SUBJECTS: basic word processing, chair massage, CPR, first aid, history of massage, internships, job hunt seminars, kinesiology I & II, law & ethics, muscle testing, pregnancy massage, principles & effects of massage, small business management, sports massage.

SCHOOL STATEMENT: The Academy's primary mission is to train men and women to serve effectively in the computer, medical, business, child care, legal, and wellness fields.

#431 Allied Medical & Technical Careers
104 Woodward Hill Rd.
Edwardsville, PA 18704
(717) 288-8400

Contact school for program information.

#432 The Alternative Conjunction Clinic and
School of Massage Therapy
716 State Street
Lemoyne, PA 17043
(717) 737-6001

HOURS OF TRAINING: 504.

DURATION OF COURSE: 28 weeks, day and evening programs available.

COST: $4,739 includes books, charts, study aids, oils & lotions, bolster and misc. supplies. Payment plan without interest is available.

FINANCIAL AID: OVR, SETCO, Veteran's Administration, JTPA.

YEAR FOUNDED: 1994.

PREPARATION FOR OUT-OF-STATE LICENSING EXAM: Florida, Iowa.

GRADUATES PER YEAR (APPROX.): 50 to 100.

MODALITIES AND SUBJECTS: advanced therapeutics, allied spa services, chair massage & marketing, CPR/first aid, designer massage, esalen, history taking, HIV/AIDS, kinesiology, law & ethics, lymphatic drainage, marketing & business practices, massage theory, medical massage, muscle testing, myofascial release, neuromuscular therapy, pregnancy massage, reflexology, russian massage, sports massage, trigger point therapy.

SCHOOL STATEMENT: We are a medically and clinically-based massage therapy program. Our students become competent, confident therapists using modalities that are synergistic, for maximum healing potential.

#433 Aura Rose, A. Rose Therapeutics
352 E. 6th Av.
Conshohocken, PA 19428
(610) 834-8140

HOURS OF TRAINING: 42.

DURATION OF COURSE: 8 weeks for basic course.

COST: $630 including $60 per class and Reiki I Certification.

YEAR FOUNDED: 1985.

MODALITIES AND SUBJECTS: Edgar Cayce lymphatic massage, Reiki, deep tissue, chakra balancing, oriental theory, reflexology, intuitive and energy theory, sports massage.

SCHOOL STATEMENT: The program can be tailored to individual needs and interests. Students may continue open-ended training after completing the basic course. Emphasis is on technique.

#434 **Berks Technical Institute**
2205 Ridgewood Road
Wyomissing, PA 19610
(610) 372-1722 or 1-800-821-4662

HOURS OF TRAINING: 915 (600 in-class hours).

DURATION OF COURSE: 9 months, day & evening programs available.

COST: $8,597, including books and fees. Payment plan without interest is available.

FINANCIAL AID: Student Loans, Plus (Parent) Loans, Pell Grants.

YEAR FOUNDED: school 1987, massage program 1995.

ACCREDITATIONS/APPROVALS: ACCSCT.

GRADUATES PER YEAR (APPROX.): 45.

MODALITIES AND SUBJECTS: acupressure, aromatherapy, business principles & practices, chair massage, CPR, cranio-sacral therapy, first aid, massage therapy externship, myofascial release, neuromuscular therapy, polarity, reflexology, shiatsu, sports massage, touch for health, trigger point therapy.

SCHOOL STATEMENT: The program mainly focuses on Swedish Massage using both classroom instruction and clinical experience. The program is designed to train entry level professional massage therapists.

#435 **Career Training Academy**
Main Campus
950 Fifth Ave.
New Kensington, PA 15068
(724) 337-1000

Additional Location
ExpoMart, 105 Mall Boulevard, suite 300W
Monroeville, PA 15146
(412) 372-3900

HOURS OF TRAINING: 300, 600, 900, 1,500.

DURATION OF COURSE: 300 hours 5 months, 600 hours 9.5 months, 900 hours 11.5 months, 1,500 hours 19 months, courses offered days and evenings.

COST: 300 hours $1,900, 600 hours $3,800, 900 hours $5,700, 1,500 hours $7,600. Payment plan without interest is available.

FINANCIAL AID: Pell Grants, Federal Direct Subsidized Loans, Federal Direct Unsubsidized Loans.

YEAR FOUNDED: 1986.

ACCREDITATIONS/APPROVALS: ACCSCT, IMSTAC, COMTA/Accredited.

GRADUATES PER YEAR (APPROX.): 175.

MODALITIES AND SUBJECTS: acupressure, AIDS awareness, applied kinesiology, aromatherapy, basic shiatsu, business principles, chair massage, clinic, cranio-sacral therapy, diversity in the workplace, first aid/CPR, infant massage, kinesiology, lymphatic drainage, marketing, medical massage, myofascial release, myotherapy, neuromuscular therapy, nutrition, orthopedic assessment, pathology (intro & advanced), polarity, practicum, pregnancy massage, principles of wellness, psychology, public speaking, reflexology, shiatsu, somatic therapy, sports massage, therapeutic modalities, therapeutic touch, touch for health, trigger point (upper & lower).

SCHOOL STATEMENT: We are an institution of specialized learning with an educational environment that is both unique and traditional. Staff and students participate in community service projects.

#436 **Central PA School of Massage, Inc.**
336 South Fraser Street
State College, PA 16801
(814) 234-4900

HOURS OF TRAINING: 175 or 900.

DURATION OF COURSE: 175 hours 7 weeks full-time or 4 months part-time; 900 hours 30 weeks full-time, up to 4 years part-time, day & evening & weekend programs available.

COST: 175 hours $1,277.25, 900 hours $8,550 both include all texts, workbooks, lab fees, sheets, towels, oils, lotions & creams.

FINANCIAL AID: JTPA, OVR, in-house financing.

YEAR FOUNDED: 1994.

GRADUATES PER YEAR (APPROX.): 75.

MODALITIES AND SUBJECTS: acupressure, applied kinesiology, aromatherapy, bioenergetics, body-mind, business development, chair massage, chi gong, connective tissue bodywork, cranio-sacral therapy, energy around us, equine sports massage, ethics, first aid & CPR & HIV awareness, healing touch, infant massage, intro. to chiropractic assisting, kinesiology, lymphatic drainage, medical massage, meditation techniques, myofascial release, myotherapy, neuromuscular therapy, pathology, pregnancy massage, range of motion, record-keeping, reflexology, reiki, shiatsu, soap charting, somatic therapy, sports massage, tai chi, therapeutic touch, trigger point therapy, watsu, yoga therapy.

SCHOOL STATEMENT: Medically based training in massage and chiropractic assisting. 1/6 student-teacher ratio. 100% placement rate, 98% graduation rate, 97% pass rate at national boards.

#437 **East-West School of Massage Therapy**
504 Park Road North
Wyomissing, PA 19610
(610) 375-7520

HOURS OF TRAINING: 520 hours.

DURATION OF COURSE: 8 months days, 11 months evenings.

COST: $4,750 including texts. Payment plan without interest is available.

FINANCIAL AID: Office for Vocational Rehabilitation, Penn Card (Berks County), Wayne County JTPA, Poconos SDA.

ACCREDITATIONS/APPROVALS: IMSTAC.

YEAR FOUNDED: 1995.

GRADUATES PER YEAR (APPROX.): 25.

MODALITIES AND SUBJECTS: acupressure, applied kinesiology, aromatherapy, chair massage, polarity, pregnancy massage, reflexology, shiatsu, sports massage introduction.

SCHOOL STATEMENT: Our goal is to provide quality education using a variety of techniques while awakening the unlimited creative potential within each student.

#438 **Healing Hands School of Massage**
3522 Primrose Rd.
Philadelphia, PA 19114
(215) 676-9891

515 White Horse Pike
Haddon Heights, NJ 08035
(609) 546-7471

HOURS OF TRAINING: 50, 180, 550.

DURATION OF COURSE: 3 months, 5 months, 14 months, afternoon, evening & weekend programs available.

COST: $500, $1,800, $5,600.

FINANCIAL AID: Working scholarship, private finance company loans.

YEAR FOUNDED: 1978.

GRADUATES PER YEAR (APPROX.): 20–24.

MODALITIES AND SUBJECTS: business, ethics, hydrotherapy & chinese liniments, lymphatic drainage, medical massage, movement therapy, myofascial release, neuromuscular therapy, nutrition & herbs, oriental & western physiology, polarity, professional self-care, reflexology, shiatsu, women's health issues, yoga therapy.

SCHOOL STATEMENT: For 20 years, our school excels at preparing serious students to enter this profession. We're dedicated—small classes, enjoyable, experiential learning, seasoned instructors, beautiful setting.

#439 Health Options Institute
1410 Main St.
Northampton, PA 18067
(610) 261-0880

HOURS OF TRAINING: 62 to 500 (total 700 hours offered; students choose 500).

DURATION OF COURSE: 12 weeks to 2 years; courses offered days, evenings or weekends.

COST: $820 to $6,000 (including books and videos).

YEAR FOUNDED: 1984.

GRADUATES PER YEAR (APPROX.): 250.

MODALITIES AND SUBJECTS: acupressure, aromatherapy, chair massage, client communication skills, coordination patterns, cranial-sacral, deep muscle massage, feldenkrais, geriatric massage, group practical, medical setting massage, neuromuscular therapy, nuat thai, pre and post natal massage, polarity, postural integration, private practical, professional practice concepts, reflexology (Ingham), reiki, sports massage, therapeutic touch, trager, wetzig full potential.

SCHOOL STATEMENT: The school promotes massage as one of many ways of healing our separation from God and ourselves. The school seeks to empower its students.

#440 J. H. Thompson Academies
2910 State Street
Erie, PA 16508
(814) 456-6217

Contact school for program information.

#441 Lancaster School of Massage
317 North Queen
Lancaster, PA 17602
(717) 293-9698

HOURS OF TRAINING: 500.

DURATION OF COURSE: 6 months days, 9 months evenings.

COST: $4,800 including books and CPR.

YEAR FOUNDED: 1991.

GRADUATES PER YEAR (APPROX.): 40.

MODALITIES AND SUBJECTS: awareness & communication skills, body mechanics, business practices, cranio-sacral therapy, ethics, kinesiology, neuromuscular therapy, polarity, reflexology, sports massage, structural integration.

#442 Lehigh Valley Healing Arts Academy
5412 Shimerville Rd.
Emmaus, PA 18049
(610) 965-6165

HOURS OF TRAINING: 500.

DURATION OF COURSE: 12 months minimum, evenings and weekends.

COST: $5,250 includes books and charts.

FINANCIAL AID: Monroe County Job Partnership Training, Private

Industry Council.

MODALITIES AND SUBJECTS: acupressure, applied anatomy, applied kinesiology, aromatherapy, body-mind, business practices, carpal tunnel release, chair massage, cranio-sacral therapy, deep tissue sculpting, ethics, feldenkrais, fundamentals of energy, healing touch, herbology, insight, jin shin do, lymphatic drainage, massage theory and practice, meditation and inner journeys, myofascial release, neuromuscular therapy, oriental 5-element studies, polarity, postural integration, reflexology, reiki, shiatsu, somatic exercises, sports massage, subtle energy studies, therapeutic touch, touch for health, trager, trigger point therapy, yoga therapy, CPR.

SCHOOL STATEMENT: We teach students to work with more than flesh and bones. Self-care is stressed with emphasis on body usage. The school with heart.

#443 Massage Arts and Sciences Center of Philadelphia
1515 Locust St., 2nd floor
Philadelphia, PA 19102
(215) 985-0674

HOURS OF TRAINING: 185 or 528.

DURATION OF COURSE: 185 hours 18 weeks, 528 hours 36 weeks; day and evening programs available.

COST: 185 hours $3,500, 528 hours $6,000.

YEAR FOUNDED: 1984.

GRADUATES PER YEAR (APPROX.): 50.

MODALITIES AND SUBJECTS: anatomy of movement for bodyworkers, aromatherapy, body mechanics, business studies, connective tissue studies, CPR & first aid, ethics, joint movements and stretches, myofascial release, pathology, polarity, reflexology, shiatsu fundamentals and theory, sports massage, trigger point therapy.

SCHOOL STATEMENT: Massage Arts provides its students with the highest quality hands-on and academic education and promotes the highest standards of professionalism in the field.

#444 Mt. Nittany School of Massage
P.O. Box 8
Lemont, PA 16851
(814) 238-1121

HOURS OF TRAINING: 675 (512 in-class hours).

DURATION OF COURSE: 17 months part-time, day and weekend programs available.

COST: approx. $5,700.

FINANCIAL AID: Vocational rehabilitation, State job retraining.

YEAR FOUNDED: 1995.

GRADUATES PER YEAR (APPROX.): 20.

MODALITIES AND SUBJECTS: acupressure, applied techniques for elderly & pregnant & those with cancer or HIV/AIDS, aromatherapy, business issues, chair massage, communication skills, connective tissue massage, ethics, flower essences, foot reflexology, hydrotherapy, kinesiology, marketing & self-promotion, medical massage, movement re-education, neuromuscular therapy, pathology, pregnancy massage, polarity, reflexology, shiatsu, sports massage, subtle energy body, tai chi, technique integration, touch for health.

SCHOOL STATEMENT: Our holistic approach to massage and learning combines caring teachers, innovative teaching methods and a supportive environment to create opportunities for personal and professional transformation.

#445 Northeastern School of Medical Massage, Inc.
2525 West Main St. – 2nd floor
Norristown, PA 19403
(610) 631-5188

HOURS OF TRAINING: 100 to 600 (100 to 500 in-class hours).

DURATION OF COURSE: approximately 45 weeks, day & evening & weekend programs available.

COST: 600-hour program $5,700 plus $250 to $350 fees, books and materials.

FINANCIAL AID: Scholarships or discounts, PLUS loans, Beneke Financial Group and Monterey Financial Services.

YEAR FOUNDED: 1991.

GRADUATES PER YEAR (APPROX.): 80.

MODALITIES AND SUBJECTS: acupressure, aromatherapy*, care planning & medical record-keeping, chair massage*, connective tissue massage, CPR & first aid, cross-fiber friction, externship & clinical internship, geriatric massage, hydrotherapy, infant massage*, lymphatic drainage*, massage theory & history, medical & injury assessment skills, medical hygiene, medical massage (Peri-Medical® method), myofascial release, myotherapy, nutritional approaches to health maintenance & disease, pathophysiology, pregnancy massage, professional & business ethics, psychology, reflexology*, trigger point therapy, verbal & expository communication skills. Advanced programs: neuromuscular therapy, corrective bodywork techniques. (*continuing education.)

SCHOOL STATEMENT: Program taught by nurses, college level material in Comprehensive program, graduate level material in Advanced. Prepares students to address soft tissue problems and medical conditions.

#446 Owens Institute of Massage & Wholistic Sciences, Inc.
Regional Administrative Office
P.O. Box 1812
Media, PA 19063
1-800-99-OWENS 1-800-996-9367

HOURS OF TRAINING: 500.

IN-CLASS HOURS: 100 to 500.

DURATION OF COURSE: 6 months, 9 months or 12 months.

DAY/EVENING/WEEKEND: day, evening, weekend or combination.

COST: $3,045 (includes books).

FINANCIAL AID: $600 scholarship available to most students.

YEAR FOUNDED: 1986.

PREPARATION FOR OUT-OF-STATE LICENSING EXAM: Delaware.

GRADUATES PER YEAR (APPROX.): 200.

MODALITIES AND SUBJECTS: business practice and management, psychological-mental-spiritual success integration.

UNIQUE ASPECTS OF SCHOOL OR CURRICULUM: The student personally tailors a schedule to meet his or her needs. Curriculum is approved for credit toward Westbrook University's wholistic health arts and sciences certification and degree programs.

CONTINUING EDUCATION: reflexology, on-site, aromatherapy, Reiki, Touch for Health, therapeutic touch.

#447 Pennsylvania Institute of Massage Therapy
93 S.W. End Boulevard, #102
Quakertown, PA 18951-1150
(215) 538-5339

HOURS OF TRAINING: 521.

ACCREDITATIONS/APPROVALS: IMSTAC.

#448 Pennsylvania School of Muscle Therapy
994 Old Eagle Rd, ste. 1005
Wayne, PA 19087-1802
(610) 687-0888
www.psmt.com

HOURS OF TRAINING: 521.

DURATION OF COURSE: 9 months, day, evening and weekend programs available.

COST: $5,723.90. Payment plan without interest is available.

FINANCIAL AID: Veteran's Administration.

YEAR FOUNDED: 1980.

ACCREDITATIONS/APPROVALS: COMTA, IMSTAC.

GRADUATES PER YEAR (APPROX.): 150.

MODALITIES AND SUBJECTS: aromatherapy, business and professional ethics, chair massage, CPR/first aid, digestive & circulatory system massage, evaluation & correction of the muscular system through advanced techniques, hydrotherapy, infant massage, myofascial release, neuromuscular therapy, palpation, pathology, Pfrimmer Deep Muscle Therapy, pregnancy massage, reflexology, shiatsu, sports massage, structural evaluation.

SCHOOL STATEMENT: We train dedicated individuals to provide professional quality massage therapy, promote health and well-being, and bring due recognition to the art and science of massage.

#449 Pittsburgh School of Massage Therapy
10989 Frankstown Ave.
Penn Hills, PA 15235
(800) 860-1114

HOURS OF TRAINING: basic 308; advanced 308 (total 616) (in-class hours not specified).

DURATION OF COURSE: each program 22 weeks, day & evening & weekend classes available.

COST: $2,200 each program.

FINANCIAL AID: partial scholarships are available

YEAR FOUNDED: 1986.

GRADUATES PER YEAR (APPROX.): 85.

MODALITIES AND SUBJECTS: alexander, aromatherapy, bioenergetics, business practices, chair massage, cranio-sacral therapy, ethics, geriatric massage, hydrotherapy, myofascial release, neuromuscular therapy, ortho-bionomy, pregnancy massage, professional synthesis, reflexology, somatic psychology, sports massage certification.

SCHOOL STATEMENT: The Pittsburgh School is a student-centered organization committed to promoting the art, science and profession of massage therapy through excellence in education and training.

#450 Professional School of Massage
131 East Maple Ave.
Langhorne, PA 19047
(215) 750-0700

Contact school for program information.

#451 School of Body Therapies
931 Langhorne – Yardley Rd.
Langhorne, PA 19047
(215) 752-7666

Contact school for program information.

**#452 Synergy Therapeutic Massage Center
& Training School
P.O. Box 160
Blue Ridge Summit, PA 17214
(Classroom:13593 Monterey Lane)
(717) 794-5778**

HOURS OF TRAINING: 100 or 500.

DURATION OF COURSE: 100 hours 12½ weeks, 500 hours 12½ to 18 months; day & evening & weekend programs available.

COST: $5,000 plus $300 books and $150 fees. Payment plan without interest is available.

FINANCIAL AID: JPTA.

YEAR FOUNDED: 1997.

GRADUATES PER YEAR (APPROX.): 12–24.

MODALITIES AND SUBJECTS: alexander, applied kinesiology, aromatherapy, bioenergetics, body mechanics, breathing & energy, chair massage, chi gong, cranio-sacral therapy, emotional release, ethics & procedures & policies, feldenkrais, functional assessment, geriatric massage, hydrotherapy, infant massage, integration bodywork lab, joint mobilization, lymphatic drainage, meditation, muscle energy, muscle kinesiology & flower remedies, myofascial release, oriental energetics, ortho-bionomy, passive positioning, polarity, postural integration, pregnancy massage, reflexology, reiki, samyama, shiatsu, somatic therapy, sports massage, student clinic, therapeutic touch, yoga therapy, zero balancing.

SCHOOL STATEMENT: The mission of Synergy is to educate and train individuals to utilize touch for health and well-being of the physical, emotional, mental and spiritual self.

**#453 Valley Forge Institute of Muscle Therapy
808 Valley Forge Rd., suite 105
Phoenixville, PA 19460
(610) 935-3554**

Contact school for program information.

RHODE ISLAND

State licensing requires 500 hours at COMTA-approved school or 1,000 hours.

National Certification Exam accepted.

  Board: (401) 222-2827, ext. 112

SOUTH CAROLINA

State licensing requires 500 hours.

National Certification Exam accepted.

  Board: (803) 896-4830

SCHOOLS:

**#454 Charleston School of Massage
778 Folly Road
Charleston, SC 29412
(803) 762-7727**

HOURS OF TRAINING: 500.

DURATION OF COURSE: 6 months, day and evening programs available.

COST: $5,000 including textbooks.

FINANCIAL AID: Grants and bank loans.

YEAR FOUNDED: 1997.

MODALITIES AND SUBJECTS: acupressure, aromatherapy, body imaging enhancement™, chair massage, energy techniques, examination procedures, facial massage, hydrotherapy, introduction to other bodywork methods, marketing & business & statutes, myofascial techniques, neuromuscular therapy, nutritional approaches, reflexology, shiatsu, sports massage. In addition to the 500-hour training, certifications are offered in oriental techniques, myofascial techniques, day spa therapies, sports massage, aromatherapy and energy techniques.

SCHOOL STATEMENT: We teach the art and science of therapeutic massage in a creative environment, training successful therapists who promote wellness of body, mind and sprit.

**#455 DoveStar Holistic Technology School
4C Northridge Dr.
Hilton Head Island, SC 29926
(803) 342-3361**

HOURS OF TRAINING: 500 (in-class hours not specified). Classes held in Hilton Head & Florence, SC.

DURATION OF COURSE: 6 months.

COST: $4,120.

**#456 The European Institute of
Complementary Therapies
1 Corpus Christie, 115 Executive Center
Hilton Head Island, SC 29928
(803) 842-9355**

HOURS OF TRAINING: 700.

DURATION OF COURSE: 25 weeks, evenings and weekends.

COST: $6,000. Payment plan without interest is available.

FINANCIAL AID: Scholarships or discounts available.

YEAR FOUNDED: 1996.

GRADUATES PER YEAR (APPROX.): 12.

MODALITIES AND SUBJECTS: Therapeutic Massage and Bodywork (500 hours), Clinical Aromatherapy (200 hours); acupressure, chair massage, G5 vibratory, geriatric massage, healing touch, infant massage, lymphatic drainage, neuromuscular therapy, pregnancy massage, reflexology, reiki, therapeutic touch.

SCHOOL STATEMENT: To further the interests of complementary therapies nationally and internationally through the higher education of qualified students and therapists wishing to improve knowledge and skills.

**#457 New Life Center
P.O. Box 7614
Myrtle Beach, SC 29578
(843) 361-7735**

500-hour program including acupressure and reflexology and yoga and meditation. Contact school for program information.

**#458 Pinewood School of Massage
1000 N. Pine St., suite 2B
Spartanburg, SC 29303
(864) 582-7558**

HOURS OF TRAINING: 500 (350 in-class hours).

COST: $4,950.

YEAR FOUNDED: 1990.

ACCREDITATIONS/APPROVALS: IMSTAC.

GRADUATES PER YEAR (APPROX.): 64.

MODALITIES AND SUBJECTS: acupressure, alexander, aromatherapy, chair massage, CPR, cross fiber, energy exchange, feldenkrais, hellerwork, hydrotherapy, lymphatic drainage, marketing & business & ethics, myofascial release, pregnancy massage, rolfing, shiatsu, stretches, trigger point therapy. Advanced classes are held in myofascial release, therapeutic, aromatherapy.

SCHOOL STATEMENT: We teach the art of Swedish Massage for relaxation. We also introduce many other techniques, such as Therapeutic, Reflexology, Myo-fascial Release, Aromatherapy, and many more.

#459 South Carolina Massage Institute
1216 Washington St., suite 86
Columbia, SC 29201
(803) 933-0200

HOURS OF TRAINING: 500 day & evening classes available.

COST: $5,000 includes textbooks and choice of massage table or massage chair.

MODALITIES AND SUBJECTS: business practicum, chair massage, communications skills, ethics, oriental massage techniques.

SCHOOL STATEMENT: Our goal is to have you graduate from the program as a competent and confident massage therapist. We also provide continuing education.

#460 Southeastern School of Neuromuscular and Massage Therapy, Inc.
7410 Northside Dr., suite 105
North Charleston, SC 29420
(803) 569-7444
www.se-massage.com

HOURS OF TRAINING: 500.

DURATION OF COURSE: 6 months full-time, one year part-time; morning or evening classes.

COST: $5,300.

YEAR FOUNDED: 1997.

GRADUATES PER YEAR (APPROX.): 50-100.

MODALITIES AND SUBJECTS: business, clinical neuromuscular & structural bodywork (certification included in 500-hour program), ethics, hydrotherapy, laws & rules. Advanced program: 100-hour certification in Clinical Neuromuscular and Structural Bodywork by Kyle C. Wright (local instructors vary).

SCHOOL STATEMENT: Specializing in the training of the clinical therapist who typically works for or is referred to by physicians and other health care practitioners.

#461 Southeastern School of Neuromuscular and Massage Therapy, Inc.
3007 Broad River Road
Columbia, SC 29210
(803) 798-8800
www.se-massage.com

HOURS OF TRAINING: 500.

DURATION OF COURSE: 6 months full-time, one year part-time; morning or evening classes.

COST: $5,300.

YEAR FOUNDED: 1998.

GRADUATES PER YEAR (APPROX.): 50–100.

MODALITIES AND SUBJECTS: business, clinical neuromuscular & structural bodywork (certification included in 500-hour program), ethics, hydrotherapy, laws & rules. Advanced program: 100-hour certification in Clinical Neuromuscular and Structural Bodywork by Kyle C. Wright (local instructors vary).

SCHOOL STATEMENT: Specializing in the training of the clinical

therapist who typically works for or is referred to by physicians and other health care practitioners.

#462 Southeastern School of Neuromuscular and Massage Therapy , Inc.
850 South Pleasantburg Drive, suite 105
Greenville, SC 29607
(864) 421-9481
www.se-massage.com

HOURS OF TRAINING: 500.

DURATION OF COURSE: 6 months full-time, one year part-time; morning or evening classes.

COST: $5,300.

YEAR FOUNDED: 1997.

GRADUATES PER YEAR (APPROX.): 50-100.

MODALITIES AND SUBJECTS: business, clinical neuromuscular & structural bodywork (certification included in 500-hour program), ethics, hydrotherapy, laws & rules. Advanced program: 100-hour certification in Clinical Neuromuscular and Structural Bodywork by Kyle C. Wright (local instructors vary).

SCHOOL STATEMENT: Specializing in the training of the clinical therapist who typically works for or is referred to by physicians and other health care practitioners.

SOUTH DAKOTA

No State licensing.

SCHOOLS:

#463 Carrie's Kadesh and School of Massage Theory and Practice
112 E. 3rd Ave.
Mitchell, SD 57301
(605) 996-3916

HOURS OF TRAINING: 1,100 (860 in-class hours).

COST: $4,550 including adm. Fee, screening & testing, books, charts, etc.

GRADUATES PER YEAR (APPROX.): 8–24 (4–12 per class).

MODALITIES AND SUBJECTS: acupressure, aromatherapy, business & professionalism & ethics, color therapy, contraindications & effects of massage, CPR & first aid, craniology, deep tissue, health & hygiene, hydrotherapy, infant massage, iridology, kinesiology, light therapy, magnetic therapy, medical terminology, reflexology (zone therapy), sports massage, yoga.

#464 Sioux Falls School of Massage Therapy
317 South Cleveland Ave.
Sioux Falls, SD 57103
(605) 338-3607

HOURS OF TRAINING: 200 (100 in-class hours, 100 clinical).

COST: $2,254 including books, school shirt & registration fee.

YEAR FOUNDED: 1995.

GRADUATES PER YEAR (APPROX.): 25.

MODALITIES AND SUBJECTS: chair massage, deep tissue, ortho-bionomy, pregnancy massage, reflexology, shiatsu, sports massage. Continuing education seminars are also offered.

#465 South Dakota School of Massage Therapy, Inc.
902 W. 22nd St.
Sioux Falls, SD 57105
(605) 334-4422

HOURS OF TRAINING: 550 (500 in-class hours).

DURATION OF COURSE: 6 months; day, evening and weekend classes offered.

COST: $4,500 including textbooks. Payment plan without interest is available.

YEAR FOUNDED: 1987.

PREPARATION FOR OUT-OF-STATE LICENSING EXAM: contact school

GRADUATES PER YEAR (APPROX.): 40.

MODALITIES AND SUBJECTS: acupressure/shiatsu, applied kinesiology, aromatherapy, chair massage, clinical practice, CPR/first aid, deep tissue, disease process, emotional release work, foot/hand reflexology, hydrotherapy, introduction to sports massage, kinesiology, pathology, personal growth, polarity, rebirthing, sports massage, TMJ, yoga therapy.

SCHOOL STATEMENT: The school promotes a holistic approach to learning in an environment which stresses basic values and promotes development of a sense of who we are.

TENNESSEE

State licensing requires 500 hours education from state-accredited school.

National Certification Exam accepted.

Board (615) 532-5083

SCHOOLS:

#466 Alpha Health Institute
1200 Kenesaw Ave.
Knoxville, TN 37919
(423) 525-6683

HOURS OF TRAINING: 650 (in-class hours not specified).

COST: $6,399 including Oakworks massage table.

FINANCIAL AID: Vocational Rehabilitation.

GRADUATES PER YEAR (APPROX): 15–20.

MODALITIES AND SUBJECTS: asian traditions, body/mind, chair massage, cranio-sacral therapy, esalen/relaxation, facial massage, geriatric massage, human rhythms, integrated bodywork, kinesiology, marketing & business skills, medical & rehabilitation, muscle energy, myofascial facilitation, neuromuscular massage therapy, pre and post-surgical massage, pregnancy massage, professional development & dynamics, project health care, proprioceptive neuromuscular facilitation, public speaking, reflexology, somatic movement, sports massage, strain/counterstrain, therapeutic boundaries & fuction, traditional energy.

#467 Bodyworks School of Massage
541 Carriage House Dr.
Jackson, TN 38305
(901) 664-4891

HOURS OF TRAINING: 508 (plus clinic hours).

DURATION OF COURSE: 35 weeks, day and evening programs available.

COST: $4,272 including books, oil, bottle & holster.

YEAR FOUNDED: 1989.

MODALITIES AND SUBJECTS: advanced bodywork, business & marketing, chair massage, clinical practices, esalen, exercise & fitness & massage, medical massage, myofascial release, neuromuscular therapy, reflexology, trigger point therapy, yoga therapy.

SCHOOL STATEMENT: BSM works diligently to assist students in achieving occupational skills; to instill the desire for a lifetime of learning; to be prepared for professional career.

#468 Core Institute of Tennessee
9220 Park West Blvd.
Knoxville, TN 37923
(423) 694-4220

HOURS OF TRAINING: 586 (536 in-class hours).

DURATION OF COURSE: 6 months, day & evening programs available.

COST: $5,895 including table, books, anatomy lab fee, insurance and oil. Payment plan without interest is available.

FINANCIAL AID: Scholarships or discounts available.

YEAR FOUNDED: 1996.

GRADUATES PER YEAR (APPROX.): 50.

MODALITIES AND SUBJECTS: allied modalities, aromatherapy, bindegewebsmassage, body-mind, chair massage, community outreach, core myofascial therapy, esalen medical massage, hydrotherapy, myofascial release, neuromuscular therapy, reflexology, sports massage, student clinic, tennessee law, watsu, yoga.

SCHOOL STATEMENT: The Core Institute is dedicated to promoting and modeling wellness through touch; professionalism through education; knowledge through inquiry and research; and caring through community service.

#469 Cumberland Institute for Wellness Education
500 Wilson Pike Circle, suite 121
Brentwood, TN 37027
(615) 370-9794

HOURS OF TRAINING: Massage therapist 500 hours, continuing ed. 343 hours.

DURATION OF COURSE: minimum 9 months, maximum 27 months, day and evening courses available.

COST: $7,140 including all textbooks. Payment plan without interest is available.

FINANCIAL AID: 10% prepayment discount, State Vocational Rehabilitation (military and non-military).

YEAR FOUNDED: 1987.

GRADUATES PER YEAR (APPROX): 40 to 60.

MODALITIES AND SUBJECTS: acupressure & meridian massage, applied kinesiology, aromatherapy, bodywork ethics, business marketing, chair massage, cranio-sacral therapy, esalen massage, internship, introduction to massage, kinesiology & applied anatomy, lymphatic drainage, massage for injury, medical massage, myofascial release, neuromuscular therapy, postural integration, reflexology, shiatsu, spinal-orthopathic-syndesmobilization, sports massage, terminology & pathology & documentation, therapist-client dynamics, touch dynamics.

SCHOOL STATEMENT: Cumberland Institute provides a holistic training approach, presenting the student with over 350 years of faculty experience—resulting in a 97% graduate success rate.

#470 East Tennessee School of Massage Therapy
Sequoyah Place, Hwy. 68, suite 3
Sweetwater, TN 37874
(423) 337-3221

HOURS OF TRAINING: 500.

DURATION OF COURSE: 6 months, evenings.

COST: $2,800 including books, registration and massage table. Payment plan without interest is available.

FINANCIAL AID: Scholarships or discounts available.

YEAR FOUNDED: 1997.

MODALITIES AND SUBJECTS: aromatherapy, athletic massage,

body-mind, chair massage, consultation & preparation, effects & indications & contraindications, exercise & nutrition, externship, first aid & CPR, healing touch, infant massage, kinesiology, lymphatic drainage, massage in nursing & health care, pregnancy massage, specialized massage, sports massage, the business of massage, the practice of massage past & present, touch for health, trigger point therapy.

SCHOOL STATEMENT: Education is the Beginning of Success.

#471 Institute of Therapeutic Massage & Movement, Inc.
1161 Murfreesboro Rd., suite 405
Nashville, TN 37217
(615) 360-8554

HOURS OF TRAINING: 500.

DURATION OF COURSE: 7½ months, day or evening programs available.

COST: $5,186.52 including books and application fee. Payment plan without interest is available.

YEAR FOUNDED: 1995.

GRADUATES PER YEAR (APPROX.): 90.

MODALITIES AND SUBJECTS: assisted stretching, biomechanics, business planning & practices, chair massage, CPR, esalen, ethics, feldenkrais, HIV/AIDS, hydrotherapy, infant massage, insurance, introduction to swedish application, lymphatic drainage, medical massage, myofascial release, neuromuscular therapy, pathology, posture, pregnancy massage, reflexology, sports massage, structural integration, structural kinesiology, TN law, trigger point therapy, yoga.

SCHOOL STATEMENT: ITMM = Educating Mind and Body.

#472 The Massage Institute of Memphis
3445 Poplar Ave. #4
Memphis, TN 38111
(901) 324-4411

HOURS OF TRAINING: 550 (500 in-class hours).

DURATION OF COURSE: days 6 months, evenings/weekends 12 months.

COST: $4,800 tuition plus approximately $870 for books, massage table, supplies, hydrotherapy trip to Hot Springs, and application fee.

FINANCIAL AID: Veteran's Administration.

YEAR FOUNDED: 1987.

PREPARATION FOR OUT-OF-STATE LICENSING EXAM: Arkansas.

GRADUATES PER YEAR (APPROX.): 20.

MODALITIES AND SUBJECTS: aromatherapy, basic massage theory and practice, business, law and ethics, chair massage, clinical practicum, CPR/first aid, electrotherapy, heliotherapy, hydrotherapy, hygiene, kinesiology, pathology, reflexology, sports massage, trigger points, universal precautions, AIDS/HIV and bloodborne pathogens.

SCHOOL STATEMENT: We teach client-centered, holistic massage, emphasizing wellness, self care and disease prevention for both therapist and client, while integrating the sciences and intuition.

#473 Middle Tennessee Institute of Therapeutic Massage
394 West Main, suite A-15
Hendersonville, TN 37075
(615) 826-9500 or 826-9501

HOURS OF TRAINING: 500 (450 in-class).

DURATION OF COURSE: one year, day & evening & weekend programs available.

COST: $5,600 including $600 for all texts.

YEAR FOUNDED: 1995.

GRADUATES PER YEAR (APPROX.): 75.

MODALITIES AND SUBJECTS: acupressure, applied kinesiology, aromatherapy, body-mind, business & marketing, chair massage, client therapist relations, CPR/first aid, cranio-sacral therapy, esalen, infant massage, kinesiology (basic & advanced), lymphatic drainage, medical terminology, muscle sculpting lab, myofascial release, neuromuscular therapy, nutrition, pathology, pharmacology, polarity, pregnancy massage, reflexology, shiatsu, sports massage, touch concepts, touch for health, trigger point therapy.

SCHOOL STATEMENT: Providing a nurturing educational environment leading to the greatest personal and professional growth possible, and giving each student the tools to be a successful therapist.

#474 Natural Health Institute
209 10th Ave. South, suite 540
Nashville, TN 37203
(615) 242-6811

Contact school for program information.

#475 Tennessee Institute of Healing Arts, Inc.
5779 Brainerd Road
Chattanooga, TN 37411
(800) 735-1910 or (615) 892-9882

HOURS OF TRAINING: 1,000 (920 in-class hours).

DURATION OF COURSE: one year, day and evening programs offered

COST: $8,125 includes books, fees and miscellaneous.

YEAR FOUNDED: 1989.

ACCREDITATIONS/APPROVALS: authorized by Tennessee Higher Education Commission, ACCSCT, approved for veterans' training.

PREPARATION FOR OUT-OF-STATE LICENSING EXAM: Florida.

GRADUATES PER YEAR (APPROX.): 48.

MODALITIES AND SUBJECTS: body-mind, chair massage, CPR and first aid, documented practice, geriatric massage, HIV/AIDS, hydrotherapy, illness care massage, marketing and business, medical massage, neuromuscular therapy, nutrition, pathology, pregnancy massage, professional ethics, rules and history of massage, russian massage technique, self-care, statutes, student clinic.

SCHOOL STATEMENT: Students who successfully complete all phases of the program will also be certified in neuromuscular therapy through the International Academy of Neuromuscular Therapy, St. Petersburg, Florida.

#476 Tennessee School of Massage
4726 Poplar #4, Memphis, TN 38117
Classroom: 556 Colonial, Memphis, TN 38117
(901) 767-8484

HOURS OF TRAINING: 500.

DURATION OF COURSE: 9 months, day and evening programs available.

COST: $4,200 plus $130 books, $40 uniform, $50 application fee. Payment plan without interest is available.

FINANCIAL AID: Rehab. aid, some vocational grants.

YEAR FOUNDED: 1988.

ACCREDITATIONS/APPROVALS: approved by Tennessee Higher Education Commission.

GRADUATES PER YEAR (APPROX.): 40.

MODALITIES AND SUBJECTS: applied kinesiology, aromatherapy,

basic acupressure, business, chair massage, community skills (psychology), ethics, healing touch, hydrotherapy, infant massage, kinesiology, lymphatic drainage, medical massage, nutrition, polarity, pregnancy massage, reflexology, shiatsu, sports massage, therapeutic touch.

SCHOOL STATEMENT: Training emphasizes Swedish style, relaxing deep tissue massage and sports massage techniques, along with hydrotherapy and wholistic wellness principles. Holistic learning center under development.

TEXAS

State Licensing/registration: 300 hours (250 hours plus 50 hours internship).

National Certification Exam not accepted.

Board: (512) 834-6616

SCHOOLS:

#477 The Academy for Massage Therapy Training
1409 North Main Ave.
San Antonio, TX 78212
(210) 224-8111

Contact school for program information.

#478 Academy of Healing Arts
531 Londonderry Ln. #120
Denton, TX 76205
(940) 566-1880

HOURS OF TRAINING: 300 (250 in-class hours).

DURATION OF COURSE: 14 weeks days or 6 months evenings & weekends.

COST: $2,100 includes all required books and supplies except carry bag. Payment plan without interest is available; $100 discount for prepayment

YEAR FOUNDED: 1993

GRADUATES PER YEAR (APPROX): 40

MODALITIES AND SUBJECTS: business practices, clinical practice, ethics, health and hygiene, hydrotherapy, internship, joint range of motion.

SCHOOL STATEMENT: Student/teacher ratio of not more than 12:1 allows for individual attention.

#479 Alvin Community College
3110 Mustang
Alvin, TX 77511
(281) 331-6111

Contact school for program information.

#480 A New Beginning School of Massage
2525 Wallingwood Dr., suite 1501
Austin, TX 78746
(512) 306-0975

Contact school for program information.

#481 Asten Center of Natural Therapeutics
797 Grove Rd., suite 101
Richardson, TX 75081
(972) 669-3245

HOURS OF TRAINING: basic 300, advanced 250.

DURATION OF COURSE: basic 5 to 12 months; advanced 5 to 12 months, day, evening and Sunday programs available.

COST: basic $2,630, advanced $2,456, includes textbooks. Payment plan without interest is available, discounts for prepayment in full & for 2 or more family members.

FINANCIAL AID: Texas Rehabilitation Commission, Private Lender (TRC), Texas Commission for the Blind.

YEAR FOUNDED: 1983.

ACCREDITATIONS/APPROVALS: COMTA/approved.

GRADUATES PER YEAR (APPROX.): 65–100.

MODALITIES AND SUBJECTS: business practices & ethics, chair massage, clinical treatment for 12 specific injuries, elderly & pregnancy massage, health & hygiene, hydrotherapy, infant massage, internship, lymphatic drainage, medical massage, polarity, reflexology, sports massage, trigger point therapy (all courses may be taken individually as continuing education).

SCHOOL STATEMENT: We at the Asten Center strive to prepare each person to recognize and achieve their dreams and highest goals through the practice of Massage Therapy.

#482 Austin School of Massage Therapy (ASMT)
2600 W. Stassney Ln.
Austin, TX 78745
(512) 462-3005 or 1-800-276-2768
www.asmt.com

Additional locations:
Amarillo, College Station, Dallas, El Paso, Fort Worth, Lubbock, Midland, San Angelo, San Antonio, Waco

HOURS OF TRAINING: 300.

DURATION OF COURSE: 3-month summer intensive or 6 months or 9 months, day & evening & weekend programs available.

COST: $2,650 including 3 textbooks, polo shirt, videotape, business cards, student notebook.

FINANCIAL AID: Scholarships or discounts available, JTPA, Texas Commission for the Blind, Texas Rehabilitation Commission, VA.

YEAR FOUNDED: 1985.

ACCREDITATIONS/APPROVALS: IMSTAC.

GRADUATES PER YEAR (APPROX.): 900.

MODALITIES AND SUBJECTS: body-mind, business practices, chair massage, health & hygiene, hydrotherapy, internship, professional ethics, trigger point therapy. Advanced classes: anatomy, myofascial release, neuromuscular therapy, sports massage. Additional certifications: personal trainer, holistic health, lifestyle consultant.

SCHOOL STATEMENT: Performance-based training challenges the student to perform at a high standard of professionalism. The program emphasizes Skills Evaluation, Teams, Outreach, and Practical Applications.

#483 Avalon School of Massage
310 W. Sterling
Baytown, TX 77520
(281) 428-1894

HOURS OF TRAINING: 300.

DURATION OF COURSE: 4 to 7 months, day & evening & weekend programs available.

COST: $2,500 including all books and supplies used in class.

YEAR FOUNDED: 1997.

GRADUATES PER YEAR (APPROX.): 20–25.

MODALITIES AND SUBJECTS: business & ethics, chair massage, esalen, health & hygiene, hydrotherapy, internship.

SCHOOL STATEMENT: Avalon School of Massage is for the student who demands the finest education as preparation for a successful career in massage therapy.

#484 Body Perfect School of Massage and Reflexology
2237 Parker Rd., suite B & C
Plano, TX 75023
(972) 596-1311

Contact school for program information.

#485 Brazosport College
500 College Dr.
Lake Jackson, TX 77566
(409) 266-3000

Contact school for program information.

#486 Castleman School of Massage
1565 West Main, suite 114
Lewisville, TX 75067
(972) 221-7717

Contact school for program information.

#487 Christian Associates
25030 I-45 N
Spring, TX 77386
(281) 367-6515

HOURS OF TRAINING: 300.

DURATION OF COURSE: days 3 months, evenings 6 months.

COST: $2,615 (includes books).

FINANCIAL AID: discounts, work exchange.

YEAR FOUNDED: 1990.

ACCREDITATIONS/APPROVALS: veterans administration, Texas rehabilitation commission, Texas commission for the blind.

GRADUATES PER YEAR (APPROX.): 50.

MODALITIES AND SUBJECTS: business practices and ethics, chair massage, health and hygiene, hydrotherapy, internship.

SCHOOL STATEMENT: Your well-being is our purpose!

#488 Colle Massage Therapy School
9331 Gulf Fwy.
Houston, TX 77017
(713) 947-2172

HOURS OF TRAINING: 300.

DURATION OF COURSE: 2½ months days, 5 months evenings, 6 months weekends.

COST: $2,500 including book, material and supplies.

FINANCIAL AID: Scholarships or discounts available.

YEAR FOUNDED: 1996.

GRADUATES PER YEAR (APPROX.): 50 to 100.

MODALITIES AND SUBJECTS: business & ethics, health & hygiene, hydrotherapy.

SCHOOL STATEMENT: Provide massage therapy students the quality of education to prepare the student for a successful career as a massage therapist.

#489 El Paso Community College
100 W. Rio Grande
El Paso, TX 79902
(915) 831-4116

HOURS OF TRAINING: 300.

COST: $928.

YEAR FOUNDED: 1996.

GRADUATES PER YEAR (APPROX.): 20.

MODALITIES AND SUBJECTS: business practices & professional ethics, health & hygiene, hydrotherapy, internship.

SCHOOL STATEMENT: This course prepares students to become Texas registered massage therapists, and practice therapeutic massage in a variety of settings, serving the needs of their clients.

#490 El Paso School of Massage
661 S. Mesa Hills, suite 100
El Paso, TX 79912
(915) 833-2935

Contact school for program information.

#491 European Institute
33 East Shady Lane
Houston, TX 77063
(713) 783-1446

Contact the school for program information.

#492 European Massage Therapy Institute
7220 Louis Pasteur, suite 140
San Antonio, TX 78229
(210) 615-8207 or (800) 458-5440

HOURS OF TRAINING: Basic Massage Therapy - 300, Advanced Massage Therapy I - 100.

DURATION OF COURSE: Basic Massage Therapy 9 months, Advanced Massage Therapy 6 months, day and evening programs available.

COST: Basic Massage Therapy $2,495.26, Advanced Massage Therapy $1,000 (prices include books, insurance, uniform, linens, carrying bag, towels and hand sanitizer). Payment plan without interest is available.

FINANCIAL AID: Texas rehabilitation, Veterans Administration, Texas Commission for the Blind.

YEAR FOUNDED: 1988

GRADUATES PER YEAR (APPROX): 90.

MODALITIES AND SUBJECTS: aromatherapy, business practices, clinical internship program, health and hygiene, hydrotherapy, kinesiology, manual lymphatic drainage (basic and advanced), medical terminology, muscle toning facial massage, paraffin treatments & painful joints, pathology, postural analysis, practicum, reflexology.

SCHOOL STATEMENT: European Massage Therapy Institute promotes a practical, hands-on method, utilizing its trademarked Chiromassage. The strengths of E.M.T.I. lie in assessment skills and precision techniques.

#493 Fort Worth School of Massage
2929 Cleburne Road
Fort Worth, TX 76110
(817) 923-9944

HOURS OF TRAINING: 300.

DURATION OF COURSE: 3 months days, 6 months evenings, 8 months Saturdays.

COST: $2,300 including books. Payment plan without interest is available.

FINANCIAL AID: Scholarships or discounts available.

YEAR FOUNDED: 1997.

GRADUATES PER YEAR (APPROX.): 60–72.

MODALITIES AND SUBJECTS: business practices & professional ethics, health & hygiene, hydrotherapy, internship.

SCHOOL STATEMENT: Touch is transformational and empowering. FWSM will provide the opportunity to learn and grow through massage: effecting positive change in people and the world.

#494 Giving Tree Cottage
1808 South St.
Nacogdoches, TX 75964
(409) 560-6299

HOURS OF TRAINING: 300.

DURATION OF COURSE: 6 months, evenings.

COST: $2,500 includes books, linens, towels, oil, dry brush, notebook. Cost of student insurance additional. Payment plan without interest is available.

FINANCIAL AID: Scholarships or discounts available.

YEAR FOUNDED: 1995.

GRADUATES PER YEAR (APPROX.): 14.

SCHOOL STATEMENT: We believe in caring more than others think is wise, risking more than others think is safe, and expecting more than others think is possible.

#495 Greater Beaumont School of Massage
229 Dowlen, Suite 15A
Beaumont, TX 77706
(409) 866-8661

Contact school for program information.

#496 Hands-On Therapy School of Massage
625 Gatewood
Garland, TX 75043
(972) 240-9288

1101 E. 5th
Tyler, TX 75701
(903) 535-7733

2880 LBJ Freeway, suite 501
Dallas, TX 75234
(972) 484-8180

HOURS OF TRAINING: 300 (State requirement) or 500.

DURATION OF COURSE: 6 months, day and evening programs available.

COST: 300 hours $2,300; 500 hours $3,550. Payment plan without interest is available.

FINANCIAL AID: scholarships available.

ACCREDITATIONS/APPROVALS: Veteran's Administration.

YEAR FOUNDED: 1991.

MODALITIES AND SUBJECTS: business practices, health and hygiene, hydrotherapy, internship.

SCHOOL STATEMENT: The school emphasizes personal growth and the psychological aspects of bodywork.

#497 Health Masters
101 Franklin
Houston, TX 77002
(713) 228-8499 or 529-3296

HOURS OF TRAINING: 300.

DURATION OF COURSE: approximately 6 months; day, evening and weekend programs offered.

COST: $2,500 including books and supplies.

FINANCIAL AID: Veteran's Administration, Texas Rehabilitation Commission.

ACCREDITATIONS/APPROVALS: University of Houston Graduate Program

YEAR FOUNDED: 1990.

GRADUATES PER YEAR (APPROX): 50.

MODALITIES AND SUBJECTS: aromatherapy, business & ethics, chair massage, health & hygiene, human hydrotherapy, infant massage, pregnancy massage, reflexology, shiatsu.

SCHOOL STATEMENT: Health Masters School of Massage Therapy is committed to excellence in providing a training program for the massage therapy student in a safe, nurturing environment.

#498 Institute of Cosmetic Arts
1105 Airline
Corpus Christi, TX 78412
(512) 991-8868 or 991-1352

HOURS OF TRAINING: 300.

DURATION OF COURSE: 10½ weeks days or 9 months evenings.

COST: $3,108 including books and notebook.

FINANCIAL AID: Texas Rehabilitation, Texas Commission for the Blind, Texas Workforce Commission for the Deaf.

YEAR FOUNDED: 1982.

GRADUATES PER YEAR (APPROX.): 30 to 40.

MODALITIES AND SUBJECTS: business, hydrotherapy, hygiene, internship.

SCHOOL STATEMENT: We encourage a strong basic massage program. Our business management training is as important as the therapy program. Our ratio 10 students per instructor.

#499 The Institute of Natural Healing Sciences
4100 Felps Drive, suite E
Colleyville, TX 76034
(817) 498-0716

HOURS OF TRAINING: 300 or 600 (in-class hours not specified).

DURATION OF COURSE: 300 hours 4 months days, 8 months evenings; additional 300 hours 8 months evenings.

COST: 300 hours $2,430. Payment plan without interest is available.

FINANCIAL AID: scholarships, Texas Rehabilitation Commission, JTPA.

YEAR FOUNDED: 1985.

ACCREDITATIONS/APPROVALS: COMTA/approved.

GRADUATES PER YEAR (APPROX.): 60.

MODALITIES AND SUBJECTS: aromatherapy, business practices, chair massage, cranio-sacral therapy, designer massage, health & hygiene, hydrotherapy, myofascial release, neuromuscular therapy, polarity, radiance technique, reflexology, shiatsu, sports massage, thai massage, trigger point therapy.

SCHOOL STATEMENT: We focus on body, mind and spirit. Students are accepted just as they are, allowing for change. We aim to turn out exceptional, caring therapists.

#500 In-Touch School of Massage
50 Briar Hollow, suite 280 West
Houston, TX 77027
(713) 961-1669

HOURS OF TRAINING: 300 basic, 250 advanced.

DURATION OF COURSE: basic: day or evening class 5 months, weekend class 4 months.

COST: basic $2,500 plus $140 books and supplies; advanced programs $10 per hour, workshops $12 per hour.

FINANCIAL AID: Texas Rehabilitation Commission, Texas Commission for the Blind.

YEAR FOUNDED: 1991.

MODALITIES AND SUBJECTS: Basic: business practices & professional ethics, hydrotherapy, human health & hygiene, internship. Advanced: advanced business concepts, aquatic rehabilitation, chair massage, clinical pathology of the human condition, ethics & massage therapy, exercise & training & the immune system, kinesiology, medical terminology, nutrition & metabolism & the digestive system, pain assessment & neuromuscular massage therapy, pain mechanisms of the lower back, personal fitness training, regulation & integration of the nervous & endocrine systems, sports massage.

SCHOOL STATEMENT: In-Touch School provides educational opportunities to empower individuals so they may achieve their highest potential and thereby enhance the quality of life.

#501 The Lauterstein-Conway Massage School and Clinic
4701-B Burnet Road
Austin, TX 78756
(512) 374-9222 or 1-800-474-0852

HOURS OF TRAINING: 300 (one semester), 550 (two semesters) 750 (three semesters).

DURATION OF COURSE: Semester one 6 to 9 months, semesters two and three 6 months each. Day, evening and evening/weekend programs available.

COST: $2,450 per semester for semesters one and two, $2,200 for semester three, plus required texts.

FINANCIAL AID: approved by Texas Rehabilitation Commission.

YEAR FOUNDED: 1989.

ACCREDITATIONS/APPROVALS: COMTA/Accredited.

GRADUATES PER YEAR (APPROX.): 300.

MODALITIES AND SUBJECTS: acupressure, aromatherapy, business practices and ethics, chair massage, clinical applications in bodywork, cranio-sacral work, deep massage, advanced anatomy and physiology, human health and hygiene, integrative bodywork, internship, movement skills, myofascial release, pregnancy massage, professionalism, psychology of bodywork, reflexology, shiatsu, sports massage, structural bodywork, advanced structural bodywork, trager, zen shiatsu, zero balancing.

SCHOOL STATEMENT: Our mission is to run the school in a manner as healing as the subjects we teach. We emphasize the integration of structure and energy.

#502 Massage Education Institute
3195 Calder
Beaumont, TX 77702
(409) 832-3020

Contact school for program information.

#503 Massage Institute
5639 Bell Ave.
Dallas, TX 75206
(214) 826-0500

HOURS OF TRAINING: 300 basic plus 300 advanced.

DURATION OF COURSE: 4 to 7 months, day or evening/weekend programs available.

COST: $2,250 including books, linens, intern shirt, oils/lotion. Payment plan without interest is available.

FINANCIAL AID: Work study, Veteran's Administration, Texas Rehabilitation Commission.

YEAR FOUNDED: 1995.

GRADUATES PER YEAR (APPROX.): 50+.

MODALITIES AND SUBJECTS: aromatherapy, body-mind, business practices & ethics, chair massage, clinical internship, cranio-sacral therapy, health & hygiene, hydrotherapy, myofascial release, pregnancy massage, reiki, shiatsu, somatic therapy, sports massage, trigger point therapy, yoga.

SCHOOL STATEMENT: Relaxed atmosphere with small classes to provide individualized attention and group rapport. Strong academic and clinical foundation balanced with nurturing innate ability of the individual.

#504 Massage Therapy Clinic & School
2045 Space Park Drive, suite 100
Nassau Bay, TX 77058
(281) 333-0400
www.wxs.com/spaofnassau

HOURS OF TRAINING: 300 (Level I), 500 (Level II) or 600 (Mastery Plus).

DURATION OF COURSE: Level I, 12 to 24 weeks (days or evenings or weekends); Level II and Mastery Plus, 2 weekends per month for 10 to 18 months.

COST: Level I $2,550, Level II $4,055, Mastery $5,250.

FINANCIAL AID: Scholarships, Texas Rehabilitation Commission, GI Bill, Texas Commission for the Blind.

YEAR FOUNDED: 1990.

GRADUATES PER YEAR (APPROX.): 120.

MODALITIES AND SUBJECTS: aromatherapy, business practices & professional ethics, chair massage, day spa, deep tissue, human health & hygiene, hydrotherapy, infant massage, internship, medical massage, myofascial release, pain release, polarity, pregnancy massage, reflexology, shiatsu, sports massage, trigger point therapy.

SCHOOL STATEMENT: MTCS offers superior massage therapy training, using the latest techniques coupled with traditional methods, so students may offer the most beneficial therapy to their clients.

#505 Midland College
3600 N. Garfield
Midland, TX 79701
(915) 685-6440

HOURS OF TRAINING: 300.

DURATION OF COURSE: 4 months, evening & weekend programs available.

COST: $1,150 includes books and insurance.

FINANCIAL AID: JTPA.

YEAR FOUNDED: 1996.

GRADUATES PER YEAR (APPROX.): 20 to 48.

MODALITIES AND SUBJECTS: business practices & ethics, health & hygiene, hydrotherapy.

SCHOOL STATEMENT: Midland College is dedicated to education and serves the citizens in offering quality education provided by qualified faculty.

#506 MIND BODY Naturopathic Institute
10911 West Avenue
San Antonio, TX 78213-1537
(210) 342-7444

HOURS OF TRAINING: 300.

DURATION OF COURSE: approx. 9 months, evenings & Sat. a.m.

COST: $2,400 including books, supplies, linen, lotion. Payment plan without interest is available.

FINANCIAL AID: Texas Rehabilitation Commission.

YEAR FOUNDED: 1988.

GRADUATES PER YEAR (APPROX): 50+.

MODALITIES AND SUBJECTS: aromatherapy, body-mind, business & ethics, chair massage, colon hydrotherapy, cranio-sacral therapy, ear candling, health & hygiene, hydrotherapy, internship, live cell analysis, lymphatic drainage, neuro-linguistics, reflexology, sports massage, yoga therapy.

SCHOOL STATEMENT: Combining MIND-BODY-SPIRIT and natural healing as taught through naturopathic principles.

#507 Mirabella Education Center & Day Spa
820 Nederland Ave.
Nederland, TX 77627
(409) 721-5959

HOURS OF TRAINING: 300.

COST: $2,000.

GRADUATES PER YEAR (APPROX.): 56.

MODALITIES AND SUBJECTS: business ethics & professional ethics, health & hygiene, hydrotherapy, internship.

#508 MRC School of Massage
2990 Richmond, suite 142
Houston, TX 77098
(713) 522-1423

HOURS OF TRAINING: 300.

DURATION OF COURSE: 5 months days, 6½ months evenings.

COST: $2,400 including most books and all supplies; discounts for pre-payment and for morning class.

FINANCIAL AID: discounts are available, approved for financial aid by Texas Rehabilitation Commission, Texas Commission for the Blind.

YEAR FOUNDED: 1989.

GRADUATES PER YEAR (APPROX.): 100.

MODALITIES AND SUBJECTS: business practices, carpal tunnel, deep tissue, health and hygiene, hydrotherapy, infant massage, internship, pregnancy massage, professional ethics, reflexology.

#509 Neuromuscular Concepts Massage Therapy School
8607 Wurzbach Road, Bldg. R, suite 150
San Antonio, TX 78240
(210) 558-3112

Contact school for program information.

#510 North Texas School of Swedish Massage
2335 Green Oaks Blvd. West
Arlington, TX 76016
(817) 446-6629

HOURS OF TRAINING: 300.

DURATION OF COURSE: 3, 6 or 9 months, mornings, evenings or weekends.

COST: $2,659 (includes books). Payment plan without interest is available.

FINANCIAL AID: discount for payment in full at start of class, Texas Comm. for the Blind, Texas Rehab. Commission.

YEAR FOUNDED: 1994.

GRADUATES PER YEAR (APPROX.): 60-80.

MODALITIES AND SUBJECTS: business and ethics, health and hygiene, hydrotherapy, internship.

#511 Phoenix School of Holistic Health
6610 Harwin #256
Houston, TX 77036

2611 FM 1960 West #H-100
Houston, TX

1500 Marina Bay Drive, Baily Center Building
Clear Lake Shores, TX
(713) 974-5976

HOURS OF TRAINING: 300.

COST: $2,450 includes handout packets.

YEAR FOUNDED: 1986.

MODALITIES AND SUBJECTS: body mobilization, business, health & hygiene, holistic massage^{sm} hydrotherapy, internship, professional ethics.

SCHOOL STATEMENT: The Phoenix School of holistic health is a nationally recognized holistic learning center founded to provide fundamental and advance training in the holistic arts.

#512 The Relax Station School of Massage Therapy
1409 Kingwood Dr.
Kingwood, TX 77339
(281) 358-0600
www.TheRelaxStation.com

HOURS OF TRAINING: 300.

DURATION OF COURSE: day 10 weeks, evenings 22 weeks, summer 8½ weeks (all plus internship).

COST: $2,966.50 includes books, oils, cremes, paraffin. Payment plan without interest is available.

FINANCIAL AID: Texas Rehabilitation Commission.

YEAR FOUNDED: 1995.

GRADUATES PER YEAR (APPROX): 54.

MODALITIES AND SUBJECTS: business practices and professional ethics, health and hygiene, hydrotherapy (chirojet, aromaspa, floatation tank, paraffin, ice treatments), internship.

SCHOOL STATEMENT: Our school atmosphere is friendly, caring and tailored to the individual. Small classes, personal attention, one-on-one, direct access to instructors and director.

#513 St. Phillips Community College
1801 Martin Luther King Drive
San Antonio, TX 78203
(210) 531-3200 or 531-4807

Contact school for program information.

#514 School of Natural Therapy
4309-B N. 10th
McAllen, TX 78504
(956) 630-0928

HOURS OF TRAINING: 300.

COST: $2,909 including all books & supplies.

YEAR FOUNDED: 1989.

GRADUATES PER YEAR (APPROX.): 60.

#515 Sterling Health Center and Massage School
15070 Beltwood Parkway
Addison, TX 75244
(972) 991-9293
www.flash.net/~sterchc

HOURS OF TRAINING: 300 plus optional 200-hour advanced course.

DURATION OF COURSE: 4 months to one year, day & evening & weekend programs available.

COST: $1,975 plus $225 estimated cost for books and supplies. Payment plan without interest is available.

FINANCIAL AID: Discount for payment in advance, Texas Rehabilitation Commission, Veteran's Administration.

YEAR FOUNDED: 1991.

GRADUATES PER YEAR (APPROX.): 75.

MODALITIES AND SUBJECTS: business practices & ethics, chair massage, human health & hygiene, hydrotherapy, infant massage, internship, pregnancy massage, reflexology, shiatsu, sports massage, trigger point therapy.

SCHOOL STATEMENT: To provide excellence in professional service, education and training to our students and the community.

**#516 Texas Healing Arts Institute, L.C. (THAI)
        The School of Massage Therapy
        2704 Rio Grande, suite 11
        Austin, TX 78705
        (512) 236-THAI or 477-1826
        www.thaisom.com**

HOURS OF TRAINING: 300, two 20-hour advanced programs on myofascial release.

DURATION OF COURSE: 4 months or 6 months, day & evening & weekend programs available.

COST: $1,750, $235 each for advanced programs.

FINANCIAL AID: Texas Rehabilitation Commission.

YEAR FOUNDED: 1997.

GRADUATES PER YEAR (APPROX.): 100.

MODALITIES AND SUBJECTS: acupressure, chair massage, craniosacral therapy, esalen, myofascial release (physiology of pain part one: lower body & part two: upper body), neuromuscular therapy, reflexology, trigger point therapy.

SCHOOL STATEMENT: THAI is dedicated to providing pragmatic and innovative instruction to individuals pursuing an education in massage therapy and bodywork.

**#517 Texas Massage Therapy Corp.
        3617 Red Bluff
        Pasadena, TX 77503
        (713) 472-0383**

Contact school for program information.

**#518 Therapeutic Body Concepts
        6162 Wurzbach
        San Antonio, TX 78238
        (210) 684-6563**

Contact school for program information.

**#519 Wellness Skills, Inc.
        6102 E. Mockingbird Lane, suite 401
        Dallas, TX 75214
        (214) 828-4000
        www.wellnessskills.com**

Classes also offered at:

**#520 Wellness Skills, Inc.
        6301 Airport Freeway
        Fort Worth, TX 76117
        (817) 838-3800**

HOURS OF TRAINING: 300 (semester I) or 500 (semester I plus 200 hours advanced programs).

DURATION OF COURSE: Semester I: 4 months or 7 months part-time, or one course at a time; Semester II: 4 to 8 months. Day program and evening/weekend program available.

COST: Semester I: $2,485 (discounts up to $300 are available); 100-hour advanced programs $885 each.

YEAR FOUNDED: 1985.

ACCREDITATIONS/APPROVALS: Texas Rehabilitation Commission, Texas Commission for the Blind, Veteran's Administration.

GRADUATES PER YEAR (APPROX.): 250.

MODALITIES AND SUBJECTS: acupressure, aromatherapy, business practices and ethics, chair massage, clinical anatomy & physiology, clinical internship, health and hygiene, hydrotherapy, massage for the medical setting, pathology, polarity, reflexology, session design, shiatsu, sports massage, therapeutic touch, trigger point therapy, yoga therapy.

**#521 Williams Institute School of Massage
        810 S. Mason Rd., suite 290
        Katy, TX 77450
        (281) 392-9212**

HOURS OF TRAINING: 300.

DURATION OF COURSE: 6 to 6½ months, day and evening programs available.

COST: $2,650 including books and estimated cost of supplies. Payment plan without interest is available.

YEAR FOUNDED: 1993.

MODALITIES AND SUBJECTS: business practices & ethics, human health & hygiene, internship, pregnancy massage, reflexology, shiatsu.

SCHOOL STATEMENT: Providing the highest standards in massage therapy education.

**#522 The Winters School
        4625 Southwest Freeway #142
        Houston, TX 77027-7100
        (713) 626-2200**

HOURS OF TRAINING: Basic Program 300, Associate Program 250, various workshops.

DURATION OF COURSE: Basic program 4 to 8 months, Associate Program 5 to 6 months; day, evening and weekend programs available.

COST: $2,500 plus $100 to $150 for supplies.

YEAR FOUNDED: 1984.

ACCREDITATIONS/APPROVALS: Texas Rehabilitation Commission, Veterans Administration

GRADUATES PER YEAR (APPROX.): 85.

MODALITIES AND SUBJECTS: business development, chair massage, deep tissue somatics, health, hydrotherapy, internship, polarity, reflexology, session design, shiatsu.

SCHOOL STATEMENT: Our programs provide graduates with professional satisfaction as they serve the public while enhancing their own academic, spiritual and financial growth.

NON-SCHOOL INSTRUCTORS

In addition to certifying massage schools, the State of Texas also certifies instructors who may teach independent of a school.

The following individuals are certified as massage instructors by the State of Texas. Contact them for program information:

Connor, Joanna, HC RT. 70, Box 614, Concan TX 78838 (830) 232-6384

Decuir, Carole, 6390 Phelan, Beaumont, TX 77706 (409) 860-4944

Graves, Michael, 3930 Kirby Dr., suite 205, Houston, TX 77098 (713) 528-2097

Jones, Bruce, 2537 S. Gessner, #120, Houston, TX 77063
(713) 771-4007

Lane-George, J. Christine, 2007 Hwy 332, Lake Jackson, TX 77566
(409) 798-9172

Magee, Harlin, 1910 Justin Ln., Austin, TX 78757
(512) 451-0846

Trevino, Olivia, 120 E. Park #8, Pharr, TX 78577
(210) 783-5303

Vetrone, Dee, 29526 Brookchase, Spring, TX 77386
(281) 298-5156

UTAH

State Licensing: 600 hours or 1,000-hour apprenticeship.

National Certification Exam accepted for portion of written exam.

Board: (801) 530-6551

SCHOOLS:

#523 Awakening Spirit Massage School
421 S. 400 E
Salt Lake City, UT 84111
(801) 532-5018

Contact school for program information.

#524 Myotherapy College of Utah
1174 E. 2700 S., suite 4
Salt Lake City, UT 84106
(801) 484-7624 or
1-800- 432-5968 (1-800-HEAL-YOU)

HOURS OF TRAINING: 780.

DURATION OF COURSE: day class 9 months, evening class 15 months

COST: $6,685 including books, fees and table.

FINANCIAL AID: scholarships available as well as Pell grants and FFELP loans.

YEAR FOUNDED: 1987.

GRADUATES PER YEAR (APPROX): 100.

ACCREDITATIONS/APPROVALS: ACCSCT, Utah Department of Rehabilitation, Veterans' Administration.

MODALITIES AND SUBJECTS: acupressure, acutherapy, applied anatomy, applied kinesiology, aromatherapy, body-mind, chair massage, chi gong, clinical pathology, clinical practice, common pathology, cranio-sacral therapy, cryotherapy, feldenkrais, functional anatomy, geriatric massage, hydrotherapy, infant massage, joint pathology, myofascial release, nutrition, organo body balancing, oriental meridians/shiatsu, personology, polarity, practice building, pregnancy massage, psychology for the massage therapist, reflexology, reiki, segmental massage, shiatsu II, specialized massage, spinal touch therapy I and II, sports massage I and II, survey of bodywork, tai chi, therapeutic principles, therapeutic touch, touch for health, trigger point therapy, tuina.

SCHOOL STATEMENT: Our program offers a positive, supportive atmosphere to promote greater personal awareness and wellness of the student, the practitioner and their clients.

#525 Ogden Institute of Massage Therapy
3500 Harrison Blvd.
Ogden, UT 84403
(801) 627-8227

HOURS OF TRAINING: 610 (518 in-class hours).

DURATION OF COURSE: one year, evenings.

COST: $6,000 including table, books, lab fees, clinic shirt.

YEAR FOUNDED: 1997.

GRADUATES PER YEAR (APPROX.): 20.

MODALITIES AND SUBJECTS: acupressure, applied kinesiology, aromatherapy, body mechanics, business & marketing, chair massage, chiropractic assisting, CPR, cranio-sacral therapy, deep tissue therapy, feldenkrais, health & wellness, infant massage, injury massage, law & ethics, lymphatic drainage, myofascial release, oriental bodywork, pregnancy massage, shiatsu, sports massage, touch for health, trigger point therapy.

SCHOOL STATEMENT: To prepare students entering the Alternative Healthcare field with necessary knowledge and skills, both business and massage therapy, to successfully practice this healing art.

#526 Sensory Development Institute
1871 W. Canyon View Drive
St. George, UT 84770
(435) 652-9003

HOURS OF TRAINING: 604.

DURATION OF COURSE: 10½ months (days).

COST: $6,000 including books and table.

YEAR FOUNDED: 1997.

GRADUATES PER YEAR (APPROX.): 40.

MODALITIES AND SUBJECTS: acupressure, advanced therapeutic massage, aromatherapy, business management & marketing, chair massage, CPR & first aid, cranio-sacral therapy, infant massage, neuromuscular therapy, nutrition & wellness, polarity, pregnancy massage, rebirthing, reflexology, reiki, sensory development, shiatsu, spa treatments, sports massage, state exam reviews, trigger point therapy, trimonics (spinal balance).

SCHOOL STATEMENT: Our philosophy of instruction is to provide students with a solid foundation of basic therapeutic massage, along with many hours of hands-on experience.

#527 Utah College of Massage Therapy
25 South 300 East
Salt Lake City, UT 84111
(801) 521-3330

HOURS OF TRAINING: 712

DURATION OF COURSE: six months days, one year evenings.

COST: $5,112 day program or $4,812 evening program including course manuals and clinic uniform.

FINANCIAL AID: Pell grants, Federal Family Education Loan Program, Vocational Rehabilitation, Veterans' Benefits.

YEAR FOUNDED: 1986.

ACCREDITATIONS/APPROVALS: COMTA/Accredited, ACCET.

MODALITIES AND SUBJECTS: Esalen, shiatsu, acupressure, Touch for Health, trigger point therapy, sports massage, Russian sports massage, injury massage, proprioceptive neuromuscular facilitation, craniosacral bodywork, on-site, infant massage, deep tissue bodywork, Feldenkrais, body mechanics, medical terminology, pathology, educational kinesiology, Russian classical massage, hydrotherapy, qi gong, t'ai chi, yoga, anatomical massage, body energy techniques, client prospecting, reflexology, first aid/CPR, AIDS awareness, professional development.

VERMONT

No State licensing.

SCHOOLS:

#528 Body Music
35 King St.
Burlington, VT 05401
(802) 860-2814

HOURS OF TRAINING: 400 (296 in-class hours).

DURATION OF COURSE: six week-long modules over a two-year period.

COST: $2,800 includes texts. Payment plan without interest is available.

FINANCIAL AID: Vermont Student Assistance grants available to Vermont residents.

YEAR FOUNDED: 1989.

GRADUATES PER YEAR (APPROX.): 12.

MODALITIES AND SUBJECTS: Resonant Kinesiology Training Program: developmental patterns, evolutionary movement, experiential anatomy & kinesiology, inclusive attention, language patterns, perception, structure of emotions, vibration.

SCHOOL STATEMENT: Advanced training for experienced bodyworkers, teachers, therapists and health professionals, learning to use inclusive attention, touch, movement and sound to evoke learning and health.

#529 Nippon Shiatsu Daigaku
Box 330J RR2 (Fred Hougton Rd)
Putney, VT 05346
(802) 387-5594

HOURS OF TRAINING: 100 to 1000.

DURATION OF COURSE: 30 weeks to 2 years or more, day & weekend programs available.

FINANCIAL AID: Scholarships, VT Student Assistance Corp.

YEAR FOUNDED: 1950 (private instruction; the school's director has been teaching shiatsu since 1950 and was a founder of the AOBTA).

GRADUATES PER YEAR (APPROX.): 25 to 30

MODALITIES AND SUBJECTS: acupressure, applied kinesiology, chair massage, chi gong, cranio-sacral therapy, hoshino, integrative eclectic shiatsu, jin shin do, lymphatic drainage, pregnancy massage, shen, sports massage, tui na.

SCHOOL STATEMENT: The school teaches and trains students to practice Integrative/Eclectic Shiatsu for the purpose of promoting spiritual, mental and physical health within people professionally.

#530 Universal Institute of Healing Arts
RFD 3, Box 5285
Montpelier, VT 05602
(802) 229-4844 or in VT 1-800-773-4844

HOURS OF TRAINING: 170 (one evening per week).

COST: $2,600 over 3 years.

YEAR FOUNDED: 1982.

GRADUATES PER YEAR (APPROX.): 5.

MODALITIES AND SUBJECTS: alignment assessment & treatment, bodywork strategies, business practices, chakra system & meridians & aura, crystal healing, deep tissue proprioception & therapy, dynamic body assessment, emergency relief, energy release, ethical issues, high sense perception, injury assessment & treatment, moxabustion, self-care, sensitivity & awareness development, shiatsu meridian clearing & treatment, sotai, stretching, symptomatic treatment, visual body assessment, wellness, yin/yang energy.

SCHOOL STATEMENT: Heal yourself in some way and you may help another.

#531 Vermont Institute of Massage Therapy
10 Cottage Grove Ave
So. Burlington, VT 05403
(802) 862-1111

HOURS OF TRAINING: 550.

DURATION OF COURSE: 12 months days, 18 months evenings.

COST: $3,700.

FINANCIAL AID: State aid through Vt. Student Asst. Corp. Interest-free payment plan available.

YEAR FOUNDED: 1986.

GRADUATES PER YEAR (APPROX.): 25 to 30.

MODALITIES AND SUBJECTS: acupressure, advanced massage, applied kinesiology, aromatherapy, chair massage, deep relaxation techniques, infant massage, pregnancy massage, pressure points, quantum physics, reflexology, small business preparation.

SCHOOL STATEMENT: Comprehensive format preparing effective massage therapists to work in harmony for the physical and emotional well-being of themselves and their clients.

#532 Vermont School of Professional Massage
14 Merchant Street
Barre, VT 05641
(802) 479-2340 or 1-800-287-8816

HOURS OF TRAINING: 600.

DURATION OF COURSE: 9 months, days.

COST: $3,800 includes books and practicum materials. Payment plan without interest is available.

FINANCIAL AID: Vermont Student Assistance Corp. Non-Degree Grants.

YEAR FOUNDED: 1989.

GRADUATES PER YEAR (APPROX.): 10.

MODALITIES AND SUBJECTS: bindegewebsmassage, business practices, ethics, massage theory, medical massage, medical terminology, myofascial release, neuromuscular therapy, office procedures, practicum, trigger point therapy.

SCHOOL STATEMENT: This family oriented 600 hour structured program prepares our graduates for careers in the health profession of Massage Therapy and enables one to sit for the NCETMB.

VIRGINIA

State Licensing requires 500 hours of education.

National Certification Exam accepted.

  Board (Board of Nursing): (804) 662-9909

SCHOOLS:

#533 Advanced Fuller School of Massage
3500 Virginia Beach Blvd., #100
Virginia Beach, VA 23452
(757) 340-7132

HOURS OF TRAINING: 250 to 800.

DURATION OF COURSE: 5½ to 12 months, day & evening & weekend classes available.

COST: 250 hours $1,720; 500 hours $3,460 (both include books).

FINANCIAL AID: Veteran's Administration, Internship Program, Dept. of Rehab., Dept. of Blind.

YEAR FOUNDED: 1983.

GRADUATES PER YEAR (APPROX.): 80.

MODALITIES AND SUBJECTS: acupressure, applied kinesiology, aromatherapy, body mechanics, body-mind, business management & professional ethics, chair massage, CPR/first aid, cranio-sacral therapy, hydrotherapy, infant massage, medical massage, myofascial and deep tissue techniques, myotherapy, neuromuscular therapy, oriental massage, ortho-bionomy, pregnancy massage, qi gong, range of motion, reflexology, sports massage, therapeutic stretches, touch for health.

ADVANCED PROGRAMS: Up to 300 hours of advanced training may be taken as individual courses — advanced anatomy and physiology, aromatherapy certification, mind/body integrative therapy, marketing/business practice, hydrotherapy, advanced sports massage, injury assessment and therapy, myofascial release, oriental massage, reflexology certification, medicinal herbs/aromatherapy/nutrition, integration of clinical skills. 300-hour advanced certificate is awarded for completion of all advanced course work.

SCHOOL STATEMENT: Our proven program challenges students to be the best. After the 250-hour basic, you receive $20 per massage intern pay while completing certification requirements.

#534 American Institute of Massage
3900 Monument, suite B
Richmond, VA 23230
(804) 254-3977

Contact school for program information.

#535 American Spirit Institute
473 McLaws Circle
Williamsburg, VA 23185
(757) 220-8000

Contact school for program information.

#536 Applied Kinesiology Studies
1671 Cedar Hollow Way
Reston, VA 20194
(Classroom: 692 Pine, Herndon)
(703) 471-9332

HOURS OF TRAINING: 500 (in-class hours not specified).

DURATION OF COURSE: 9 months, day and evening programs available.

COST: $3,125 including books. Payment plan without interest is available.

FINANCIAL AID: Veteran's Administration.

YEAR FOUNDED: 1992.

GRADUATES PER YEAR (APPROX.): 45.

MODALITIES AND SUBJECTS: acupressure, alexander, applied kinesiology, aromatherapy, chair massage, cranio-sacral therapy, myofascial release, polarity, pregnancy massage, reflexology, reiki, rolfing, shiatsu, sports massage, touch for health, trager.

SCHOOL STATEMENT: Basic Swedish Massage, with introduction to other modalities listed above.

#537 Blue Ridge Massage and Yoga School
201 S. Main Street
Blacksburg, VA 24060
(540) 552-2177

HOURS OF TRAINING: 500.

DURATION OF COURSE: 12 months or 18 months.

COST: $3,400 plus textbooks, table, supplies and application fee. Payment plan without interest is available.

YEAR FOUNDED: 1990.

MODALITIES AND SUBJECTS: alexander technique for bodyworkers, benefits & contraindication, comprehensive & holistic healthcare, eastern & western massage, ethical responsibilities, history, legal requirement, massage theory, myofascial release, osteopathic massage & bodywork, reflexology (certification), yoga.

SCHOOL STATEMENT: The School exists to train massage therapists in a comprehensive course of bodywork techniques that enable practitioners to be of service to the human condition.

#538 Cayce/Reilly School of Massotherapy
P.O. Box 595 / 67th Street And Atlantic Ave.
Virginia Beach, VA 23451
www.are-cayce.com
(757) 437-7202

HOURS OF TRAINING: 600 (578 in-class hours).

DURATION OF COURSE: approximately 6½ months, courses offered days or evenings.

COST: Tuition $4,500, application fee $35.00, books $350.00, supplies $150.00. Payment plan without interest is available.

FINANCIAL AID: Veterans benefits, Dept. of Visually Handicapped, Dept of Rehabilitative services, State employment Commissions, Tuition Reduction.

YEAR FOUNDED: 1987.

ACCREDITATIONS/APPROVALS: COMTA/Accredited.

GRADUATES PER YEAR (APPROX.): 80.

MODALITIES AND SUBJECTS: body/mind/spirit, Cayce home remedies, Cayce/Reilly massotherapy, chair massage, cranio-sacral therapy, dreams & meditation, foot reflexology, healing touch, hydrotherapy therapeutic touch, intermediate massage, integrative massage, introduction to alexander techniques, introduction to jin shin do, lymphatic drainage, neuromuscular therapy, pregnancy massage, professional business & ethics, sports massage, therapeutic massage, therapeutic touch, zero balancing.

SCHOOL STATEMENT: We seek individuals who wish to develop not only as massage therapists and also as healers truly desiring to integrate body, mind and spirit.

#539 Daniels Institute for Holistic Health, Inc.
2329 Franklin Road, S.W.
Roanoke, VA 24016
(540) 344-3538

Contact school for program information.

#540 Natural Touch School of Massage Therapy
291 Park Ave.
Danville, VA 24541
(804) 799-0060

1204 Main St.
Lynchburg, VA 24504
(804) 845-3003

HOURS OF TRAINING: 500.

DURATION OF COURSE: 25 weeks days or 18 months evenings.

COST: $4,500 plus $200 books and $150 materials. Payment plan without interest is available.

FINANCIAL AID: South Central Private Industry Council (804) 392-2300.

YEAR FOUNDED: 1994.

GRADUATES PER YEAR (APPROX.): 16-20.

MODALITIES AND SUBJECTS: applied kinesiology, bioenergetics, body-mind, body psychology, business & ethics, classical massage, cranio-sacral therapy, deep tissue, energy, esalen, functional assessment, healing touch, hydrotherapy, myofascial release, neuromuscular therapy, polarity, rebirthing, shiatsu, somatic therapy, sports massage, stretching, therapeutic touch, trigger point therapy, yoga therapy.

SCHOOL STATEMENT: From a solid foundation of A&P, we teach therapeutic bodywork, with an energetic awareness of the body's inner wisdom, to awaken the healer within.

#541 The Piedmont School of Professional Massage, Inc.
12712 Directors Loop
Woodbridge, VA 22192
(703) 492-2024

HOURS OF TRAINING: 500.

DURATION OF COURSE: 10 months, day or evening program available.

COST: $3,970 includes 2 texts, 1 workbook, set of massage tools. Payment plan without interest is available.

FINANCIAL AID: Discount for prepayment.

YEAR FOUNDED: 1995.

GRADUATES PER YEAR (APPROX.): 22.

MODALITIES AND SUBJECTS: aromatherapy, business, chair massage, chi gong, CPR/first aid, esalen, ethics, history, holistic health, hydrotherapy, indications & contraindication, intro. to allied professions, intro to specialized techniques, legalities, lymphatic drainage, nutrition, postural analysis, pregnancy massage, reflexology, reiki, shiatsu, sports massage, stretching & exercise, therapeutic touch, trager, trigger point therapy.

SCHOOL STATEMENT: Our program is professionally oriented. Graduates become entry level professionals able to meet the needs of business, the health care and personal service industries.

#542 RAV School of Professional Studies
Pembroke Three, suite 300
Virginia Beach, VA 23462
(757) 499-5447

1001 Boulders Pkwy., suite 305
Richmond, VA 23225

5501 Backlick Rd., suite 250
Springfield, VA 22151

HOURS OF TRAINING: 600.

DURATION OF COURSE: 6 months days, 15 months evenings.

COST: $5,237 including books and application fee.

FINANCIAL AID: Discount for full payment within the first week of class, Pell Grants, Stafford Loans, PLUS loans.

YEAR FOUNDED: 1975.

ACCREDITATIONS/APPROVALS: Accrediting Council for Independent Colleges and Schools.

GRADUATES PER YEAR (APPROX.): 50.

MODALITIES AND SUBJECTS: advanced massage, applied kinesiology, aromatherapy, body-mind, chair massage, fundamental massage, hydrotherapy, introduction to business, jin shin do, medical terminology, professionalism & ethics, reflexology, shiatsu, sports massage.

SCHOOL STATEMENT: Massage Program is designed to ensure the graduate will have met the Virginia State requirements to sit for the state certification exam.

#543 Richmond Academy of Massage
2004 Bremo Rd., suite 102
Richmond, VA 23226
(804) 282-5003

HOURS OF TRAINING: approx. 800 (approx. 500 in-class).

DURATION OF COURSE: 12 months evenings and some Saturdays.

COST: $3,850 including books. Payment plan without interest is available.

FINANCIAL AID: VA Dept. of Rehab., Capital Area Training Consortium, Veteran's Administration.

YEAR FOUNDED: 1987.

PREPARATION FOR OUT-OF-STATE LICENSING EXAM: Oregon.

GRADUATES PER YEAR (APPROX): 45.

MODALITIES AND SUBJECTS: acupressure, AMMA, chair massage, geriatric massage, medical massage, pregnancy massage, reflexology, shiatsu, sports massage, therapeutic massage theory & practical, trigger point therapy.

SCHOOL STATEMENT: Structured for those wishing to make a full-time career in Massage Therapy. Emphasis on self-awareness, personal growth, and attention to detail. National Exam Eligibility.

#544 Richmond School of Health and Technology
P.O. Box 2111
Richmond, VA 23218-2111
(Classroom: 421 E. Franklin, 3rd floor)
(804) 780-0167

HOURS OF TRAINING: Basic 100 hours, Intermediate 200 hours, Advanced 200 hours.

DURATION OF COURSE: Each program lasts 6 months; day and evening classes available.

COST: Basic $750, Intermediate $1,050, Advanced $1,050 plus $50 per program for textbooks and lab fee.

FINANCIAL AID: Scholarships or discounts available.

YEAR FOUNDED: 1997.

MODALITIES AND SUBJECTS: acupressure, amanae, AMMA, applied kinesiology, aromatherapy, aston-patterning, berrywork, bioenergetics, body logic, body-mind, bowen technique, chair massage, chi gong, cranio-sacral therapy, designer massage, esalen, feldenkrais, hakomi bodywork, healing touch, hellerwork, hoshino therapy, jin shin do, looyenwork, medical massage, myofascial release, myotherapy, neuromuscular therapy, polarity, postural integration, radiance technique, reflexology, reiki, shiatsu, shen, somatic therapy, sports massage, therapeutic touch, touch for health, trigger point therapy, tui na, watsu.

SCHOOL STATEMENT: This comprehensive program prepares graduates for state certification. Emphasis on mind/body/spirit connection and bio-energy techniques (e.g., acupressure, polarity, reflexology, reiki, shiatsu, etc.).

#545 Virginia Academy of Massage Therapy
5314 George Washington Memorial Hwy.
Yorktown, VA 23692
(757) 872-0934

Contact school for program information.

#546 Virginia School of Massage
2008 Morton Drive
Charlottesville, VA 22903
(804) 293-4031 or 1-888-599-2001

HOURS OF TRAINING: 500 (in-class hours not specified).

DURATION OF COURSE: 18 months, day & evening programs available.

COST: $4,350.

YEAR FOUNDED: 1989.

GRADUATES PER YEAR (APPROX.): 80.

MODALITIES AND SUBJECTS: alexander technique, applied kinesiology, body-mind, chair massage, cranio-sacral therapy, healing touch, myofascial release, myotherapy, polarity, postural integration, reflexology, shiatsu, sports massage, structural integration, therapeutic touch, zero balancing.

SCHOOL STATEMENT: VSM provides a comprehensive academically challenging program. All subjects taught from holistic perspective, emphasizing the transformational aspects of bodywork.

WASHINGTON

State Licensing: 500 hours.

National Certification Exam accepted.

Board: (360) 586-6351

APPROVED OUT-OF-STATE SCHOOLS:

American Institute (ID); American Institute, Costa Mesa CA; Atlanta School of Massage; Bancroft School of Massage, (MA); Bonnie Prudden, Tucson AZ (see Trigger Point); Boulder School of Massage (CO); Cascade Institute (OR); Central Ohio School; Chicago School of Massage; Colorado Institute of MT; Colorado School of Healing Arts; Connecticut Center for Massage; Crystal Mountain (NM); Desert Institute (AZ); East-West College (OR); Feldenkrais Guild, P.O. Box 489, Albany OR; Hawaiian Islands School; Health Enrichment (MI); Heartwood (CA); International Professional School (San Diego, CA); Moscow School (ID); Mueller College (CA); Myotherapy Institute (UT); National Holistic Inst (CA); New Center (NY); New Mexico Academy of Healing Arts; New Mexico School of Natural Therapeutics; Oregon School of Massage; Pennsylvania School of Muscle Therapy; The Rolf Institute, Boulder CO; Scherer Academy (NM); South Dakota School of Massage Therapy; Suncoast (FL); Swedish Institute (NY); Utah College of Massage Therapy.

SCHOOLS:

#547 Alexandar School of Natural Therapeutics
4032 Pacific Ave.
Tacoma, WA 98408
(253) 473-1142

HOURS OF TRAINING: 650.

COST: $6,300.

YEAR FOUNDED: 1979.

GRADUATES PER YEAR (APPROX): 60.

MODALITIES AND SUBJECTS: aromatherapy & herbal & facial & body spa treatments, body psyche & advanced deep body work, business practices & management, chair massage, clinical applications, fundamental of oriental medicine, human behavior & client interaction, hydrotherapy, indications & contraindication, insurance & law & recordkeeping, living kinesiology & body mechanics, muscle anatomy & kinesiology, pathophysiology, reflexology, remedial exercises, sports massage I & II, student clinic.

SCHOOL STATEMENT: The ASNT is committed to provide an innovative and creative program in the natural healthcare field, specifically in the instruction of massage and bodywork modalities.

#548 Bellevue Massage School
16301 NE 8th, suite 210
Bellevue, WA 98008
(425) 641-3409

HOURS OF TRAINING: 513.

DURATION OF COURSE: 6½ months, day & evening & weekend programs offered.

COST: $5,230.

FINANCIAL AID: Discount for prepayment, L & I Providers (Dept. of Labor Industries).

YEAR FOUNDED: 1977.

GRADUATES PER YEAR (APPROX): 60.

MODALITIES AND SUBJECTS: acupressure, AIDS education, aromatherapy, body-mind, business skills & marketing, carpal tunnel prevention & education, chair massage, CPR/first aid, cranio-sacral therapy, deep tissue, emotional stress release, healing touch, holistic self-care healing, hydrotherapy, infant massage, insurance billing, jin shin do, kinesiology, lomilomi, lymphatic drainage, maniken, medical massage, myofascial release, ortho-bionomy, palpation, pathology, postural balancing, pregnancy massage, professional ethics, reflexology, reiki, shiatsu, soma bodywork, sports massage, student clinic, therapeutic touch, touch for health, trager, treatment massage, trigger point therapy, yoga therapy.

SCHOOL STATEMENT: Small classes for individual attention, an innovative, unique program that encourages students to use massage and other modalities to enhance their lives and the lives of others physically, mentally, emotionally and spiritually. Credit may be awarded for prior massage education.

#549 The Bodymind Academy
1247 – 120th Ave. NE, suite K
Bellevue, WA 98005
(425) 635-0145

HOURS OF TRAINING: 639 (619 in-class).

DURATION OF TRAINING: 9 months, day or evening/weekend programs available.

COST: $6,387 includes books and manuals.

FINANCIAL AID: Veteran's Administration, WA State Workforce Training, DVR, Labor and Industries Retraining Programs.

YEAR FOUNDED: 1990.

GRADUATES PER YEAR (APPROX): 40.

MODALITIES AND SUBJECTS: abuse and the body, AIDS trainings, aromatherapy, case study internship program, chair massage, client assessment and charting, cranio-sacral therapy, deep tissue, emotional release during massage, ethics, first aid/CPR, injury treatment, insurance billing, kinesiology, laws, learning processes, lymphatic drainage, medical massage, medical terminology, myofascial release, neuromuscular therapy, palpation, pregnancy massage, proprioceptive neuromuscular facilitation, practice management & professionalism, reciprocal inhibition, reiki, self-care, shiatsu, sports massage, trigger point, tui na. Advanced programs: The school also offers certification Advanced programs: shiatsu, counseling hypnotherapy, breathwork and fitness & nutrition. Completion of all five core programs is the first step toward certification as a BodyMind Practitioner.

SCHOOL STATEMENT: The training incorporates emotional sensitivity, medical knowledge and bodywork modalities into a healing process that is grounded in experiencing touch as a catalyst for healing.

#550 The Brenneke School of Massage
160 Roy St.
Seattle, WA 98109
(206) 282-1233

HOURS OF TRAINING: 650 or 1,000 (in-class hours not specified).

DURATION OF COURSE: one year (either program), day and evening programs available.

COST: 650 hours $6,350; 1,000 hours $9,500.

FINANCIAL AID: scholarships, tuition waiver, Pell grants, Stafford Loans, PLUS loans, DVR, Commission for the Blind, Veterans Administration, Employment security, Labor and Industries Retraining program.

YEAR FOUNDED: 1974.

GRADUATES PER YEAR (APPROX): 150.

ACCREDITATIONS/APPROVALS: COMTA/Accredited, ACCSCT, Washington Workforce Training and Education Coordinating Board, approved for CEU's for Certified Athletic Trainers.

PREPARATION FOR OUT-OF-STATE LICENSING EXAM: Ohio.

MODALITIES AND SUBJECTS: AIDS education, aromatherapy, bindegewebsmassage, body-mind, business skills, cadaver anatomy, chair massage, chi gong, common running injuries, connective tissue massage, cranio-sacral therapy, feldenkrais, field experience/externship, first aid/CPR, hanna somatics, healing touch, hellerwork, herbology, infant massage, intermediate & advanced massage techniques, introduction to oriental massage, kinesiology, loku lomi, lomilomi, massage labs, medical massage, lymphatic drainage, myofascial release, myotherapy, naturopathic hydrotherapy, neuromuscular therapy, pathology, polarity, pregnancy massage, professional development, reflexology, reiki, shiatsu, somatic therapy, sports massage, teaching clinic, therapeutic touch, treatment clinic, trigger point therapy, ways of learning.

SCHOOL STATEMENT: We offer a supportive, non-competitive environment for learning. Emphasis on body-mind connection, injury treatment and health maintenance. Individual interests supported through elective classes.

#551 Brian Utting School of Massage
900 Thomas St.
Seattle, WA 98109
(206) 292-8055 or 1-800-842-8731

HOURS OF TRAINING: 1,000.

DURATION OF COURSE: 14 to 15 months, day and evening programs available.

COST: $10,150 to $11,055, including books, massage table, licensing fees, optional electives and miscellaneous expenses.

YEAR FOUNDED: 1982.

ACCREDITATIONS/APPROVALS: COMTA/Accredited, Veterans' Administration, Workforce Retraining.

PREPARATION FOR OUT-OF-STATE LICENSING EXAM: Oregon.

GRADUATES PER YEAR (APPROX.): 120.

MODALITIES AND SUBJECTS: acupressure, bindegewebsmassage, business skills and marketing, cadaver anatomy, chair massage, circulatory massage, communication skills, connective tissue massage, cranio-sacral therapy, deep tissue techniques, hydrotherapy, hygiene, injury evaluation and treatment, kinesiology, lymphatic drainage, medical massage, movement, myofascial release, myotherapy, neuromuscular therapy, pathology, postural integration, pregnancy massage, professional ethics, reflexology, self-care, shiatsu, sports massage, structural integration, student clinic, trager, trigger point therapy.

SCHOOL STATEMENT: Our mission is to produce outstanding massage practitioners with a deeper sense of their humanity.

#552 Cedar Mountain Center for Massage, Inc.
2700 NE Andresen Road
Vancouver, WA 98661
(360) 696-2210

HOURS OF TRAINING: 700 (550 in-class hours).

DURATION OF COURSE: one year, day and evening programs are available.

COST: $6,550 plus books $300. Payment plan without interest is available.

YEAR FOUNDED: 1984.

ACCREDITATIONS/APPROVALS: private vocational school association.

PREPARATION FOR OUT-OF-STATE LICENSING EXAM: Oregon.

GRADUATES PER YEAR (APPROX.): 60.

MODALITIES AND SUBJECTS: AMMA, aromatherapy, clinic practice, communication skills, connective tissue massage, deep tissue, educational kinesiology, history of massage, hydrotherapy, hygiene, independent study, internship, kinesiology, pathology, reflexology, shiatsu, touch for health.

SCHOOL STATEMENT: We focus on educating students to become "thinking therapists", preparing them to meet the challenge of clients' health needs in a creative and appropriate way.

#553 Gabriel Institute
22515 100th Place, Southwest
Vashon Island, WA 98070
(206) 463-1200

Contact school for program information.

#554 Inland Massage Institute, Inc.
W. 1717 Francis Ave., suite 103
Spokane, WA 99205
(509) 328-3116

HOURS OF TRAINING: 650.

COST: $4.600 plus $500 books and fees.

YEAR FOUNDED: 1988.

GRADUATES PER YEAR (APPROX.): 65.

#555 New Perspectives Institute
Northwest Hellerwork
3210 NE 167th St.
Lake Forest Park, WA 98155
(206) 368-8145 or (800) 243-5194

HOURS OF TRAINING: 1,250 (840 in-class hours).

DURATION OF COURSE: 6 2-week intensives over a period of 18 months.

COST: $12,900.

YEAR FOUNDED: 1979.

ACCREDITATIONS/APPROVALS: WA State Workforce Training, Ed. Coordinating Board.

GRADUATES PER YEAR (APPROX.): 16.

MODALITIES AND SUBJECTS: Hellerwork is a system of structural bodywork that integrates movement education, energetics and dialogue. It is based on the inseparability of body, mind and spirit, and it emphasizes self-awareness and balance. Graduates of this training are prepared for the Washington Massage Licensing Exam and are also certified Hellerwork Practitioners (see listing in Bodywork section).

#556 Northwest School of Massage
1727 S. 341st Place, suite D
Federal Way, WA 98003
(253) 838-6225

519 hours, 6 months. Contact school for program information.

#557 Peninsula College Massage Therapy Program
1502 East Lauridsen Blvd.
Port Angeles, WA 98362
(360) 417-6569
www.pc.ctc.edu

HOURS OF TRAINING: 850 to 1,000 (800 to 950 in-class hours).

COST: in-state $3,496; out-of-state $7,727 (including books, massage table, supplies, state exam fee and licensing fee.

YEAR FOUNDED: 1995.

GRADUATES PER YEAR (APPROX.): 20.

MODALITIES AND SUBJECTS: chair massage, clinic practicum, communications, deep tissue, first aid & CPR, HIV/AIDS, hydrotherapy, injury treatment & evaluation, kinesiology, movement & body mechanics, neuromuscular therapy, pathology, professional development, professional ethics, professional placement, shiatsu.

SCHOOL STATEMENT: Weaving together a broad scope of approaches, our curriculum strives to assure graduates a high-quality holistic vase from which to launch a massage career.

#558 Port Townsend School of Massage
       P.O. Box 1055
       Port Townsend, WA 98368
       (360) 385-6183

HOURS OF TRAINING: 545 (530 in-class).

DURATION OF COURSE: 9 months days or 14 months weekends.

COST: $5,535 including textbooks and anatomy lab.

YEAR FOUNDED: 1996.

GRADUATES PER YEAR (APPROX.): 28.

MODALITIES AND SUBJECTS: acupressure, aromatherapy, chair massage, clinical treatments, deep tissue, hydrotherapy, kinesiology, lymphatic drainage, medical massage, pathology, polarity, professional practice, reiki, sports massage, student clinic, therapeutic touch.

#559 Renton Technical College Massage Program
       3000 Northeast Fourth St.
       Renton, WA 98056
       (425) 235-2352

Contact school for program information.

#560 Seattle Massage School
       7120 Woodlawn Ave. NE
       Seattle, WA 98115
       (206) 527-0807

       5005 Pacific Highway E, suite 20
       Fife, WA 98424
       (253) 926-1435

       2721 Wetmore Ave.
       Everett, WA 98201
       (425) 339-2678
       www.seattlemassageschool.com

COST: $8,990.

YEAR FOUNDED: 1974.

GRADUATES PER YEAR (APPROX.): 200.

MODALITIES AND SUBJECTS: AIDS education, business skills, chair massage, chronic pain, deep tissue techniques, first aid & CPR, hospital internship, hydrotherapy, kinesiology I–IV, massage theory & practice I–IV, pregnancy massage, professional development I–IV, sports massage, student clinic, student project.

SCHOOL STATEMENT: To promote touch as a positive force in the world through massage education. To support people in creating meaningful work in the massage field.

#561 Soma Institute of Neuromuscular Integration
       730 Klink Rd.
       Buckley, WA 98321
       (360) 829-1025
       www.soma-institute.com

HOURS OF TRAINING: 568.

DURATION OF COURSE: 6 months weekends.

COST: $9,500.

FINANCIAL AID: Workforce Training & Educational Coordinating Board.

YEAR FOUNDED: 1978 (1986 current owner).

GRADUATES PER YEAR (APPROX.): 12 to 16.

MODALITIES AND SUBJECTS: Foundation training in massage, plus Soma program certification for neuromuscular integration bodywork; medical applications of soma, somatic education.

SCHOOL STATEMENT: Soma creates change in the bodymind through a ten session format. Change is evident in physical well-being, optimum functioning and emotional self reliance.

#562 Spectrum Center School of Massage
       1001 N. Russell Rd.
       Snohomish, WA 98290
       (classroom: 12506 18th St. NE, Lake Stevens)
       (425) 334-5409 or (800) 801-9451

HOURS OF TRAINING: 756 (656 in-class hours).

DURATION OF COURSE: 10 months, day and evening programs available.

COST: $6,000 plus $1,100 for fees, books, table, etc.

YEAR FOUNDED: 1981.

ACCREDITATIONS/APPROVALS: Dept. of Labor and Industries, Division of Vocational Rehabilitation, Veterans Administration, Commission for the Blind.

GRADUATES PER YEAR (APPROX.): 34 to 36.

MODALITIES AND SUBJECTS: business practices, chair massage, clinical treatments, deep tissue/ advanced techniques, human behavior, hydrotherapy, indications and contraindications, kinesiology, lymphatic drainage, massage theory and practice, medical terminology, orientation, pathology, polarity, pregnancy massage, sports massage, student clinic, study skills, AIDS.

SCHOOL STATEMENT: All teachers have extensive teaching experience. Small class size enables students with various learning styles to receive personalized instruction.

#563 Tri-City School of Massage
       26 E. Third Ave
       Kennewick, WA 99336
       (509) 586-6434
       (school located in Southeast Washington)

HOURS OF TRAINING: 850 (600 in-class hours).

DURATION OF COURSE: six months.

COST: $4,400 includes books.

YEAR FOUNDED: 1968.

ACCREDITATIONS/APPROVALS: COMTA/approved.

GRADUATES PER YEAR (APPROX.): 20–40.

MODALITIES AND SUBJECTS: acupressure, AIDS awareness, applied anatomy, body mechanics, business & professional ethics, chair massage, clinical application, connective tissue, health & hygiene, hydrotherapy, infant massage, iridology, kinesiology, lymphatic drainage, magnetic therapy, medical gymnastics, pathology, polarity, positional release, pregnancy massage, reflexology, shiatsu, skilled touch, sports massage, thesis.

SCHOOL STATEMENT: Our goal is to present a comprehensive set of principles and tools from which the student can choose when faced with a particular problem.

WEST VIRGINIA

State licensing requires attendance at COMTA-approved or state-approved school

Board: WV Massage Therapy Licensing Board, P.O. Box 8038, S. Charleston, WV, 25303 (304) 736-0621

SCHOOLS:

#564 Mountain State School of Massage
P.O. Box 4487
Charleston, WV 25364
(304) 926-8822
www.mtnstmassage.com

HOURS OF TRAINING: 750 (650 in-class) or 700 (home study, 315 in-class hours).

DURATION OF COURSE: 750 hours six months, days; 700 hours 16 months.

COST: 750 hours $5,600 + textbooks; 700 hours $5,200 including textbooks.

FINANCIAL AID: Discounts available.

YEAR FOUNDED: 1995.

GRADUATES PER YEAR (APPROX.): 25.

MODALITIES AND SUBJECTS: awareness & communication skills, chair massage, connective tissue, CPR/first aid & preventing communicable diseases, ethics, hydrotherapy, infant massage, kinesiology, massage law & business practices, neuromuscular therapy, pathology, polarity, pregnancy massage, reflexology, shiatsu, sports massage.

SCHOOL STATEMENT: MSSM is dedicated to providing quality education, combining a comprehensive approach to training with an intuitive focus to the art and science of massage therapy.

WISCONSIN

State licensing: 500 to 600 hours (to be determined). See page 130.

SCHOOLS:

#565 A SpiriTouch Institute
6225 University Ave., Suite 202
Madison, WI 53705
(608) 236-9042

HOURS OF TRAINING: 600 (in-class hours not specified).

COST: $4,800.

YEAR FOUNDED: 1997.

GRADUATES PER YEAR (APPROX.): 66.

SCHOOL STATEMENT: ASI's intention is to help students open their hearts, learn the skills of a respected, growing profession, and hring their spirit through to touch lives.

#566 The Balanced Touch Institute, Inc.
N-7576 Timber Dr.,
Rib Lake, WI 54470
(715) 427-3369

HOURS OF TRAINING: 650 (500 in-class hours).

DURATION OF COURSE: 2 years, one evening per week.

YEAR FOUNDED: 1988.

GRADUATES PER YEAR (APPROX.): 16 every two years.

MODALITIES AND SUBJECTS: business practices, ethics, kinesiology, massage theory and practice, stress reduction techniques, therapeutic touch.

SCHOOL STATEMENT: The two-year, once-a-week schedule allows students the opportunity to integrate massage practice into their lives prior to graduation.

#567 Blue Sky Educational Foundation
220 Oak Street
Grafton, WI 53024
(414) 376-1011

HOURS OF TRAINING: 700 (500 in-class hours).

DURATION OF COURSE: 10 months; day, evening and weekend programs available.

COST: $5,975 including books and materials.

YEAR FOUNDED: 1985.

ACCREDITATIONS/APPROVALS: IMF, City of Milwaukee.

GRADUATES PER YEAR (APPROX): 100.

MODALITIES AND SUBJECTS: advanced massage techniques for lower back, allied health sciences review, ayurvedic facial massage, chair massage, clinical pathology in the massage practice, clinical preceptorship, facial massage, hatha for health professionals, healing touch, healthy cooking,. infant massage, introduction to business world, introduction to massage, juicing for health, learning strategies, lymphatic drainage, medical terminology & writing progress notes, movement therapy, muscles and bones, myofascial release, natural medicine, neuromuscular therapy I, II, III, IV & V, polarity I & II, pregnancy massage, reflexology, reiki, somatic therapy I & II, sports massage I, II & III, tai chi, therapeutic techniques & specialty areas, touch for health I, II & III, world of natural medicine, yoga therapy.

SCHOOL STATEMENT: Blue Sky is a non-profit organization committed to a sustainable future and to emotional, physical and spiritual well-being.

#568 Capri College
6414 Odana Road
Madison, WI 53719
(608) 274-5390 or (800) 747-8953
www.capricollege.com

HOURS OF TRAINING: 650 (in-class hours not specified).

DURATION OF COURSE: 29 weeks (one week vacation), evenings and weekends.

COST: $4,350 tuition; $5,330 including textbooks, table, carrying case, head cradle, bolster and table warmer.

FINANCIAL AID: Pell Grants, Stafford and PLUS loans, Federal SEOG grant.

ACCREDITATIONS/APPROVALS: ACCSCT, Accrediting Comm. of Career Schools & Colleges of Technology.

YEAR FOUNDED: Capri College (Iowa) 1966; Madison program 1994.

GRADUATES PER YEAR (APPROX): 30.

MODALITIES AND SUBJECTS: anatomiken hands-on anatomy, business management & marketing, chair massage, CPR & first aid, emotional release work, feldenkrais, intake & assessment intensive, ortho-bionomy, personal communication, shiatsu intensive, therapeutic touch, touch for health, trager.

SCHOOL STATEMENT: Capri offers a solid foundation in swedish massage, body mechanics, anatomy and marketing, emphasizing personal growth to promote mind body integration for practitioner and client.

#569 Chi Energy Massage and Body Work School
4222 Milwaukee St., suite 12 (Door #4)
Madison, WI 53714
(608) 244-1715

HOURS OF TRAINING: 662 (512 in-class hours).

DURATION OF COURSE: 18 to 24 months, one day and two evenings per week plus weekends.

COST: $3,230 plus approx. $700 books and approx. $500 massage table, $30 application fee.

FINANCIAL AID: Discounts available and credit for previously taken classes, GI bill.

YEAR FOUNDED: 1996.

GRADUATES PER YEAR (APPROX.): 5.

MODALITIES AND SUBJECTS: acupressure, applied kinesiology, aromatherapy, body-mind, chair massage, chi energy massage & bodywork, chi gong, cranio-sacral therapy, healing touch, holistic health, infant massage, jin shin do, joint tension release, lymphatic drainage, medical massage, meridian therapy, myofascial release, myotherapy, neuromuscular therapy, ortho-bionomy, polarity, postural integration, pregnancy massage, reflexology, reiki, shiatsu, somatic therapy, structural integration, therapeutic touch, touch for health, trigger point therapy, tui na.

SCHOOL STATEMENT: Instead of learning one technique, now you can simultaneously learn the whole body correlation of many Natural and Complementary Holistic Healing Arts and Techniques.

#570 Fox Valley School of Massage
P.O. Box 615
Neenah, WI 54157
(Classroom: 2003 Meade St., Appleton)
(920) 722-3271

HOURS OF TRAINING: 500 (352 in-class hours).

DURATION OF COURSE: 5 months full-time or 9 months part time, day & evening programs available.

COST: $5,000. Payment plan without interest is available.

YEAR FOUNDED: 1996.

GRADUATES PER YEAR (APPROX.): 40.

MODALITIES AND SUBJECTS: aromatherapy, chair massage, chi gong, cranio-sacral therapy, hydrotherapy, infant massage, myofascial stretching, myotherapy, neuromuscular therapy, ortho-bionomy, polarity, pregnancy massage, shiatsu, sports massage, yoga therapy.

SCHOOL STATEMENT: The school seeks students who are committed to ongoing personal and spiritual development and high academic standards. Teaching is approached from a multidimensional perspective.

#571 Lakeside School of Natural Therapeutics, Inc.
1726 N. 1st St.
Milwaukee, WI 53212
(414) 372-4345

HOURS OF TRAINING: 600.

DURATION OF COURSE: 6 months or 9 months, day & evening & weekend programs available.

COST: $5,200 plus $350 books. Payment plan without interest is available.

FINANCIAL AID: veterans' benefits.

YEAR FOUNDED: 1985.

ACCREDITATIONS/APPROVALS: COMTA/approved.

GRADUATES PER YEAR (APPROX.): 70.

MODALITIES AND SUBJECTS: acupressure, chair massage, CPR & first aid, ethics, jin shin do, kinesiology, massage theory & practice, myofascial release, pathology, professional practice, reflexology, shiatsu, sports massage, trigger point therapy.

SCHOOL STATEMENT: Lakeside School is committed to providing a quality entry level massage therapy training program, resulting in competent practitioners entering the profession of massage therapy.

#572 Milwaukee School of Massage
1661 N. Water St., suite 301
Milwaukee, WI 53202
(414) 347-1151

HOURS OF TRAINING: 500.

DURATION OF COURSE: 11 months, day and evening programs available.

COST: $4,900 including required textbooks, massage table, face rest, bolster & carrying case.

YEAR FOUNDED: 1995.

GRADUATES PER YEAR (APPROX.): 17.

MODALITIES AND SUBJECTS: acupressure, alexander, business practices & ethics, chair massage, chi gong, cranio-sacral therapy, infant massage, lymphatic drainage, myofascial release, neuromuscular therapy, oriental medicine, reflexology, reiki, shiatsu, shen, sports massage.

SCHOOL STATEMENT: Mission: 1. Prepare students for vocation in Swedish Massage Therapy. 2. Provide community citizens with affordable massage treatments.

Index

To contact the author or publisher:

Enterprise Publishing
P.O. Box 179
Carmel, NY 10512
(914) 228-0312

Ordering Information:

For single copies of this book:

> Send check or money order for $25.95
> to Enterprise Publishing at the above address
> > or
> Order with a credit card at 1-800-888-4741
> > or
> Inquire at your local bookstore.

For wholesale quantities for resale or use as a textbook:

> Massage schools and massage supply companies
> please contact the publisher at the above address.
> Wholesale information is also available on our website.

> Trade bookstores and libraries may order from:
> Independent Publishers Group, Baker & Taylor,
> Ingram and New Leaf.

To have your school or company included in future editions, please send a note to the author c/o Enterprise Publishing at the above address. Include your business name, address, and phone number.

Visit our website for updated state licensing information, discount offers and news from Enterprise Publishing:

www.CareerAtYourFingertips.com